Chinese Qigong
Outgoing—qi Therapy

Written by Bi Yongsheng

Translated by Yu Wenping

Translation revised by
John R.Black

Shandong Science and Technology Press

CHINA

The second edition 1997

ISBN 7—5331—1041—2/R · 277

Published by Shandong Science and Technology Press

16 Yuhan Lu, Jinan, 250002, China

Printed by Shandong Juxian Printing House

Distributed by China International Book Trading Corporation

35 Chegongzhuang Xilu, Beijing, 100044, China

P. O. Box 399, Beijing, China

Printed in the People's Republic of China

Foreword

The past decade has seen a new upsurge in the mass parti-cipation in Qigong exercises in the Orient. The great vitality of Qigong, with its waves spreading towards many parts of the world, has been pounding at various disciplines of science.

While medical Qigong is an important salubrious and curative means of traditional Chinese medicine, outgoing-qi therapy is a wonder of it. Owing to the miraculous curative effect, the therapy has been widely accepted. The physiolog-ical effect produced by outgoing-qi (waiqi) on the human body has aroused attention of scientists both at home and abroad.

Having summarized the experiences in guiding-qi massage (Tuina) and outgoing- qi treatment of diseases for many years, I published my paper *Curative Guiding-emitting-qi Technique* in *Shandong Journal of Traditional Chinese Medicine* in 1983, which has been appreciated by medical workers and Qigong fans. To meet the needs for teaching and research, I compiled successively books of *Guiding-emitting-qi Technique, Qigong Massage* and some others, which have been taken as the teaching materials of the subjects of curative Qigong and Qigong-massage in tradition-al Chinese medicine colleges of Shandong, Anhui, Jinan, etc. The present book is written right on this basis. Adhering to the philos-ophy of Qigong, *Zhouyi (the Book of Changes)* and traditional Chinese medicine, it combines outgoing-qi therapy, massage and acupuncture in one on the basis of the results of experiments and researches and the experiences in clinical application and teaching.

Divided into eight chapters, the book expounds extensively the general knowledge and the theoretical basis of outgoing—qi therapy, the points, the training of qi,the guidance of qi,the emission of qi, the diagnosis of illnesses by outgoing qi, the principle of treatment,the specific methods of treatment and the techniques for correcting the deviations occurring during Qigong practice. Introduced are also twenty methods of training and guiding qi, twenty—nine hand gestures for emitting qi and the skills of differential diagnosis and treatment of forty—five main and common diseases. To provide scientific proof, some of the results of laboratory experiments of the effect of outgoing—qi are included.

The eminent physician Zhang Jiebin (about 1563—1640) of the Ming Dynasty stated, "Without the understanding of the Change (Yi), one is not worthy of the name of an imperial physician",and "The philosophy of the Change implicates that of medicine while the practice of medicine benefits from that of the Change". Adhering to this principle, the book, as a monograph of outgoing—qi therapy, applies the three aspects——the philosophy of the Changes (Yi), the philosophy of medicine and the philosophy of qi is training qi, guiding qi, differential diagnosis and treatment and so forth. It may serve as a text book or a reference for medical professionals, Qigong fans and students of medical schools and universities.

I am most grateful to Mr Zhang Jingtao, special consultant of Shandong Provincial Government and director—general of Shandong Provincial Qigong Association, to Mr Shao

Guanyong, professor and head of the Department of Medical Palaeography of Shandong College of Traditional Chinese Medicine, and to Dai Jianguo, head of the Massage Department of Wuhu Secondary School of Traditional Chinese Medicine of Anhui Province, for their enthusiastic support and assistance in the compilation of this book. Thanks are also given to Bi Ke who helped in the demonstration of the Qigong exercises.

Bi Yongsheng

Acknowledgements

The difficulty of defining accurately the sources of one's ideas, points of view, and information is well known. The translation of this book, a book involving many ancient and modern ideas of Qigong practice, the philosophy of *Zhouyi(the Book of Changes)* and medical sciences, has been influenced by the thoughts and efforts of so many colleagues and friends that to most of them I can offer only this general acknowledgement of my indebtedness.

To Dr Zhao Shili, professor and director of Shandong Provincial Anti–epidemic Station, who has been an unfailing source of constructive advice throughout the years when the translation of this book and many of my other translations and compilations concerning Qigong, massage, preventive medicine and health education and promotion were taking shape, I express my gratitude especially. For much immediate help and suggestions in my mastery of the theory of traditional Chinese medicine and in the preparation of the translation of the text of this book, I thank Dr Yu Changzheng, professor and director of Traditional Chinese Medicine Research Institute of Shandong Province.

I am deeply grateful to Mr Sun Xigang, a senior translator and medical information specialist as well as the director of Shandong Provincial Medical Information Institute, for his kind help in the translation of the book. Finally, I would like to thank Dr Wang Yuanzhong, an epidemiological and computer scientist of Shandong Provincial Anti–epidemic Station, for his patience and efficiency with which he always provides timely assistance to my compilation of books.

Yu Wenping

Contents

Chapter One   An Introduction to Outgoing–qi Therapy

Section One   The Definition and Characteristics of Outgoing–qi Therapy

1. Definition

Qigong therapy falls into two categories: internal qi therapy and outgoing–qi (waiqi) therapy. The former, as the term implies, refers to qigong practice by patients themselves to keep fit or to cure their own illnesses,while the latter is the skill of qigong adapted to treat patients by emitting qi from their bodies.

The terminology of the latter is rather diversified. Besides outgoing–qi therapy (waiqi therapy), other terms include qigong therapy by emitting outgoing–qi, emitting–qi therapy, guiding–qi therapy, emitting–qi qigong, guiding–emitting–qi technique, distant qigong,distributing–qi therapy and, in an ancient term, "distributing qi". The therapy requires the qigong therapist to undergo a strict experience of training qi,guiding qi and emitting qi to get his intrinsic qi substantial and to facili- tate his qi circulation all over his body before he can emit his genuine qi toward the channels and collaterals, the points or a certain location of the patient's body surface to activate the patient's qi dredge the channels and collaterals ,balanced yin and yang, regulate qi and blood readjust solid and hollow internal organs (zang and fu organs), replenish deficiency and purge excess, and eventually, cure the illness. There were three general ideas of the term "distributing qi" in ancient China. One explanation was that the universe spread genuine qi to the human beings and all the things on earth. It is said in *Su Wen – Tian Yuan Ji Da Lun (Plain Questions – Great Treatise on the Universe)* that "qi of the Five Elements fills the universe which in turn spreads it to all things". Another explanation referred to the self qigong exercise through guiding qi to circulate inside the body of the practitioner. *Dao Zang Jing Hua Ling – Xi Shan Qun Xian Hui Zhen Ji (Records of Essence Preservation by Taoists – Chronicles of Gathering of the Spirit Immortals on the Western Mountain)* states, "A method of nourishing the body through distributing qi is to sit upright to facilitate the generation of qi and spread it all over the body to dredge all the channels and collaterals moisten and regulat the body". The last explanation is almost identical with the modern idea, referring to the emission of internal qi by the versed qigong masters towards the patient to cure his illness. This doctrine monopolizes a great deal of records in ancient times. *Jin Shu – Fang Ji Zhuan (The History of Jin Dynasty – Biography of Methods and Techniques)*, for example, says "Those engaged in Taoist studies and nourishment of qi are able to spread their internal qi to others when they are well nourished with qi, which is called 'distributing qi'".

In Chinese massage (Tuina) and acupuncture, stress is laid on the stimulating and regulating function of "strength" (force) to the organism, while in qigong outgoing–qi therapy, it is laid on the same function of "qi", which is often emitted by qigong therapists without the touch of his hand on the body surface of the patient. The combination of "strength" valued in Chinese massage or acupuncture and " qi" merited in qigong outgoing—qi therapy is termed in modern times as qigong—massage or qigong—acupuncture.

2.Characteristics

(1) Treating Diseases by Regulating Qi of the patient

This is the main feature of outgoing—qi therapy. A therapist cures the illnesses just by emitting his internal qi to the patient to regulate the patient's qi activities. It is believed that the disorder of the human body is mainly due to two factors: failure of the vital—qi (vital energy) and exuberance of the evil—qi (pathogenic factor).The former includes insufficiency (asthenia), disorder or stagnation of vital—qi while the latter refers to the affect by pathogenic factors in terms of wind, cold, summer—heat, dampness, dryness, fire and turbid—qi. So the therapist can treat diseases through outgoing—qi therapy, either by emitting his internal qi to the patient to replenish his vital—qi, dredge his channels and activate his qi activities to restore the normal function of the organism, or by emitting his internal qi to the patient to guide the flow of the patient's channel qi and drive the evil—qi out of his body. A patient with pain in a certain location the cause of which cannot be found by routine biochemical or mechanical examinations is a frequent clinical encounter, and treatment with modern traditional Chinese and Western methods often fails. However, detection with outgoing—qi may reveal apparent stagnation of qi at the painful region, and treatment with outgoing—qi may result in instant disappearance of the symptom.

(2) Verified Qi—emitting Methods

Many parts can be taken as qi—emitting locations and a great variety of hand gestures may be assumed. Besides the commonly used palm or finger emission of qi, qi can also be emitted from places such as the eye, and the point Tianmu (around the forehead), Shanzhong (Ren 17), Dantian (the elixir field) and Yongquan (K 1). This diversified technique provides, favourable prerequisite for treatment of diseases according to the actual conditions of the individuals, the nature of the disease and the symptoms, and is proved to be very effective.

(3) Distant Emission of Qi

In massage (Tuina), acupuncture, physiotherapy and surgical operation, effect takes only when the doctor or device touches the body of the patient, while in qigong, diseases can be cured by distant emission of outgoing—qi toward the patient; the therapist may not touch the patient's body surface at all.

(4) Requisite Competence for Emitting Qi

Baopuzi Neipian − *Zhili* (*The Internal Piece of Baopuzi* − *The Maxim*) says, "The human being lives in a world of qi and qi exists in the human being; the Heaven, Earth and all the things in the universe cannot exist without qi". Every living person has qi of the human being, and everyone can practise distributing qi. However, emission of outgoing—qi needs the prerequisites of experience and competence of qigong practice. As stated in *Zun Sheng Ba Jian* − *Yan Nian Que Bing Jian* (*Eight Annotations on Health Preservation* − *Records of Longevity and Disease Prevention*) that a person can distribute his qi to treat diseases only when "he is versed in cultivation of qi and can carry out embryo respiration".

(5) Wide Range of Indications

As the functions of the internal organs,channels and collaterals,extremities, bones, muscles and the tissues of the human body are all related to the nourishment and the activities of qi, those who gain qi will live and those who lose qi will die. Diseases of the human beings are no doubt closely related with the function of qi. So outgoing—qi therapy, through regulation of qi of the patient, can heal many functional and organic diseases or relieve the symptoms. This is why qigong has so wide a range of indications.

(6) Satisfactory Curative Effect with No Side Effects

No facilities and medical equipment are needed for qigong outgoing—qi therapy. Instant curative effect may be achieved in treatment of diseases caused by disorder of qi. More important, unexpected results are frequently obtained in treatment of some knotty cases. Clinical practice for many years has proved that there is no side effect of the therapy provided that the diagnosis and qi—emitting methods are correct.

Section Two   The Origin and Development of Outgoing—qi Therapy

" Distributing—qi therapy" or outgoing—qi therapy of qigong goes back to remote antiquity. Legend has it that as early as the primitive society more than 2000 years ago there existed the "Zhuyou" specialty, which included treatment of diseases by " distributing qi" through directing qi and uttering sounds. *Yi Jing Bian Qi Lun (On Transformation of Essence in-*

to Qi), a chapter of *Su Wen (Plain Questions)* says, "In the past when they lived among birds and beasts, the ancients conducted movements to avoid cold, lived in the shade to prevent sunstroke, had no burden of family dependents and sought no officialdom. Being indifferent to fame or gain, they were resistant to pathogenic evils. So they needed no treatment internally by drugs or externally by needles. It was enough for them to transform essence into qi according to Zhuyou specialty". Again, "I learn that in ancient times that the treatment of diseases was done by transformation of essence into qi". Transformation of essence into qi is to refine essence into qi and in turn heal illnesses with qi. It is stated, in *Xuan Yuan Huang Di Zhu You Ke (The Zhuyou Specialty of the Xuan Yuan Yellow Emperor)*, that "Inhale qi from the right heel and Yongquan (K 1) into the mouth, then the teeth will feel cold. Close the mouth and utter 'xu' and 'si' in burst to spread qi onto the magic figures (Taoist drawings)"; "... like the rising sun that glitters. Inhale it into the throat then send it to the lung to get it mixed with that of the lung. Close the eyes and blink several times, then utter 'ke' and 'si' to spread qi onto the magic figures to store the glittering qi"; "Take a breath to get in qi of Heaven and then spread it onto the paper", to mention but a few. All this explains that with the methods in the specialty of Zhuyou, qi can be spread onto paper or other things, and no doubt can be spread onto the human body to treat diseases. Another technique included in the specialty of Zhuyou is to draw magic figures on the human body and then utter sounds to spread qi to it, which in fact is the direct emission of qi to the human body. To spread qi by uttering sounds is a main characteristic of the specialty of Zhuyou, with which qi is directed and emitted by uttering the five words with different phones, "si", "ke", "chui", "hu" and "xu",on the basis of the doctrine of interpromotion and interrestraint of the Five Elements (metal, wood, water, fire and earth). The philosophy is rather obscure and not yet fully understood. It should not be dismissed simply under the label of superstition. To the contrary, it should be analysed and studied on the principle of discarding the dross and selecting the essence.

Outgoing—qi treatment can not only be performed at a short distance without the qi—emitting part of the therapist touching thethe patient's body surface, but be carried out at long distances. A typical example is Ge Yue (with the Taoist name of Huang Luzi) of the Han Dynasty (206 B.C. − A.D. 220) who was quite famous for his long—distance treatment with outgoing—qi. *Shenxian Zhuan (Biographies of Spirit Immortals)* compiled by Ge Hong of the Eastern Jin Dynasty (317 − 420) holds, "A patient can be cured just by writing his name to the therapist without the therapist seeing him". Ge Hong recorded in *Baopuzi— Neipian − Shizhi (Elimination of Stasis, Internal Chapter of Baopuzi)*, "When one is bitten by poisonous insects, he may be treated with the therapist uttering 'xu' and distributing qi to his own hand (left for male victim and right for female). The condition can be cured immediately though the victim is dozens of miles away". Sun Simiao of the Tang Dynasty (618 − 907) mentioned the similar thing in his *She Yang Zhen Zhong Fang (Health Preservation Prescriptions)*,adding facts to its practice. In another chapter of *Baopuzi*, it is recorded that Shi Chun, a Taoist priest of the Period of the Three Kingdoms, was able to distribute qi to treat diseases, saying: " The Wu Kingdom had a Taoist priest Shi Chun who, whenever distributing qi to treat patients, would not eat until the disease was cured or ate once every hundred or thirty days". It is explained in the same book that bleeding from wound due to weapon can be stopped by emitting qi, and snake bite heals quickly with the same method, and the like, indicating the application of outgoing—qi therapy in the fields of trauma, weapon wound, bleeding, snake, insect or beast bite, fracture, cough and many others.

In *Jin Shu (The History of Jin Dynasty)*, an acount is made of a doctor by the name of Xing Ling who became widely known because "he cured, with outgoing qi, Lu Yi's mother of her illness flaccidity—arthralgia—syndrome from which she had suffered for more than ten years, and enabled her to walk". As a result, "There was a flow of people coming to see the wonder, either by land or by water".

During the Tang (618 — 907) and Song (960 — 1279) dynasties, the scope of outgoing—qi therapy was expanded. *Huan Zhen Xian Sheng Fu Nei Yuan Qi Jue (Master Huan Zhen's Pithe Formula for Intake of Primordial Qi)* of the Tang Dynasty has a record of "Formula of Distribution of Qi", introducing the essentials, methods and other aspects of distribution of qi. The book *Wunengzi* written by an anonymous person in the late Tang Dynasty gives an account on how Wunengzi cured his bosom friend Yuzhongzi of his precordial pain by distribution of outgoing—qi.

The Song Dynasty had more contributions to the doctrine and practice of distributing qi for treatment of diseases in books such as *Song Shi — Fang Ji Zhuan (The History of Song Dynasty — Biography of Methods and Techniques)* and *Jiu Jiang Tong Zhi (A General History of Jiujiang)*.The Ming (1368 — 1644) and Qing (1644 — 1911) dynasties saw the improvement and progress of qigong outgoing–qi therapy in its curative methods and mechanism owing to the further development of medical, Taoist and Buddhist practice of qigong. It is said in *Zun Sheng Ba Jian — Yan Nian Que Bing Jian (Eight Annotations on Health Preservation — Records of Longevity and Disease Prevention)*compiled by Gao Lian of the Ming Dynasty (1368 — 1644) that "To distribute qi for treatment of diseases, one must take in qi of the different viscera and distribute it to the related viscerum. The patient who should be asked to face a proper direction, with heart clear and pure, when qi is distributed to him. After the distribution of qi, ask the patient to swallow qi. In so doing, the ghosts and thieves (evils) will flee all by themselves and the evil–qi will be eradicated". This paragraph, as a summary, explains in detail the different steps of outgoing–qi therapy in terms of regulation of qi, diagnosis, adjustment of direction and curative methods, and effects.

Han Mao, a physician of the Ming Dynasty (1368 — 1644), wrote *Han Shi Yi Tong (Han's Book on General Medicine)*, in which he recorded the treatment of pain syndrome in the shoulder, back, extremities, joints and wrists with human qi.

*Qing Shi Gao— Yi Shu Zhuan (The Manuscript of the History of the Qing Dynasty — Biography of Arts)*has an account of Gan Fengchi, a master of martial arts in the days of Emperor Kang Xi, who treated the infectious disease tuberculosis,saying,"The son of his townsman Tan attracted tuberculosis that failed to heal with medical treatment. Gan Fengchi sat at night in a quiet room, windows closed,with his back against that of the patient and the patient recovered in forty—nine days".

Owing to the rapid development of qigong since the founding of P.R China, the theory of outgoing—qi, the method of its emission and the scope of its clinical application have gained much progress. In 1980, Zhao Guang firstly had its contribution *On Emission of Outgoing—Qi* published in the journal "Qigong", which introduced the procedures for practice of outgoing—qi emission and the measures for its detection. In 1983, we published, in *The Shandong Journal of Traditional Chinese Medicine* and *The National qigong Corpus*, the papers of *Clinical Technique of Outgoing—Qi Emission and Guidance*, expounding the specific skills and clinical applications of outgoing—qi therapy in terms of training qi, guiding qi, emitting qi and treatment, then *Reports on Correction of qigong Deviations in Sixty—eight Cases, Treatment of Twenty—two Mastitis Cases with Outgoing—qi,* and the like, presenting detailed results of clinical observations and researches. In the same year, the same topic was discussed by Ma Jiren, Lin Houxing et al in their publications of *Chinese qigong* and *Three Hundred Questions on Qigong*. Wang Yin gave an exposition of the rudiments and clinical experience of outgoing—qi therapy in his monograph *Qigong Outgoing—qi Therapy*.

A great deal of scientific experiments on the effect of outgoing—qi have been carried out in recent years.The results show that outgoing—qi can kill the Gram—positive and Gram—negative bacteria or promote their growth and multiplication in compliance with the will of the qi emitter. Acting on cancer cells, outgoing qi has a lethal dose of 30% and more. Animal experiments we made from 1986 to 1987 revealed obvious regulating function of outgoing—qi on both the Oddi's sphincter of rabbit and the cardiac muscles of toad. Similar tests were made by others on animals with cancer, which showed marked prolongation of survival time.Other results showed prominent function on the regulation of blood pressure and obvious improvement of the immunity level of the animals. In a word, abundant scientific experiments and clinical conclusions have proved that outgoing—qi therapy of qigong is a desirable curative approach in traditional Chinese medicine. With its long history, rich experience and reliable curative effect, it will certainly play an active role in health preservation and treatment of diseases.

Section Three   The Relationship between Outgoing—Qi Therapy and Massage (Tuina) and Acupuncture

Zhou Qianchuan, the eminent qigong master and scholar of traditional Chinese medicine, says in his *Diet Therapy and Deviation—rescue Techniques in qigong,* "Definitely speaking, all the well—known masters and seniors of acupuncture, bone—setting and massage of various generations have consummate attainments in qigong, or at least know qigong". He repeatedly explains the relationship between qigong and traditional Chinese medicine, especially the close link between qigong and massage, bone—setting and acupuncture. These wise remarks are conclusions made on the basis of his rich experience and penetrating analysis of data.

No doubt, outgoing-qi therapy, massotherapy and acupuncture treatment are all important means of prevention and treatment in traditional Chinese medicine.

In outgoing-qi therapy, diagnosis or treatment of diseases is confirmed or performed through "emitting qi", and its prominent feature lies in "qi" regulation; while in modern Chinese massotherapy and acupuncture, the treatment of diseases is obtained through massage manipulations and needle-puncturing and needle-manipulations, with its prominent feature lying in "strength" regulation. Both the brilliant massceurs and acupuncturists of the old days laid emphasis on practice of qigong and on the combination of qigong with manipulations of massage and acupuncture. By combining "qi regulation" with "strength regulation" in treatment, they raised the curative effect to a great extent and, this, according to Zhou Qianchuan, may be where the wisdom of "all the well-known masters and seniors of acupuncture and moxibustion, bone-setting and massage of various generations" lies.

Anmo Jing (Massage Classic) written by an anonymous person of the Qing Dynasty (1644 – 1911) says, "The pathogen enters the body by way of Shuitu (St 10). ... On pressing Shuitu (St 10), the patient may feel slight pain in the subaxillary area and numbness of the fingers; elevating the thumb, he may feel the release of hot qi from his arm and fingers". "Press the tight part with the right thumb... with two-seven (fourteen) respiratory cycles, then remove the thumb... the evil heat descends along the channels to the legs and, hot as fire, down to the two feet," and the like. In this book, respiratory cycle is expressed in two—seven (fourteen) when hotness sensation produced by hand manipulation is mentioned, which conforms to the number of yang—fire (positive fire) of the theory "Earth produces fire in two and Heaven compensates it in seven". "The turbulence" on pressing implies the feeling of evil—qi (pathogenic message) by the therapist through hand manipulations.And "hot as fire down to the two feet", refers to the sensation of qi by the patient. That is the reason why great attention is paid to the sensation of qi when the manipulation of "guiding—qi massage" applied. The manipulation described by Wang Yaru in his book *Digital Acupoint—pressing Massotherapy According to the Chart of Internal Organs'* is in fact "guiding—qi massage", for the method mentioned in this book is actually created by the Taoist priests, with which massage manipulation is carried out based on the doctrine of the transposed Five Elements. So the principle of the book is closely related to the philosophy of qigong practice of the Toaist priests. The book mentions many phenomena of smooth circulation of qi when sensation of qi by the therapist is described. For example, the sensation of the appearance of a mass or several masses, the sensation of "water flow",the sounds "zhi zhi", the sensation of successive bubble bursts and other phenomena,are all the signs indicating the beginning of the free circulation of qi. With the routine massage manipulations, these sensations of qi are difficult to get and the therapist may not be able to make a clear judgement of whether qi is circulating or stagnated. So only when the manipulations of massage are combined with those of qigong, or in other words, when "strength" is combined with "guidance of qi", can the sensation of hotness or coldness, vital qi or pathogenic qi, and freely circulating qi or stagnated qi be identified.

The same applies to the curative effect, which can only be upgraded through combination of qigong and massage. Clinically, when the treatment needs more stimulation and regulation by "strength", "strength regulation" should be taken as the main aspect with "qi regulation" as the accessary, and vice versa. Generally, it is rather difficult to distinguish "strength" and "qi". However, "qi" here means the outgoing-qi emitted, while "strength" means the power of force exerted as well as its direction and frequency, for which the therapist manipulates with his hand touching the body surface of the patient.

As the combination of qigong and acupuncture is concerned, Yang Jizhou of the Ming Dynasty (1368 – 1644) attached great importance to it in his book *Zhen Jiu Da Cheng* (*Great Compendium of Acupuncture and Moxibustion*). He held that the posture, mental activities and respiration of the therapist should conform to the principle of "three regulations" in qigong, saying that when the reinforcement manipulation was performed, the acupuncturist "must stand or sit straight, keep sedate and concentrate the mind without slackness. ... The importance of acupuncture lies in concentration of the mind". He also pointed out that the reinforcement and purgation should be carried out in compliance with the sun, the moon and the variations of qi of the universe, with the body posture proper, mind concentrated, guidance of qi by will, regulation of qi by respiration and manipulation of the needle by strength so that the genuine qi could be led to the focus of disease. *Hou Han Shu – Fang Shu Lie Zhuan* (*History of the Late Han Dyn-*

asty — Biographies of Methods and Techniques) cites a quotation from Guo Yuzhi, "The striae of skin, muscles and viscera are so fine and minute that the manipulation on them should be performed with regulation of qi. ... The effect of mind concentration on the heart and the hand is within tacit understanding but beyond words". This indicates that the needling level of an acupuncturist rests with whether he can "concentrate his attention on the heart and hand" during operation, for as a therapist, qi follows will (in the adept at qigong), and when attention is concentrated on the heart and hand, qi can be "governed" by will and the "channel qi" of the patient can then be controlled and led to the focus of the disease. *Zhen Jiu Da Cheng (Great Compendium of Acupuncture and Moxibustion)* introduces in detail the methods of training qi for acupuncturists, pointing out that the practice of qigong should be started with the training of small circle of qi (qi circulating along the Ren and Du Channels), and through strict, arduous training of qi circulation, to attain the realm in which the practitioner "feels the body and mind in Chaos as if he has entered into nihility that he does not know whether his body is for him and he is for his body and spirit is for qi and qi is called spirit; he does not intend to confine himself but he is confined; he is not able to make fetal breath but fetal breath accours automatically; water (fluid) circulates without guidance by will, fire is expelled with no suggestion; light generates in void and needle is threaded in the darkness; he knows that things are so but does not know why they are so, and he does not know whether the Ren Channel is Du or the Du Channel is Ren". If an acupuncturist can reach the realm described in the book, to perform qigong—acupuncture for treatment of diseases will be as easy as turning his hand over. So when the adept performs "lighting the mountain fire", real hotness may be induced; when he conducts "cooling the Heaven", real coolness will occur. And once he combines qi with strength in treatment of diseases, he will attain a kind of curative effect hard for common healers to come by.

It is generally considered that when qigong therapists emit qi to a patient, they do not touch the body surface of the patient, and the farther they are away from the patient, the better the curative effect and the more brilliant the therapist will be. This is actually a prejudice. In fact, an experienced qigong therapist can emit his qi into the body of the patient no matter whether he touches the patient or not. The difference lies in that emitting qi with hand away from the body surface of the patient embodies "qi regulation"; and with hand touching the patient embodies "strength regulation", which is a combination of strength and qi, or, the facilitation of strength by qi. This is the reason that we say that it is not enough for a good outgoing—qi therapist to have the experience in qigong practice and the skill of emission of outgoing—qi,moreover, he should have a profound understanding of the philosophy of the technique, have a good grasp of the skills of massage and acupuncture, and be able to combine them as an organic whole so that he can carry out treatment with high proficiency to ensure the quality of treatment and to avoid misdiagnosis and erroneous treatment of diseases.

Section Four   Indications of Outgoing—qi Therapy and Points For Attention

1. Indications

Outgoing—qi therapy is a special curative method of regulation of the organism of the patient with "qi" and "strength". As the viscera, tissues and life activities of the human body are all related to "qi", "qi" is the first to be regulated whenever functional or organic disorders of the organism occur. This lengthens the scope of indications to a certain extent, though the nature of qi and its mechanism of action await for further research. Based on clinical experimental studies in China, a conclusion may be drawn that the degree of curative effect depends on the competence and versatility of the qigong therapist and the extent of response of the patient to outgoing—qi. In patient whose channels and points are very sensitive to outgoing—qi, miraculous results are often expected even if their conditions may be rather complicated. For those whose channels and points are not so sensitive to qi, repeated stimulation and regulation are needed to raise their sensitivity and make qi activities more vigorous and synchronized so that satisfactory effect can be, as it is often, achieved.

The results of clinical application and scientific research have proved that outgoing—qi therapy is fairly effective for internal, surgical, gynecological, traumatological and pediatric complaints and those of the five sense organs, e.g., headache, stomachache, chest pain, lumbago, cough, constipation, mastitis, dysmenorrhea, common cold, cholecystitis, hypertension, angiitis, pelvic inflammation, myopia as well as qigong deviations.

2. Points for Attention

(1) As emitting outgoing—qi consumes qi and energy, the therapist may, after successive emission of qi, feel tired, dizzy, cold in the extremities and discomfort in the hepatic region and the lower abdomen. This means that he has consumed more qi and energy than could be replenished, which may impair his own health. So the qi—emitting time should not be too long and the number of patients to be treated in one day should not be too large. It is advisable to manage the treatment according to one's own qigong acomplishments and health status. Constant supplement of nutrients and fluid and frequent exposure to fresh air are helpful to replenishing energy, regulating qi activities and leading qi back to its origin.

(2) Emission of qi should be avoided by all means if the therapist has fallen ill or feels feeble, tired, starved, overfed, drunk, overjoyed, deeply grieved or indignant. Washing hands or bathing with cold water immediately after emission of qi is harmful to the health.

(3) The disordered qi or pathogenic qi of the patient may invade into the body of the therapist and interfere with his own qi activities, causing discomfort, lassitude, soreness, distention, pain and numbness of certain parts. When this occurs, the therapist should timely drive the evil—qi out of his body and regulate his own qi activity to get it normal as soon as possible. Patients suffering from cancer may affect the therapist's qi activity more seriously, so care should be taken not to carry out

too much emission of qi, or not to emit qi to these kinds of patients at all.

(4) Desirable effect can be attained only when the patient is cooperative with the therapist. The patient should try to create good conditions for outgoing—qi therapy by way of concentrating attention, regulating respiration and relax the whole body or only the part that receives qi.

Patient whose channels and collaterals are sensitive may get the sensation of qi easily or present spontaneous moving phenomenon. Some are not so sensitive at first but may become sensitive step by step along with the repetition of treatment. Anyhow, good curative effect may occur in those who has no sensation of qi or spontaneous dynamic phenomenon at all, while in some,although sensation of qi is obvious and dynamic phenomenon occurs easily, the curative effect may not be satisfactory owing to their specific conditions of health and illness. The therapist should make the patients aware of the fact that sensation of qi and spontaneous movement are not the criteria of effect lest they misunderstand the therapy and be misled.

(5) Outgoing—qi therapy is no omnipotence. While it is very effective for some diseases or for a certain type of diseases and can cure them completely, it may only relieve the symptoms of others and in such cases may serve only as an auxiliary treatment. For patients with acute diseases or in a critical condition, it is advisable to take comprehensive measures by combining traditional and westen treatment. Lavish praise on the technique and superstitious practice of it should be strictly guarded against so as to avoid delay of treatment.

(6) Qigong exercises described in Chapter Eight of this book, serving as the methods of accessory treatment, are for patients to practise 2 – 4 times a day, or following the doctor's advice.

Chapter Two   The Theoretical Basis of Outgoing–qi Therapy

Section One   The Theory of Traditional Chinese Medicine and Outgoing–qi Therapy

The Concept of Wholism

The concept of wholism, by taking the universe and the human being as one, is one aspect of the basic theory of traditional Chinese medicine and qigong. *Zang Fu Tu Dian Xue Fa (Digital Acupoint Pressing Based on Chart of the Viscera)* states, "Qi of Heaven is that of man. The Heaven is a large circle of qi and man a small circle of qi". The ancient qigong masters took not only the cosmos and nature as one whole and the human being as one whole, but also the human being and the nature as an organic whole in unity. Thus the theory taking the universe and the human being as one has been established as a system and used to guide qigong exercise and medical practice.

1. The Human Body Is an Organic Whole

Su Wen – Liu Jie Zang Xiang Lun (Plain Questions – On Appearance of the Six– section Viscera) holds that "The heart is the source of life and the derivative of spirit". *Lei Jing Tu Yi – Yiyi (Illustrated Supplementary to the Classied Canon – Application of the Book of Changes to Medicine)* by Zhang Jiebin of the Ming Dynasty (1368 – 1644) says, "The heart is the monarch of the body. ... The human body is a small universe in which all things are connected together without an iota of interspace". This explains that the human body itself is an organic whole. And the five viscera, as the centre of the whole, keep close relations with the tissues and organs of all parts of the body through the channels, qi and blood. The function of this organic setup can be seen clearly under both normal physiological and pathological conditions.

As "the monarch of the body governing consciousness and spirit", the heart occupies an important place in the life activities. Under the command of the heart, the viscera, tissues and all the organs of the human body carry on normal physiological activities. In qigong exercise and outgoing—qi therapy, great importance is attached to the function of spirit or mind concentration or will. The physiological activity of any one of the five zang—organs is conducted with the close cooperation of the other organs. For example, the spleen functions to transport and transform nutrients and the stomach works to receive food; the two together accomplish the digestive process of food. In turn, the transporting and transforming function of the spleen is carried out with the assistance of the dispersive effect of the liver, and the transfusion and distribution of the essential substance derived from water and cereals or food staff transported and transformed by the spleen rest with the physiological activities of the heart, lung and kidney. So it goes without saying that the spleen needs the coordination of the liver, heart, lung and kidney in its work for transportation and transformation. On the other hand, the zang—organs and fu—organs areinterrelated with the different tissues and the body surface. The liver, for instance, has its specific opening in the eyes. The lung is in charge of the skin and hair, the spleen is in charge of the extremities and the kidney has its specific opening in the ears. So when we carry out outgoing—qi therapy for treatment of a disease, the body as a whole rather than one organ or tissue should be taken into account in determination of the channels, points, hand gestures and manipulations for emitting qi so that desirable effect can be achieved.

2. The Relationship between Man and Nature

The concept of holism regarding the universe and the human being as one has its special emphasis on the relationship between the human being and nature. According to the ancients, the concrete incarnation of holism is "correspondence between man and universe" and "the relationship between the human body and the natural environment".

When we say "correspondence between man and universe", we mean that the life activitity of the human being is closely related to nature. *Su Wen — Yin Yang Ying Xiang Da Lun (Plain Questions — On Conclusions of Correspondence of Yin and Yang)* holds, "The essence of Heaven corresponds with the lung, of Earth with the pharynx, of wind with the liver, of thunder with the heart, of food—stuff with the spleen, and of rain with the kidney". And it is said in *Lei Jing Tu Yi — Yiyi (Illustrated Supplementary to the Classified Canon — Application of the Book of Changes to Medicine)*, "Qi of the universe is that of man; the body of man is that of universe"; "Wherever there is will, there will be qi; and as spirit goes with qi, one may correspond with Heaven, Earth, ghosts and immortals". From the above scriptures, it can be seen that man and all the things of the universe are products derived from the primordial qi, and the primordial qi spreads all over the universe amongest Heaven, Earth and man. Qi of man communicates with that of the universe, and qi of the universe influences the life activities of man. As the climate varies with the four seasons in a year, prominent changes will take place in physiology and qi activity of the human body accordingly. For example, man has more sweat and less urine in summer and vice versa in winter; the pulse becomes taut in spring, full in summer, superficial in autumn and deep in winter.

The overwhelming variation of the climate with the four seasons that goes beyond the adaptability of the human body will impel the origination, development and changes of diseases. Measles and epidemic meningitis are often prevalent in spring, malaria and epidemic encephalitis B usually occur in the wet season summer, storm may worsen heart diseases, and cloudy, rainy and wetn days often give rise to joint pain, to mention but a few.

In the long process of development, man and nature are interrelated with and interact on each other. The human being has absorbed various messages of nature, replenished himself and improved the adaptability to the environment. As a result, man has his individual ability and functions corresponding with natural environment, which, in the ancient times, was called "correspondence between man and universe". Lei Jing Tu Yi — Yiyi (Illustrated Supplementary to the Classified Canon — Application of the Book of Changes to Medicine) by Zhang Jiebin of the Ming Dynasty states, "The physique of the human body is the structure of the universe. ... The universe has twelve months, man has twelve internal organs; the universe has twelve rendezvous (hui) of the twelve stars, man has twelve channels; the universe has twelve two—hour periods of the day, man has twelve sections of the body. If this is understood, the circulation of ying—energy (nutrients) and wei—energy (resistance) and the relationship between the exterior and interior of the channels and collaterals are clear".

The theory "correspondence between man and universe" is considered as utmost important for qigongpractice and outgoing—qi therapy. The practitioner and the therapist must first be good at adaptation to the law of natural variations so as to correspond with nature, then they can have a good grasp of the methods of mind concentration, respiration regulation and qi—emitting manipulation. The ancient qigong masters believed that Heaven, Earth and man had three treasures each——the sun, the moon and the stars; water, fire and wind; and jing (essence), qi (vital energy) and shen (spirit) respectively. qigong practice is right aimed at the combination of each group of the three treasures in one so as to reinforce the essence, vital energy and spirit. Attention should also be paid to acting "in line with yin and yang", "in correspondence with the four seasons" and " in accord with the application of numbers" , as well as "avoiding pathogenic factors and evil wind". Only in this way, can one strengthen the resistance of the organism to diseases, adapt to the variable environment, and get the primordial qi substantial and circulating continuously. From this point of view, we say that the training of qi, guidance of qi, and diagnosis and treatment of diseases by outgoing—qi concretely embody the concept of wholism in terms of Heaven, Earth and man as one.

Yin and Yang

The doctrine of yin (negative) and yang (positive) is a summarization of the opposition of all things. *Neijing — Yin Yang Ying Xiang Da Lun (Canon of Internal Medicine — On Conclusions of Correspondence of Yin and Yang)* says, "Yin—yang is the law of the universe, the principle governing all things, the parents of changes, and the origin of life and death". Generally speaking, all that are hyperfunctional, exciting, hot, dynamic, strong, bright, invisible, light, upward, outward, clear and the like, belong to yang (positive). On the contrary, all that are waning, restraining, cold, static, weak, turbid, and the like, belong to yin (negative). The same opposition exists in Heaven and Earth, sun and moon, day and night, hotness and coldness, male and female, superior and inferior, outside and inside, motion and rest, fire and water, exhale and inhale, and excess and deficiency. So all things of the natural world containing two opposite components can be divided into yin and yang.

1. The Motion Law of Yin and Yang

(1) The Opposition and Interdependence of Yin and Yang

Yin and yang are not only opposite but also interdependent, without the other, neither can exist. The saying "Without yang, yin can not grow while without yin, yang can not develop", or "Yang can by no means work without yin and yin can never live without yang" fully explains the relationship between yin and yang in terms of interdependence and interconnection.

(2) The Waning and Waxing of Yin and Yang

Yin and yang are by no means in a state of absolute staticness. There exists between them constant struggle of waning and waxing. "While yin waxes, yang wanes, and vice versa". They keep, to some extent, a state of dynamic equilibrium. If the waning and waxing of yin and yang exceed the normal limit and break through the state of dynamic equilibrium, excess or deficiency of yin and yang will occur, leading to development of abnormalities.

(3) The Transformation between Yin and Yang

As the two opposite components of things, yin and yang do not always stay at a standstill. Under certain conditions, they may transform toward the opposite aspect, i.e., yang may transform into yin and yin can transform into yang. This phenomenon is clearly stated in *Su Wen − Yin Yang Ying Xiang Da Lun (Plain Questions − On Conclusions of Correspondence of Yin and Yang)*, saying "Yin in overabundance will transform into yang and yang in overabundance will transform into yin", and " Overabundance of cold may bring about false heat and overabundance of heat may bring about false cold".

2. The Application of Yin and Yang in Outgoing−qi Therapy

(1) Yin and Yang in Explanation of the Physiological Structure of the Human Body

As far as the whole human body is concerned, the upper part is yang while the lower is yin; the back is yang, the abdomen is yin; the left is yang and the right is yin; the exterior is yang and the interior is yin. So far as the internal organs of the human body are concerned, the six fu−organs (six hollow organs referring to the gallbladder, stomach, large intestine, small intestine, urinary bladder and Sanjiao or three warmers) are yang while the five zang or viscera (five solid organs referring to the heart, liver, spleen, lung and kidney) are yin. As for an individual organ, the function of the organ is yang and the substance is yin; qi is yang while the blood is yin. It is hence written in *Su Wen − Jin Gui Zhen Yan Lun (Plain Questions − Synopsis of Genuine Words of the Golden Chamber)* that "It is said that, of the human being,the lateral aspect is yang and the medial is yin; of the body, the back is yang and the abdomen is yin". According to Neijing (Canon of Internal Medicine), the human body can be divided into three pairs of yin and yang: with the navel as a horizontal demarcation line, the part above the navel (from the navel to the head) is yang and below that (from the navel to the feet) is yin; with the points Baihui (Du 20) and Huiyin (Ren 1) as a vertical demarcation line, the left half of the bodyis yang and the right is yin; the posterior half is yang and the anterior half is yin (Fig. 2−1). Qi activities of

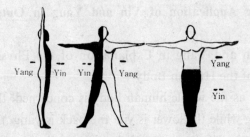

Fig. 2−1 The Yin and Yang Aspects of the Human Body

these yin−yang unities and the internal organs and tissues, in terms of evil or vital, excessive or deficient, strong or weak, as well as the direction and nature of qi can be detected with outgoing–qi at their corresponding body surfaces so that data for diagnosis and treatment can be provided. For example, strong, dense, dry and hot sensation of qi around the head may manifest in the syndrome of excess in the upper and deficiency in the lower and excess of yang and deficiency of yin, a case that requires the therapist to guide yang to descend and yin to ascend to restore the normal physiological function with yin and yang balanced and water and fire coordinated.

(2) Training Qi and Treating Diseases According to the Motion Law of Yin and Yang

As, for example, the spring and summer are regarded as yang and the autumn and winter as yin; the six two–hour periods of Zi, Chou, Yin, Mao, Chen and Si as yang and the si two–hour periods of Wu, Wei, Shen, You, Xu and Hai as yin; exhalation as yang and inhalation as yin, patients with exuberance of yang and hyperactivity of fire should practice training qi during the yin periods, facing north, and with stress laid on exhaling, while the therapist should adhere to the principle of replenishing yin to invigorate yang and leading yang to descend to supplement yin.

(3) Yin and Yang in Explanation of the Pathological Changes of the Human Body and in Diagnosis of Diseases

If the equilibrium of the dynamic state of yin and yang is disturbed, overabundance or deficiency of yin or yang will develop, and diseases will occur accordingly.Generally speaking,the over–exuberance of yang may lead to deficiency of yin, giving rise to illness; while the over–exuberance of yin may lead to deficiency of yang, similarly giving rise to illness. Hot syndrome can be the result of either overabundance of yang or deficiency of yin while cold syndrome may result from either overabundance of yin or deficiency of yang. Once the nature of yin and yang is determined, proper method of outgoing—qi emission can be selected to regulate the excess and insufficiency of yin and yang so as to cure the disease. The principle of treatment is explained in *Su Wen — Zhi Zhen Yao Da Lun (Plain Questions — Great Conclusions of Genuine Essentials)*, saying "Cold—syndrome should be treated with warm—natured drugs and heat—syndrome with cold—natured drugs"; and in *Su Wen — Yin Yang Ying Xiang Da Lun (Plain Questions — On Conclusions of the Correspondence of Yin and Yang)*, saying "Treat yin for yang diseases; treat yang for yin diseases". This means that treatment should be aimed at purging the excess to replenish the insufficiency and regulating the over—exuberance or deficiency of yin and yang so that the normal, balanced state of the body can be restored. For instance, intake of cold food or drinks may lead to overabundence of yin which in turn gives rise to cold—syndrome of spleen and stomach manifested by pain, diarrhoea, aversion to cold and cold extremities. Here outgoing—qi therapy can be preformed in line with "treating cold—syndrome with warm—natured drugs", that is, to guide hot yang qi and emit it toward the points such as Zhongwan (Ren 12) and Tianshu (St 25), and then guide the cold qi of the patient out of the body by way of Zusanli (St 36) and Yinlingquan (Sp 9), etc.

The Five Elements (Wu Xing)

The doctrine of the Five Elements was originated in the old days when people took the five substances of wood, fire, earth, metal and water as representatives to explain the attribution of things and the relationship between them. Zhang Jiebin of the Ming Dynasty (1368—1644) expounded the relationship between yin— yang and the Five Elements in his *Lei Jing Tu Yi — Wu Xing Tong Lun (Illustrated Supplementary to the Classified Cannon — General Conclusion of the Five Elements)*, stating "The Five Elements are the essence of yin and yang and yin and yang are the qi of the Five Elements; while qi will not exist without essence, essence will not act without qi. So the action of the Five Elements is the circulation of qi of yin and yang."

1. The Basic Contents of the Five Elements

(1) The Correspondence of Things with the Five Elements

The ancient medical masters made comprehensive comparisons and studies on the organs and tissues of the human body, its physiology and pathology, as well as all kinds of things of the natural world that are related to the human life, attributing them to one of the Five Elements according to their different properties, functions and forms. The following table summarizes the correspondence of the Five Elements with the human body and nature on the basis of *Neijing*(*Canon of Internal Medicine*) and related books on qigong (Table 2—1).

Table 2−1 Correspondence of the Five Elements with the Human Body and Nature

		Wood	Fire	Earth	Metal	Water
The Human Body	Five Elements	Wood	Fire	Earth	Metal	Water
	Five Zang−organs (Solid)	Liver	Heart	Spleen	Lung	Kidney
	Six Fu−organs (Hollow)	Gall−bladder	Small intestine	Stomach	Large intestine	Urinary bladder
	Five Sense Organs	Eye	Tongue	Mouth	Nose	Ear
	Five Tissues	Tendon	Vessel	Flesh	Skin	Bone
	Five Emotions	Anger	Joy	Anxiety	Grief	Fear
	Five Sounds	Shouting	Laughing	Singing	Crying	Moaning
	Five Spirit Manifestations	Spirit soul	Spirit	Intention	Material soul	Essence
	Five Material Manifestaions	Extremity	Complexion	Lip	Hair (body)	Hair (head)
Nature	Seasons	Spring	Summer	Late summer	Autumn	Winter
	Growth & Development	Germination	Growth	Trans−formation	Reaping	Storing
	Environmental Factors	Wind	Heat	Dampness	Dryness	Cold
	Five Colours	Green	Red	Yellow	White	Black
	Five Tastes	Sour	Bitter	Sweet	Acrid	Salty
	Five Orientations	East	South	Centre	West	North
	Time	Dawn	Midday	Sun setting	Sunset	Midnight
	Five Shapes	Straight	Sharp	Square	Thin	Round
	Five Stars	Sui	Yinghuo	Jinzhen	Taibai	Chen
Others	Generating Number	Three	Two	Five	Four	One
	Resultant Number	Eight	Seven	Ten	Nine	Six
	Heavenly	Jia−Yi	Bing−Ding	Wu−Ji	Geng−Xin	Ren−Kui
	Earthly Branches	Yin−Mao	Si−Wu	Chen−Wei Xu−Chou	Shen−You	Hai−Zi
	Eight Diagrams	Zhen−Xun	Li	Kun−Gen	Qian−Dui	Kan

qigong and traditional Chinese medicine attribute the organs and tissues of the human body and the phenomena of the natural world to the Five Elements, and explain the relationship among them. For example, the liver, gallbladder, tendons, and eyes are attributed to "wood" of the Five Elements, at the same time, they are related to spring, wind, green colour of nature, the numbers three and eight, Jia and Yi of the Heavenly Stems and Gen and Xun of the Eight Diagrams. This classification method, though based on the Five Elements, does not indicate wood, fire, earth, metal and water per se, rather, it is an abstract concept of the attribution of different things drawn in the light of the characteristics of the Five Elements, a method easy to apply in qigong practice and clinical treatment.

(2) The Generation, Restriction, Subjugation and Reverse Restriction of the Five Elements

The doctrine of the Five Elements explains the relationship between different things by means of generation and restriction among the Five Elements. The generation relationship of the Five Elements is: wood generates fire, fire generates earth, earth generates metal, metal generates water, and water generates wood, in endness cycles . The restriction relationship is: wood restricts earth, earth restricts water, water restricts fire, fire restricts metal, and metal in its turn restricts wood. Every element has two aspects —— generating and being generated, and restricting and being restricted. The element that generates is regarded as mother, while the element that is generated as child. Hence the relationship between generating and being generated is also termed "the relationship between mother and child". Similarly, the element that restricts is the successful side while that being restricted is the defeated side. *Lei Jing Tu Yi – Wu Xing Tong Lun (Illustrated Supplementary to the Classified Canon – General Treatise on the Five Elements)* written by Zhang Jiebin of the Ming Dynasty says, " In the process of growth and development, both generation and restriction are needed. Without generation, growth will have no origin while without restrict, growth will be rampant and turn into harm".

2. The Application of the Five Elements in Outgoing–qi Therapy

(1) In Explanation of Physiology and Pathology

The law of generation and restriction may be used to explain the inter– generating and inter–restricting relationship between the internal organs. For instance, the vital essence of the kidney (water) nourishes the liver (wood). The heat of the heart (fire) warms the spleen (earth). On the other hand, the origination of diseases of the human body is the result of the breakdown of the normal equilibrium of generation, restriction, subjugation and reverse restriction among the organs and tissues. Take disorder of the liver for example, if the illness spreads to the spleen, it is regarded as "wood usbjugating earth"; to the lung, as "wood reversely restricting metal"; to the heart, as "mother–organ involving child–organ", and to the kidney, as "child– organ involving mother–organ".

(2) In Outgoing–qi Treatment

Hyperactivity of the liver–fire may be manifested by blue complexion and congested eyes, vexation, irritability, taut pulse, dry mouth and reddened tongue. According to the generating and restricting law of the Five Elements, the syndrome can be treated, if with qigong exercise, by practising the exercise of taking essence from the moon, the exercise of nourishing the kidney to replenish yin (nourishing water to replenish wood), the exercise of uttering "xu" (purging the liver—qi), and the exercise of uttering "ke" (purging fire of the child—organ); if with outgoing—qi therapy, by taking in water—qi and emitting qi for 6 respiratory cycles during the period of Zi or Hai to help nourish the kidney—water (water restricts fire), then guide qi of the heart and small intestine out of the body for 7 respiratory cycles for purgation (purging the child to cure the mother).

The most difficult and dangerous condition is named "triple factors affecting one", which means one organ may be affected by the abnormal function of three different organs simultaneously. Take the disorder of the spleen as an example, it may be due, simultaneously, to the failure to generate the spleen— earth caused by extreme asthenia of heart—fire, the restriction of the spleen— earth caused by hyperactivity of the liver—wood, and reverse restriction of the spleen—earth caused by adverse up—flowing of kidney—water.

The Five Viscera (Wu Zang)

1. The Liver

The liver—gallbladder is attributed to wood. The liver is regarded as the Green Emperor, belonging to Zhen in the Eight Diagrams, in image of the Green Dragon, in shape of a suspending gourd, and pertaining to Jia—Yi of the Heavenly Stems and Yin—Mao of the Earthly Branches. Located below the right ribs, it stores spirit soul, its energy (qi) moves along the left side, its channels and vessels spread over the hypochondria of both sides, and its condition is reflected at the nails. The liver bears the dispersing effect and has its upper orifice in the eyes (the left is Jia and the right Yi). The gallbladder is the hollow organ of the liver and is interior—exteriorly related with the liver.

Patients with diseases of the liver may have dry eyes, pain in the hypochondria which may radiate to the lower abdomen, and changing moods, accompanied by flushed left cheek in case of excessive liver—heat, by liability to be frightened and feel cold in case of liver—deficiency, by dreaming mountains, forests and the like in case of yin exuberance, and by headache, deafness and swelling cheeks in case of adverse up—stirring of liver—qi. When liver disorders occur, there may be moving qi below the left side of the navel which feels hard on pressure, pain and fullness in the hypochondria, cramps, drowsiness, blurred vision, pterygium, etc.

In qigong treatment, patients with syndrome of deficiency and cold of the liver should practice the exercise of taking in green qi and that of nourishing the kidney (nourishing the mother to replenish the child); those with syndrome of sthenia and heat of the liver should practice the exercise of uttering "xu" and that of uttering "ke" (purging the child to treat the mother). In this respect, *Yi Shen Ji – She Sheng Xiao Xi Lun (Keep—fit Collections – On Regime Information)* by Qiu Chuji of the Yuan Dynasty (1271 – 1368) says, "In treatment of liver diseases, uttering 'xu' (exhaling) purges, while inhaling is replenishing". Hypochondriac pain and stuffiness and spasms due to derangement of the liver—qi should be treated by guiding qi back to the origin of the liver with outgoing—qi.

2. The Heart

The heart is attributed to south—fire and regarded as the Red Emperor, which pertains to Li in the Eight Diagrams. It is rosefinch in image, suspending inverted lotus stamen in shape, Bing—Ding of the Heavenly Stems and Si—Wu of the Earthly Branches. The heart is located in the centre of the chest to the left, coated by the pericardium, and is interior—exteriorly related to the small intestine. It controls blood circulation, stores the spirit, and takes charge of perspiration. The tongue is the orifice to the heart and the complexion reflects its condition.

Patients with excessive heat in the heart may have a flushed complexion, full pulse, sptum, and pain in the chest, hypochondrium, shoulder, back and arms; patients with asthenia of the heart may have radiating pain in the abdomen and dreams of weapons, flames, red clothes or other red—coloured things, flaming stoves and various terrifying events. In the case of heart disease, there is arterial impulse above the navel which often disappears upon pressing,hot sensation in the soles and palms, dry mouth, stiffness of the tongue and absent of mindedness.

qigong treatment of sthenia—heat syndrome of the heart can be conducted either by the patient himself through practising the exercise of uttering " ke" to guide water—qi (kidney—qi) to suppress fire, or by the therapist who may guide the evil—qi out of the body of the patient along the Heart Channel and the Small Intestine Channel with pulling and leading manipulations. It is stated in Yi Shen Ji — She Sheng Xiao Xi Lun (Keep—fit Collections — On Regime Information) that "Heart diseases should be treated by uttering 'ke', the charac-

ter with the sound helpful to expel of the evil—qi of the heart".
It also says, "Calm the heart—fire, rest the mind, be indifferent
to outside happenings and have light and proper amount of
food". This is a principle of treatment of asthenia syndrome,
which can be treated by practising "taking yellow qi" (replenishing the child to nourish the mother), or by pushing and guiding manipulations to reinforce the heart—qi and qi in Dantian.

3. The Lung

The lung belongs to west—metal and is regarded as the
White Emperor and pertained to Dui in the Eight Diagrams. It
is the White Tiger in image, suspended chine stone in shape,
pertaining to Geng—Xin of the Heavenly Stems and Shen—You
of the Earthly Branches. The lung, located in the chest,
connect, above with the air passages, and has its orifice in the
nose. The lung, the air passages and the nose are given the collective term of the pulmonary series. The Lung Channel is connected below lower with the large intestine and is interior—
exteriorly related with it. In charge of respiration, it controls qi
(vital energy),skin and hair,regulates the metabolism of body
fluids and is responsible for keeping qi pure and descendant.

Patients with lung disease may have pale complexion, dry
hair, dyspnea, hyposmia, stuffy nose, dryness and itching of the
skin, and discomfort and pain in the chest and back. The patient may dream of sexual acts with beauties or meeting with
long narrow funeral flags, armour, sun and moon, clouds and
cranes, and nobles. Heat syndrome of the lung may be manifested by flushed right cheek; asthenia—syndrome by shortness
of breath and failure to regulate breath;dryness— syndrome by
dry throat; and wind syndrome by perspiration and aversion to

wind which may be improved in the morning and aggravated in the afternoon and evening.

In qigong treatment of sthenia—heat syndrome of the lung, it is advisable for the patient to practise the exercises of uttering "si" and "chui" and, for the therapist, to guide the evil—qi of the patient out of the body along the Lung Channel and the Large Intestine Channel with pushing, pulling and guiding manipulations.Qiu Chuji of the Yuan Dynasty stated in his *Yi Shen Ji — She Sheng Xiao Xi Lun (Keep—fit Collections — On Regime Information)*, "phlegm in the lung should be drawn out by uttering 'si', and unintentional uttering of 'si' is a sign of disorder". For treatment of asthenia syndrome of the lung, either self— practice of qigong or outgoing—qi therapy should be aimed at replenishing the spleen (the mother) to nourish the lung and guiding qi back to its origin, the lung.

4. The spleen

The spleen is attributed to earth of the Five Elements, Kun—Gen of the Eight Diagrams, Wu—Ji of the Heavenly Stems and Chou, Chen, Wei and Xu of the Earthly Branches. It is sickle shaped, connecting with the stomach by way of the membrane. Its main functions are transporting, distributing and transforming nutrients,transporting nutrients or qi upwards,and controlling blood circulation and the activities of the extremities and muscles. Lips reflect the condition of the spleen. The mouth is the orifice to the spleen.One of the characteristics of the spleen is its preference to dryness and aversion to dampness. Failure of the normal transporting and transforming functions of the spleen may lead to poor appetite, abdominal distention, loose stool, or edema and retention of phlegm. The sinking of qi of the middle—jiao due to deficiency of the spleen is liable to cause shortness of breath, disinclination to talk, persistent diarrhoea, prolapse of anus or uterus, gastroptosia, etc. Failure of the spleen to control blood circulation because of deficiency may be manifested by bloody stool, metrorrhagia and metrostaxis, and subcutaneous hemorrhage. Qiu Chuji holds in his *Yi Shen Ji — She Sheng Xiao Xi Lun (Keep—fit Collections — On Regime Information)*, "Spleen diseases should be treated by uttering 'hu', which is effective for removing evil and noxious qi accumulated in the spleen, and helpful to digestion". To treat insufficiency of the middle—jiao, the therapist should emit outgoing—qi to Zhongwan (Ren 12) and Huangting (the Lower Dantian) for reinforcement; asthenia—heat syndrome of the spleen should be treated by guiding qi along the Spleen Channel and the Stomach Channel with pulling and leading manipulations to expel the evil—qi of the spleen and stomach.

5. The Kidney

The kidney is attributed to north—water and regarded as the Black Emperor. The two kidneys lie respectively on the two sides of the spinal column, opposite to the navel. It is dark purple in colour, belongs to Kan of the Eight Diagrams, Ren and Kui of the Heavenly Stems and Hai and Zi of the Earthly Branches and is interior—exteriorly related with the urinary bladder. The kidney stores essence, controls the bones and produces bone marrow, governs water metabolism and fire from Mingmen (Du 4, gate of life) and regulates respiration. The ear and the two yin (the anus and the external genital and urethral orifice) are the orifice to the kidney, and the kidney—energy flows to the brain.

Kidney disease is characterized by dark complexion, withered teeth, big abdomen, heavy body, dyspnea, perspiration, and moving qi below the navel which may be eliminated by pressure. Heat syndrome is manifested by flushed cheeks; deficiency syndrome by pain in the middle of the waist. According to Qiu Chuji, the author of *Yi Shen Ji — She Sheng Xiao Xi Lun (Keep—fit Collections — On Regime Information)*, "Kidney disease should be treated by purgation through uttering 'chui' and by reinforcement through laying stress on inspiration. The sluggishness and stagnation of kidney—qi can be relieved gradually by uttering 'chui' with force". That means qigong practice of the exercise uttering "chui" is effective for dredging the kidney—qi and can improve its sluggishness and stagnation, which belongs to the sthenia syndrome. The deficiency syndrome should be treated by replenishing the kidney through inhaling qi into the kidney and the waist. Decline of fire from Mingmen,(Du 4) should be treated by emitting outgoing—qi to the Lower Dantian and Mingmen (Du 4) with pushing and rotating manipulations, so as to invigorate kidney—qi and replenish the fire from the gate of life.

Essence, Vital Energy and Spirit
(Jing, Qi and Shen)

Essence (jing), vital energy (qi) and spirit (shen) constitute the essential substances for the vital activities of the human body. This theory is underlined by Lin Peiqin (1839) of the Qing Dynasty, who wrote in his *Lei Zheng Zhi Cai(Classified*

Treatment) that "The treasures the body stores are nothing but essence, vital energy and spirit".

1. Essence (Jing)

According to the understanding of the medical doctors and qigong masters of various generations, essence (jing) can be classified as congenital and acquired.

(1) Congenital Essence (Primordial Essence)

Inherited from parents, congenital essence constitutes the original substances of the human body, being the material basis for growth, development and reproduction. *Ling Shu — Jing Mai (Miraculous Pivot — Channels and Vessels)* says, "Essence exists at the beginning of life".

(2) Acquired Essence

It refers to essence derived from food. The spleen and stomach transform food into essence and then transport it through the channels and vessels to nourish the five viscera (solid organs) and irrigate the six fu—organs (hollow organs). Acquired essence is the material basis for the functional activities. Infused into the internal organs, it is called in traditional Chinese medicine "essence from the five viscera and six hollow organs".

Congenital and acquired essence are interdependent and mutual promotive. Only with the nourishment of the acquired, can the congenital be enriched and play its role. On the other hand, without the function of the congenital, the acquired can by no means be transformed.

Much emphasis is laid on the role of essence in qigong therapy. A common practice is called "transforming essence into qi", which requires painstaking effort of the practitioner in training. To raise the quality of training, one should abide by the principle of being moderate in sexual life in order to preserve essence (turbid essence).

2. Vital Energy (Qi)

As it is the basic substance and the dynamic force for maintaining normal life activities of the human body, vital energy (qi) implicates two aspects, material and functional. It is also classied into congenital and acquired. Congenital vital energy (qi) is also named primordial vital energy (qi), which is inherited from parents and derived from congenital essence. Acquired vital energy (qi) refers to the combination of the pure vital energy (qi) one receives from air and the food essence transformed into by the spleen and stomach. In the light of its distribution and function, vital energy (qi) can be further divided into four kinds: primordial qi, pectoral qi, nourishing qi and defensive qi.

(1) Primordial Qi (Yuan—qi)

Also called original qi, congenital qi, kidney—qi and genuine qi, this kind of qi includes congenital yang—qi and yin—qi. It is innate or inborn, and is the original motive force for maintaining the normal growth and development of the human body and for activating and promoting the functional activities of the internal organs. This is what *Ling Shu — Ci Jie Zhen Xie (Miraculous Pivot — Acupuncture in Regulation of the Healthy and Pathogenic Factors)* says, "The genuine qi is obtained from Heaven and is combined with food essence to nourish the body".

(2) Pectoral Qi (Zong—qi)

Pectoral qi is a combination of the fresh air inhaled by the lung and the food essence derived by the spleen and stomach from food. It is formed in the lung and accumulated in the chest, bearing the function of helping the lung in respiration and assisting the heart in blood circulation. So it is stated in *Ling Shu — Ci Jie Zhen Xie (Miraculous Pivot — Acupuncture in Regulation of the Healthy and Pathogenic Factors),* "If pectoral qi fails to descend, blood in the vessels will congeal and stagnate".

(3) Nourishing Qi (Ying—qi)

Nourishing qi is one kind of the substances derived from food essence. It enters the vessels to join the blood as one component and, as the name implies, produces blood and nourishes the whole body along with the circulation of blood.

(4) Defensive Qi (Wei—qi)

Defensive qi is one part of the substances composing yang—qi (positive qi) of the human body. It originates in the Lower—jiao (the Lower Warmer), is enriched in the Middle—jiao (the Middle Warmer) and distributed in the Upper— jiao. It is innate, coming from yang—qi (positive qi) stored in the kidney, as the saying holds, "Defensive qi comes from the Lower—jiao". In the process of its functional activities, it relies on the continuous replenishment of food essence in the Middle—jiao. Defensive qi circulates not inside but outside and along the channels and vessels to all parts of the body to warm and nourish the internal organs and the skin and hair, and to regulate the opening and closing of the points and sweat pores.

(5) Qi of qigong

This kind of qi is called "internal qi" or "external qi" (outgoing—qi) of qigong. It is a combination of primordial qi, pectoral qi, nourishing qi and defensive qi, which, through practice of the three regulations (posture, respiration and mind concentration), develops its special function with increased energy, and can gather, disperse and conduct exchanges with qi outside the body.

1) Qi and Qi Field

After qi of qigong has been trained and refined, it will become strong and be able to circulate inside the body, forming a certain "field" as that formed by the flow of electricity. It can exchange with, response to and activate qi of nature. Everyone has qi and his own qi field; the individual difference lies in the degree of perception to qi and the amount of its energy. The direction, intensity and frequency of the flow of the internal and external qi influence the physiological activities of the human body all the time.

There exists a regular system of internal qi within the human body, which is composed mainly by channels, collaterals and their points. This internal qi system is closely related to the thinking activities of the brain. Though it can not be observed by the eyes through anatomy as can be done for internal organs, nerves, muscles and other tissues under modern conditions of scientific experiment, the shape, nature, rhythm, direction and tensity of this system as well as of the internal and external qi can be perceived by the qigong adept who is especially sensitive to perception of qi. And because of this, Li Shizhen, a distinquished pharmacologist and scientist of the Ming Dynasty (1368 - 1644) holds in his book *Qi Jing Ba Mai Kao*(*Research on the Eight Extra- Channels*), "The inner scene and channels can only be perceived by those who can see things by inward—vision."

2) The Circulation of Qi

Internal qi circulates in the channels and collaterals in the direction of the course of the Twelve Channels, being in order and interior—exteriorly related to them. The course of the Twelve Regular Channel is: the Three Yin Channels of Hand run from the chest to the hand, the Three Yang Channels of Hand from the hand to the head, the Three Yang Channels of Foot from the head to the foot, and the Three Yin Channels of Foot from the foot to the abdomen and chest (Fig. 2—2).

Through training of the three regulations, the internal qi will be able to circulate not only along the course of the channels, but also against them or along several channels at the same time toward one direction to one area and, inducting or being inducted by qi of the natural world, to form a qi field. For example, if the right side of the body is yang (positive) and the left is yin (negative), the ascending of qi at the left and descending of it at the right with

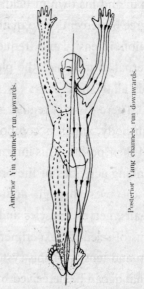

Fig. 2—2   The Course of the Yin and Yang Channels

response to qi of the natural world will form a left—descending and right— ascending qi field outside the body (Fig. 2—3).

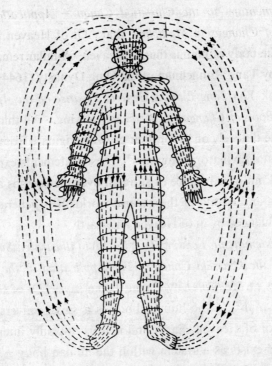

Fig. 2-3 The Qi Field of the Human Body

External qi refers to the outgoing internal qi emitted by the experienced qigong practitioner under the control of his will. This kind of qi takes form and changes its shape, nature, circulating direction and frequency following the will of the practitioner.

3) The Characteristics of Qi

The following characteristics are summarized based on the conclusion made by the ancients and the author's personal experiences in practice, observation and experimental studies.

Universality: Zhang Jiebin of the Ming Dynasty (1368-1644) held in his book *Lei Jing Tu Yi - Yiyi (Illustrated*

Supplementary to the Classified Canon − Application of the Book of Changes to Medicine) that "Qi of Heaven is that of man; the body of man is that of Heaven". Similar remarks were made by Tang Rongchuan of the Qing Dynasty (1644−1911) in his book *Yiyi Tong Lun (A General Treatise on the Application of the Book of Changes to Medicine)*, saying, "All things in the universe that rely on qi for their growth originate from qi of the congenital divinatory diagrams". These statements explain that qi is a kind of substance existing all over the cosmos and in all animals and plants of the natural world. It is generated from and influenced by qi of Heaven and Earth.

Systematism: *Lei Jing Tu Yi − Yiyi (Illustrated Supplementary to the Classied Canon − The Application of the Book of Changes to Medicine)* by Zhang Jiebin says, "Qi of Heaven is that of man. ... The human body is a small universe". This means qi of Heaven, Earth and man is not only inter−linked, but also exists as a system within the human body − "a small universe". Like the respiratory, circulatory and digestive systems, the system of qi has its own organizational structure and law of activity, bearing the responsibility of regulating the functions of the organs and tissues and the adaptability to the outside environment of qi, so as to absorb qi beneficial to the human body and expel that harmful to it.

Transmissibility: Qi has the nature of extending, disseminating, diffusing and flowing. It circulates endlessly and periodically.

Excitation: When the outgoing−qi of the therapist acts on the channels and points of the patient, it can stimulate and activate the patient's muscles and tissues to arouse movement and sensation, which may last for a certain period of time.

Synchronism: Qi posseses the nature of synchronism. When the frequency and nature of outgoing—qi are similar to those of the patient's qi, resonance and synchonism may be triggered and the patient's qi activities can be activated and regulated rapidly. In patiens or practitioners who are not so sensitive to qi, this reflect may also be obtained after repeated treatment with outgoing qi or after some qigong practice.

Sensitivity : People vary in sensitivity to qi. Those with high sensitivity may receive outgoing—qi immediately or be liable to be influenced by qi of animals, plants and other things of the outside world. Those with low sensitivity may have difficulty to perceive qi. And in some, though they do not perceive qi, they may be influenced by qi all the same.

Controlment : Qi of the human body can be controlled. This is easy for the adept of qigong. However it is not all the case. As mentioned in *Ling Shu — Jiu Zhen Shi Er Yuan (Miraculous Pivot—Nine Kinds of Needles and Twelve Source—points)* "He who understands the pivot of qi can regulate qi readily, while he who does not understand the pivot can not regulate qi at all".

3. Spirit (Shen)

Spirit, or vitality, is a general term for the life processes of the human body. It refers to the appearance of mentality, consciousness and the external conditions of essence (jing) and vital energy (qi) of the internal organs. The life activity of the human body depends on essence (jing) and vital energy (qi) as its material basis. It can be said that spirit is developed from essence and qi. For example, *Ling Shu — Ben Shen (Miraculous*

Pivot — The Original Spirit) says, "The intercourse between two kinds of essence produces spirit". *Ling Shu — Ping Ren Jue Gu (Miraculous Pivot — The Fast by Normal Man)*holds that "Spirit is the essence of grain and water (food)". So, that which derives from congenital essence is taken as yuan shen (primordial spirit or mentality), which further develops with the nourishment of the essence of food, while that which bears thinking and conciousness is taken as shi shen (perceptual spirit).

4. The Relationship between Essence, Vital Energy and Spirit and qigong Practice

Shou Shi Chuan Zhen (Portraiture of Longevity) written by Xu Wenbi of the Qing Dynasty (1644 — 1911) states, "Essence is what nourishes the body; qi is what circulates throughout the body; and spirit is what governs the body". And "Primordial essence is innate true essence, not reproductive essence; primordial qi is energy in the void, not inhaled air; and primordial spirit is original soul, not that of thinking. The so—called primordial essence, primordial vital energy and primordial spirit are those congenital which originate before birth, while the productive essence (turbid essence), air inhaled and thinking and consciousness (perceptual spirit) are acquired, which develop after birth".

The concept of essence, vital energy and spirit is different. However, they are inter—linked and mutual promotive. Of the three, essence is fundamental, vital energy is motive and spirit is dominant.

The training and regulating of essence, vital energy and spirit are of great importance in qigong practice and outgoing—qi therapy. There existed in ancient times methods of accumulating and refining essence, invigorating and regulating qi and preserving spirit, which are commonly called "refining essence into qi", "refining qi into spirit" and the like. Specificaly speaking, qigong practice is to train the acquired turbid essence, the perceptual spirit and the inhaled air in order to replenish the primordial so that life can be prolonged and diseases can be prevented and cured.

The Channels and Collaterals

Channels and collaterals are the passageways or routes by which the points per se, the points and internal organs, the internal organs and sense organs (eye, ear, nose, tongue, etc.), and the internal organs per se are interlinked with each other. Only by circulating along the channels and collaterals and linking with qi of the outside world through the skin and points, can the human qi play its normal role. The passageways of the channels and collaterals, together with the function of qi, constitute a particular channel—qi system within the human body, a system according to which and on which outgoing—qi therapy is carrird out so that qi activities can be facilitated, dredged and regulated, and evil—qi can be expelled.

The network of channels and collaterals consists of channels, collaterals and their affiliated parts such as tendon channels and skin zones. Channels include the Twelve Regular Channels running through the muscles and flesh of the body, the twelve branches of the regular channels and the Eight Extra Channels not being considered as regular. The collaterals refer to the Fifteen Reticular Branch Conduits of Channels (All the Twelve Regular Channels, the Du Channel, the Ren Channel and the Great Reticular Conduit of the Spleen have one of these conduits), the horizontal collaterals and the minute collaterals. The Twelve Tendon Channels do not run into the internal organs, while the Twelve Skin Zones are linked only to the channels. All these constitute a communicative network within the body and between the body and the outside world.

1. The Twelve Regular Channels

As the Three Yin Channels and Three Yang Channels of Hand and Foot are the principal part of the channel doctrine, they are given the name of "The Twelve Regular Channels", which include the Lung Channel of Hand—Taiyin, the Heart Channel of Hand—Shaoyin, the Pericardium Channel of Hand—Jueyin (the Three Yin Channels of Hand); the Large Intestine Channel of Hand—Yangming, the Small Intestine Channel of Hand—Taiyang, the Sanjiao Channel of Hand—Shaoyang (the Three Yang Channels of Hand); the Spleen Channel of Foot—Taiyin, the Kidney Channel of Foot—Shaoyin, the Liver Channel of Foot—Jueyin (the Three Yin Channels of Foot); and the Stomach Channel of Foot—Yangming, the Urinary Bladder Channel of Foot—Taiyang, the Gallbladder Channel of Foot—Shaoyang (the Three Yang Channels of Foot).

At the extremities, the yin channels run along the medical aspect, while the yang channel along the lateral aspect. As the medial aspect of the extremities are divided into anterior, middle and posterior sides, the yin channels running along these sides are called Taiyin, Jueyin and Shaoyin respectively. The lateral aspect is also divided into the above three sides, and the yang channels running along them are called yangming, shaoyang and taiyang accordingly. At the torso and head, the three yang channels of hand and foot are distributed along the anterior, lateral and posterior sides of the head and torso, while the three yin along the chest and abdomen (Fig. 2—4).

Each of the Twelve Regular Channels pertains to a certain viscerum. The yang channels pertain to the hollow organs and communicated with the solid while the yin channels pertain to the solid and communicated with the hollow. This forms an interior—exterior (yin—yang) relationship of communication. All the channels are inter—linked with each other and bear the responsibility of a thorougfare, along which spread the points—— the locations for qi and blood to circulate to the surface of the body.

The motion of qi and blood within the Twelve Regular Channels is circulative and continuous, starting from the Lung Channel of Hand—Taiyin, passing through all the others to the last—— the Liver Channel of Foot—Jueyin, and then to the Lung Channel of Hand—Taiyin again to restart the cycle. The terminus of one channel connects with the starting point of another, forming an endless cycle in the order of: the Lung Channel of Hand—Taiyin → the Large Intestine Channel of Hand—Yangming →the Stomach Channel of Foot—Yangming →the Spleen Channel of Foot—Taiyin →the Heart Channel of Hand—Shaoyin → the Small Intestine Channel of Hand—Taiyang → the Urinary Bladder Channel of Foot—Taiyang →the Kidney Channel of Foot—Shaoyin →the Pericardium Channel of Hand—Jueyin, → the Sanjiao Channel

of Hand—Shaoyang → the Gallbladder Channel of Foot
Shaoyang → the Liver Channel of Foot—Jueyin → the Lung
Channel of Hand Taiyin.

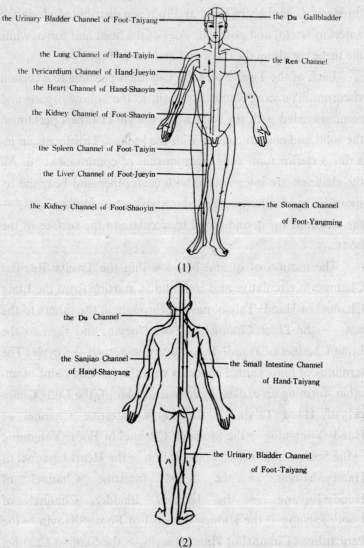

the Urinary Bladder Channel of Foot-Taiyang — the **Du** Gallbladder

the Lung Channel of Hand-Taiyin —
the Pericardium Channel of Hand-Jueyin — the **Ren** Channel
the Heart Channel of Hand-Shaoyin —

the Kidney Channel of Foot-Shaoyin —

the Spleen Channel of Foot-Taiyin —

the Liver Channel of Foot-Jueyin —

the Kidney Channel of Foot-Shaoyin — the Stomach Channel
of Foot-Yangming

(1)

the **Du** Channel —

the Sanjiao Channel —
of Hand-Shaoyang — the Small Intestine Channel
of Hand-Taiyang

the Urinary Bladder Channel
of Foot-Taiyang

(2)

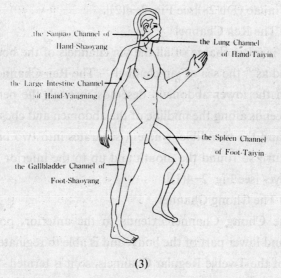

the Sanjiao Channel of Hand Shaoyang

the Lung Channel of Hand-Taiyin

the Large Intestine Channel of Hand-Yangming

the Spleen Channel of Foot-Taiyin

the Gallbladder Channel of Foot-Shaoyang

(3)

Fig. 2-4 The Distribution of the Fourteen Channels

2 The Eight Extra Channels

"The Eight Extra Channels" is a general term for the Du, Ren, Chong, Dai, Yinwei, Yangwei, Yinqiao and Yangqiao Channels. They have neither direct connection nor interior-exterior relationship with the internal organs. Generally speaking, their physiological function is to regulate qi and blood of the Twelve Regular Channels.

(1) The Du Channel

The Du Channel is regarded as "the sea of yang channels" because it governs all the yang channels of the body. It originates in the lower part of the abdomen, makes its downward way through the perineum, and then ascends along the middle of the spinal column to the brain, where it continues to ascend to the vertex and descend along the midline of the head to the apex of nose, then the point Renzhong (Du 26) and lastly the point Yinjiao (Du 28)[see Fig. 2—4(2)].

(2) The Ren Channel

As it takes charge of all the yin channels of the body, it is regarded as " the sea of yin channels". The Ren Channel originates in the lower abdomen, descrads through the perineum, then ascends along the midline of the abdomen and chest to the throat and the mandible, where it separates into two branches which turn so round the mouth and up to the inferior regions of the eyes [see Fig. 2—4(1)].

(3) The Chong Channel

The Chong Channel extends to the anterior, posterior, upper and lower part of the body, and is able to regulate qi and blood of the Twelve Regular Channels, so it is termed "the sea of the Twelve Regular Channels". This channel originates in the lower abdomen, descends and emerges at the perineum, and then ascends through the spinal column. The superficial branch of it passes through the point Qichong (St 30), meets the Kidney Channel of Foot—Shaoyin, and ascends along both sides of the umbilicus to the throat, where it goes round the lips (Fig. 2—5).

(4) The Dai Channel (The Belt Channel)

Running transversely round the waist like a belt, the Dai Channel binds and joints all the channels of the body. It starts from the lower border of the hypochondrium and runs transversely round the waist (Fig. 2—6).

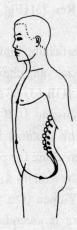

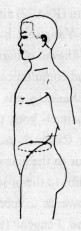

Fig. 2–5 The Chong Channel   Fig. 2–6 The Dai Channel

(5) The Yinwei Channel

The Yinwei Channel lies in the interior and serves to maintain and communicate all the yin channels in the interior of the body. This channel starts from Zhubin (K 9, a point of the Kidney Channel running along the medial aspect of the shank), ascends along the midline of the internal aspect of the lower extremities to the lower abdomen, where it passes Fushe (Sp 13) and Daheng (Sp 15) and the

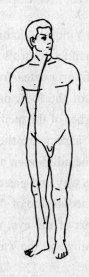

Fig.2–7   The Yingwei Channel

ribs to Qimen (Liv 14, a point of the Liver Channel) up to the chest. It then turns to go obliquely to the neck to join the points Tiantu (Ren 22) and Lianquan (Ren 23) (Fig. 2—7).

(6) The Yangwei Channel

The Yangwei Channel lies superficially and serves to maintain and communicate the superficial yang channels of the body. The channel starts from Jinmen (UB 63) of the Urinary Bladder Channel, goes upward to Yangjiao (UB 35) of the Gallbladder Channel, ascends along this channel to Bishu (a point inferior to the iliac crest) and then along the posterior aspect of the libs to the posterior end of the axillary fold, then the shoulder upwards to meet the points Yamen (Du 15), Fengfu (Du 16) and Fengchi (GB 20), where it ascends along the Gallbladder Channel to the vertex, and ends at Yangbai (GB 14) (Fig. 2—8).

(7) The Yinqiao Channel

This channel controls the yin of the left and right sides of the body. It originates from the point Rangu (K 2) at the medial side of the foot, passes through Zhaohai (K 6) to the superior borber of the medial malleolus, where it ascends along the medial aspect of the lower limb, passes through the perineum, the adbdomen and chest to Quepen (St 12). Then it continues its way and passes the anterior aspect of Renying (St 9) and the medial side of the zygomatic region and reaches the inner canthus of the eye, where it meets with the Channel of Hand—Taiyang and the Yangqiao Channel (Fig. 2—9).

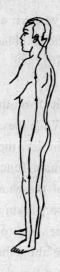

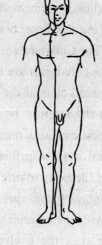

Fig. 2—8 The Yangwei Channel   Fig. 2—9 The Yinqiao Channel

(8) The Yangqiao Channel

This channel controls the yang of the left and right sides of the body. It originates at the point Shenmai (UB 62) below the external malleolus, makes its way upward along the lateral aspect of the lower limb to Juliao (femur, UB 29), which is located above the iliac bone, to the posterior aspect of the hypochondrium. Via the should and neck, it goes up to Dicang (St 4) at the corner of the mouth, then passes Juliao (St 3)

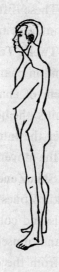

Fig. 2—10   The Yangqiao Channel

and Chengqi (St 1) to Jingming (U B 1), where it ascends into the hairline, goes behind the ear, meets the Gallbladder Channel and ends at Fengchi (G B 20) (Fig. 2–10).

3. The Collaterals

The collaterals are the branch conduits from the channels. They spread all over the body like a net. While the channels belong to the interior, lie deeper and are thicker, the collaterals are superficial and much thinner. The main function of the collateral is to transfuse qi and blood of the channels to all parts of the body to nourish the tendon, bone, skin and the five sense organs (nose, eye, lip, tongue and ear), and to link the interior with the exterior. The large one are altogether fifteen in number, i.e., the twelve from the Twelve Regular Channels respectively, plus the other three from the Du, Ren and Spleen Channels. These fifteen collaterals are all horizontal, connecting the internal and superficial channels.

4. The Twelve Tendon Channels

The tendon channels are of tendon–flesh nature affiliated to the system of channels and collaterals. They lie along the four extremitis, the body surface, the chest and abdomen. They do not enter the internal organs. Physiologically they mainly coordinate the movement of the limbs and bones.

5. The Skin Zones

The Skin Zones are the superficial parts of the system of the channels and collaterals. Although the channels lie within the flesh and muscles, not superficially near the skin, the collaterals from the channels go everywhere. Qi and blood at the skin part right rely on the collaterals for nourishment. So physiologically, the body surface is divided into twelve zones based on different channels and their collaterals. These divisions are called the Twelve Skin Zones.

6. The Application of the Theory of Channels and Collaterals to Outgoing—qi Therapy

Without knowing the doctrine of channels and collaterals, a qigong therapist can neither conduct the practice of training qi, guiding qi and emitting qi nor can he carry out differential treatment of patients, just as the old saying holds, "Without the understanding of the viscera, channels and collaterals, mistake will follow whenever one starts to talk or act".

(1) Guiding qigong Practice

Zhen Jiu Zhi Nan (*A Guidebook on Acupuncture and Moxibustion*) says "He who intends to learn acupuncture must take up exercises first. ...the skill of sitting in quiescence, to realize the circulation of qi along the channels and collaterals and the opening and closing of points so that he can have a good ground in acupuncture practice and can be clear—minded in determination of points. Otherwise he may have no idea of where to operate." This means qigong practice can help to understand the circulation of the channel qi within the human body, for it actually can facilitate a smooth flow of qi and blood along all the channels and collaterals, or in other words, the circulation of qi can be controlled by will.

The Eight Extra Channels, especially the Du and Ren Channels, are of utmost importance in qigong practice. Zhang Ziyang, lived in Song Dynasty (420—479), explained this in his book *Ba Mai Jing*(*The Eight Extra Channels*), saying, "The Eight Extra Channels of the common people are of yin nature and are closed. Only the spirit immortals have theirs burst open with yang—qi (positive energy). So they get the knack. The Eight Extra Channels are the root of the main congenital channels and the ancestor of qi. "Li Shizhen (1578) stated in his Qi Jing Ba Mai Kao(Reserch on the Eight Extra Channels), "The Ren Channel and Du Channel are the prime meridians of the human body, the routes along which the qigong adepts make the yang—fire and yin—materials go up and down, and the home where the Kan—water and Li—fire have their intercourse." The practitioners generally refer to the sensation of channel qi flowing along the Ren and Du Channels as the "small circle of qi" and that along the Ren and Du channels as well as the Twelve Regular Channels as the "large circle of qi".

(2) Guiding Emission of Qi

The Training of guiding qi and emitting outgoing—qi comprises the training of qi circulation within the channels and collaterals, tendon collaterals and skin zones. Only when one is able to control the circulation, the coming in and going out and the spread and convergence of qi voluntarily, can he carry out emission of outgoing—qi.

The channels and their branches, the extra channels, the tendon channels and the skin zones altogether compose a qi circulation whole or a channel—collateral —qi system of the human body. This system interlinks the interior and the exterior, the upper and the lower, the left and the right, and extremities, bones, internal organs and all tissues of the human body, making the human body a complete, systematic organic whole,a structure closely bound up with " qi" of the natural world by way of the skin zones and points, and a three—in—one combination of the "three gifts" ——Heaven, Earth and man.

So the practitioner of qigong can, besides training the circulation of qi of his own, absorb qi which is beneficial to his health from the natural world to replenish and facilitate qi within his body. As regards outgoing—qi therapy, it means that the therapist mobilizes and activates qi of the natural world and that of the patient with his own qi to get the patient's qi active, then regulates it with the method of purgating the excess and replenishing the deficiency, dredging the channels and leading qi back to its origin.

Section Two   Application of the Book of Changes to Medicine and Outgoing—qi Therapy

The theory of application of the Book of Changes to medicine is one of the principle guiding Qigong outgoing—qi therapy. One who knows only the science of medicine without the understanding of the Change or vice versa can speak nothing of treatment of diseases by emission of outgoing—qi, for outgoing—qi therapy is the application of a clinical combination of the philosophy of the Change, medicine and qi which requires the therapist firstly has a deep understanding of the doctrine of exchanges and changes between the universe (Heaven and Earth) and the human being, the (Taoist) theory and skills of training qi and cultivating oneself, as well as the modern physiology and pathology of the human body. Just as stated by Zhang Jiebin (1624) in his book *Lei Jing Tu Yi (Illustrated Supplementary to the Classified Canon)*, "Without the understanding of the Change one is not worthy of the name of an imperial physician." According to Zhang Jiebin, the truth of the universe lies in the creation of all things with yin—qi and yang—qi while the truth of human being lies in growth and development of bones with yin—qi and yang—qi, both being the consequence of movement, rest, waning and waxing of yin and yang. So he also stated that "the similarity of medicine and the Change in their origin is the similarity of them in their variation", "the philosophy of the Change implicates that of medicine, and the philosophy of medicine benefits from that of the Change", and "the variation of the Change rests with the universe while the application of medicine rests with the human being".

The Eight Diagrams

1. The Composition of the Eight Diagrams

Xici,a chapter of the book *Zhouyi(The Book of Changes)* states "Yi (the change) has Taiji (The Great Ultimate);Taiji articulates itself into two principles; the two principles articulate themselves into four symbols; and the four symbols articulate themselves into eight diagrams". The ancients believed that the Chaos (the nihility) when Earth was separated from Heaven was the phenomenon of Taiji (The Great Ultimate). The movement of Taiji produced the two principles of yin and yang. Yin—qi and yang—qi then developed and transformed themselves into the four symbols of Taiyin, Shaoyin, Taiyang and Shaoyang, which in turn articulated into the Eight Diagrams of Qian, Kun, Kan, Li, Zhen, Dui, Xun and Gen representing Heaven, Earth, water, fire, thunder, marsh, wind and mountain, which then divided into sixty—four diagrams and then more, in a binary system, to the infinite (Fig. 2−11).

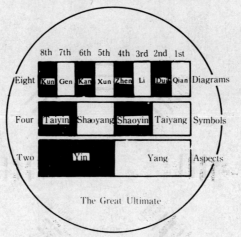

Fig. 2−11 The Sequence of the Eight Diagrams

2. The Congenital Eight Diagrams

Another term for the Congenital Eight Diagrams is Fu Xi's Eight Diagrams, with which Heaven and Earth are orientated based on Qian and Kun. In the Congenital Eight Diagrams, Heaven and Earth, wind and thunder, water and fire, and mountain and marsh are all defined as couple yin and yang opposite to each other (Fig. 2−12). This kind of diagram is taken as the body aspect which governs qi and can generate all things.

3. The Acquired Eight Diagrams

Another term for it is King Wen's Eight Diagrams, with which south and north are orientated based on Li and Kan. In the Acquired Eight Diagrams, the five orientations of east, west, south, north and centre and the five elements of metal, wood, water, fire and earth are all matched with the Eight Diagrams (Fig. 2−13). This kind of diagram is taken as the applica-

tion aspect, which controls movement and is able to form all
things.

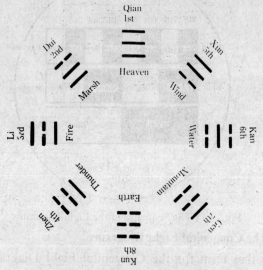

Fig. 2-12 The Congenital Eight Diagrams

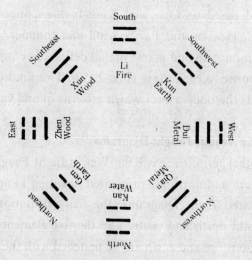

Fig. 2-13 The Aquired Eight Diagrams

4. The Essential Factors of the Eight Diagrams

The Eight Diagrams are matched with yin and yang, the Five Elements, male and female, the body, the internal organs and the number in a way of classification and analogy to summarize and explain the interrelations between all the things (Table 2-2).

Table 2-2 The Essential Factors of the Eight Diagrams

Eight Diagrams	Qian	Kun	Zhen	Xun	Kan	Li	Gen	Dui
Picture	☰	☷	☳	☴	☵	☲	☶	☱
Appearance	Three unbroken lines	Three broken lines	A vessel	One broken line below	Unbroken in the middle	Broken in the middle	An inverted bowl	One broken line above
Congenital positions	South	North	North-east	South-west	Weat	East	North-west	South-east
Aquired positions	North-west	South-west	East	South-east	North	Sorth	North-east	West
Sequence	Father	Mother	Eldest son	Eldest daughter	Middle son	Middle daughter	Youngest son	Youngest ddaughter
The body	Head	Abdomen	Foot	Thish	Ear	Eye	Hand	Mouth
Internal Organs	Large Intestine	Spleen	Gall-bladder	Liver	Kidney	Heart	Stomach	Lung
Five Elements	Metal	Earth	Wood	Wood	Water	Fire	Earth	Metal
Yin-Yang	Yang	Yin	Yang	Yin	Yang	Yin	Yang	Yin
Congenital number	One	Eight	Four	Five	Six	Three	Seven	Two
Acquired number	Six	Two	Three	Four	One	Nine	Eight	Seven

5. The Application of the Eight Diagrams

(1) The Eight Diagrams and the Configuration of the Human Body

All things, from the universe in a macroscopic concept, to animals, plants and all parts of the human body, in a specific concept, may be viewed as individual models of the Eight Congenital Diagrams. They emanate from the models and take shape of their own "bodies". As it should be, "bodies" are divided into live and dead. The live body emanates from qi, while the dead body has no qi. Things without qi will lose their vitality.

The physique of the human body is the body of the Eight Diagrams. Qian is regarded as Heaven which belongs to yang. As the head is on the top of the human body, it assumes the appearance of Heaven, with the nose as a passage for respiration and a link with the Heavenly—qi. And as all the Three Yang Channels run up and converge at the top of the head and take charge of the functional activities of the whole body, Qian should be corresponded with the head. Kun is regarded as Earth which belongs to yin. The abdomen is taken as the opposite of the head. All the Three Yin Channels converge in the abdomen which also pertains to yin, so Kun should be coupled with the abdomen. With the head as Qian and the abdomen as Kun, a yin—yang body with one yin and one yang is configurated. As to the Zhen Diagram beside Qian, it has one yang at the bottom, appearing to be yin with one yang. Tang Rongchuan of the Qing Dynasty (1644—1911) said in his works *Yiyi Xiang Jie(Detailed Explanations of Application of the Book of Changes to Medicine)*," If yang is exuberant at the Lower—jiao, the feet will be warm". Yang—qi (positive qi) of the human body originates at the lower part, so Zhen should be coupled with the foot. The Xun Diagram beside Qian is of yin nature with one yin at the bottom; yang has yin growing at its bottom and yang should be at the upper and coupled with the

Liver Channel of Jueyin. The liver is in charge of the tendons and the main tendons extend downward to the thigh, so Xun couples with the thigh to correspond with Zhen, also forcing a pair of yin and yang. Kan is regarded as water, belongs to yin and couples with the kidney. The kidney has its upper orifice in the ear which, with a thin membrane to hold yang—qi, can hear sound. Kan looks full in the middle, so it is coupled with the ear. Li is regarded as fire which belongs to yang and is related to heart—fire. Fire manifests itself in the eye. One awakens at day time when the heart—vitality comes out into the eye.So the eye should be coupled with Li.The ear and the eye, one being yin and another yang, form the main sense organs of the human body.The Gen Diagram is regarded as yang; yang comes out of yin and stays at the upper. In his works *Yiyi Xiang Jie (Detailed Explanations of Application of the Book of Changes to Medicine)*, Tang Rongchuan stated, " The lucid—yang ascends from the gallbladder into the stomach and spreads externally to the hand." The hand has the appearance of stopping things, so Gen is coupled with the hand. The Dui diagram is of yin nature, which controls the generation of fluid. With an opening at its upper line, Dui pertains to the lung. The lung—qi comes out of the mouth and nose, and fluid gushes in the mouth, so the mouth should be coupled with Dui. Gen and Dui, or the hand and the mouth, being one yin and one yang, form a pair of main functional organs.

Because every specific portion of the human body embraces the message of the whole body, this portion, even its individual cells, can be explained with the Eight Diagrams. One example is the points arranged based on the Eight Diagrams in child massage, which expresses the relationship between the eight points (diagrams) and the internal organs (Fig. 2—14). The explanation of the human body according to the Eight Diagrams concretely embodies the body aspect, application aspect, qi and movement of the Congenital and Acquired Eight Diagrams, indicating the law that the human being is linked with Heaven and Earth, and that Heaven, Earth and man are one.

(2) The Eight Diagrams and the Congenital and Acquired Qi

Tang Rongchuan of the Ming Dynasty (1644 — 1911) says in his book *Yiyi Xiang Jie (Detailed Explanations* of Application of the Book of Changes to Medicine), " At the embryonic phase, man first develops the head, which is termed in the Eight Diagrams as Qian—one, then

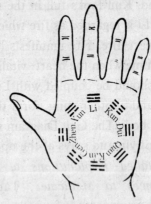

Fig. 2—14 The Eight Diagrams as Points for Child Massage (Tuina)

the lung as Dui—two, and in turn, the heart as Li—three, the liver and gallbladder as Zhen—four and Xun—five respectively, the kidney as Kan—six, the stomach and intestines as Gen—seven, and last the muscles as Kun—eight ... a process that corresponds with the image of the Eight Diagrams". From the Eight Diagrams, the process of qi transformation of the embryo can be perceived. So he said again, "During the process of development, the fetus in the first month is only a bit of yang—qi, the source of life process which corresponds with Qian—one; in the second month, qi transforms into liquid which corresponds with Dui—two and controls the body fluid; in the third month, qi and fluid combine with each other and transform into heat in correspondence with Li—three; in the fourth month, the fetus begins its movements in correspondence with Zhen—four; in the fifth month, the fetus begins its fetal respiratory movement along with maternal respiration in correspondence with Xun—five; at the sixth month, the amniotic fluid becomes sufficient in correspondence with Kan—six; at the seventh month, the fetal stomach and intestines develop in correspondence with Gen—seven; and at the eight month, the muscles and fleshes are formed, which is in correspondence with Kun—eight". So the fetus makes its original qi substantial and the physique complete in eight months in its mother's body, and attains all the fetal development in ten months. The above—mentioned may be taken as an example which, through the formation of a human fetus, explains the philosophy that the Congenital Eight Diagrams governs the body and qi. It is for this reason that when outgoing—qi therapy is applied, the correspondence relationship between yin and yang should be taken into full consideration in selection of points and channels for emission of qi, digital point—pressing or acupuncture. Only in this way, can yin and yang be well regulated and diseases be cured.

In its maternal body when its physique is not completed, the child transports, transforms and produces qi and blood mainly relying on the function of the Eight Extra—channels, while the Twelve Regular Channels are in the process of gradual development. And when the child leaves its mother's body and comes into the world of qi (atmosphere), it begins to accomplish the circulation of qi and blood relying on the Twelve

Regular Channels, while the Eight Extra—channels only function to regulate the channel qi. Or to put it differently, the
Eight Extra—channels may be considered as the body aspect
and the original qi of the Congenital Eight Diagrams, and the
Twelve Regular Channels as the application and transportation
aspects of the Acquired Eight Diagrams. And this is taken as
the principle guiding Qigong practice and treatment of clinical
cases. In Qigong practice, the opening of the circulation of qi
along the Ren and Du Channels as well as the Eight
Extra—channels and the transformation of the mouth—nasal
respiration into patent one is actually a process of transformation towards the congenital aspect. Similarly, illnesses are divided into congenital and acquired.In case of congenital
insufficiency of qi or disorder of qi activities, it is advisable to
dredge the Eight Extra—channels to regulate and consolidate
the primordial qi; while for acquired diseases of the internal organs, channels or vessels and qi, satisfactory curative effect can
only be obtained when the selection of points and the methods
of emitting qi are determined according to the characteristics of
qi circulation in the Twelve Regular Channels. No doubt, neither the congenital nor acquired factors should be neglected
owing to the fact that the origination and development of diseases may result from both the congenital and acquired factors,
the factors which are interdependent and mutually influential.

The practice of the "small circle of qi", according to the illustration of the Acquired Eight Diagrams, is called taking
Kan to fill Li, the intercourse between yin and yang, or the
coordination of water and fire. On the other hand, the practice
of the "large circle of qi" is based on the Congenital Eight Diagrams, known as the intercorse between Qian and Kun.How-

ever the alchemists always have the two diagrams Kan and Li in mind because they are positioned at Mao and You of the Earthly Branches. So the large circle of qi is also called Mao—You circle of qi.

(3) The Eight Diagrams and the Development of Male and Female

Shang Gu Tian Zhen Lun (On the True Heaven in the Ancient Times) of the book *Su Wen (Plain Questions)* says, "In female, the kidney—qi becomes substantial at the age of seven ..., and menarche begins at double—seven (age fourteen); in male, kidney—qi is full at the age of eight ..., and sexual function begins at double—eight (sixteen) when the kidney—qi is substantial ...". The reason why eight and seven are used for male and female as the base for analogizing the life process of birth, growth, adulthood and decline can be ascribed to the number in the Eight Diagrams. Kui of the Heavenly Stems corresponds with the sexual function and is regarded as water, and as the kidney is ascribed to water too, it is then taken as Kan—water in the Eight Diagrams. The Gen Diagram ☶ means young male and is given the number eight in the Acquired Eight Diagrams, Dui Diagram ☱ means young female and is given the number seven in the Acquired Eight Diagrams. Again, why it is believed that the sexual functions of male begin at double—eight (sixteen) and of female at double—seven (fourteen)? The reason lies in that in the Congenital Eight Diagrams, the number for male is counted starting from the Gen Diagram leftwards to the number sixteen while for female is counted starting from the Dui Diagram rightwards to the number fourteen, both ending just at the position of the Kan Diagram, which indicates kidney—water (Fig.

2—15). As is stated in *Yiyi Xiang Jie (Detailed Explanations of Application* of the Book of *Changes to Medicine)* written by Tang Rongchuan, "In '*Canon of Internal Medicine*', (it is recorded) the number eight for male and seven for female, but no schools give correct explanations and it is not known that before the sexual functions begin, male and female are just young boy and young girl. Actually, it should be explained in response with the Gen and Dui Diagrams, from which the number for male and female is counted respectively".

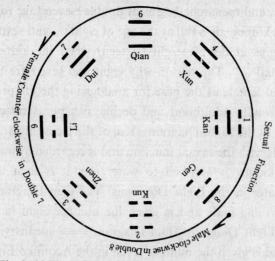

Fig. 2—15 The Relationship between the Sexual Function of Male and Female and the Eight Diagrams

The Yao Image and the Human Body

1. The Yao Image

Yao (yin or yang line) is the basic element of the picture of the diagrams. It falls into two categories: the negative yao (symbolized by the broken line——) and the positive yao (symbolized by the unbroken line——), the former representing yin and the latter representing yang. The overlap of three yao may form different trigrams of the Eight Diagrams. For example, the trigram ☴ is the overlap of the two positive yao and one negative yao, which is taken as the Xun Diagram, with two yang above one yin. Two yang and one yin can also from ☲ , the Li Diagram, and ☱ , the Dui Diagram, which have different meanings. If two diagrams (trigrams) are overlapped, then sixty—four diagrams (hexagrams) can be formed, with each diagram having six yao. Expressed in number, the positive (yang) yao is nine, and negative (yin) yao six. The order of the diagrams is arranged from the bottom to the top in six yao positions, termed respectively as bottom—yao, the 2nd—yao, 3rd—yao, 4th—yao, 5th—yao and top—yao. As it can be seen in ䷊ which is termed Tai Diagram, the picture is formed by an overlap of three negative yao (three yin lines, the Kun Diagram) and three positive yao (three yang lines, the Qian Diagram).To express its position and its attribution (yin or yang), the Tai Diagram is expressed in terms of bottom—nine, nine—two, nine—three, six—four, six—five and top—six (Fig. 2—16).

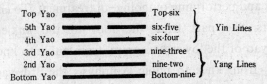

Fig. 2—16　The Tai Diagram

2. The Yao Image and the Body Partitions

Tang Rongchuan of the Ming Dynasty held in his book *Yiyi Xiang Jie (Detailed Explanations of Application of the*

Book of Changes to Medicine), "So far as the human body is concerned, ... the part from the foot to the knee is the bottom—yao, from the knee to the root of the thigh is the 2nd—yao, from the lower abdomen to the navel is the 3rd—yao, from the navel to the diaphragm is the 4th— yao, from the diaphragm to the chest and neck is the 5th—yao, and from the neck to the vertex is the top—yao". Here Tang divided the human body based on the positions of the six yao [Fig. 2—17(1)]. According to this doctrine, the lower two yao can be considered as Earth, the middle two as man, and the upper two as Heaven, meaning Qian being the head and Kun being the abdomen. Similar to the composition of yin—yang as well as the Eight Diagrams and the Five Elements, the position of the yao images is arranged in line with the principle of yin—yang encompassing yin—yang and yao image encompassing yao image, and parts closely related with the whole and man closely related with nature. The same principle is applicable to outgoing—qi therapy——the human body may be divided into two diagrams (hexagrams), the upper and the lower in the light of the relations between the upper and lower partitions for convenience of detecting qi, making diagnosis and performing outgoing—qi treatment. To enter into particulars, the part from the foot to the ankle is the bottom—yao of the lower hexagram, from ankle to knee is the 2nd—yao, from knee to pubic symphysis the 3rd—yao, from pubic symphysis to navel the 4th—yao, from navel to xiphoid process the 5th—yao, and from xiphoid process to supraclavicular notch the top—yao. As for the upper hexagram, the part from the pubic symphysis to the navel is the bottom—yao, from navel to xiphoid process the 2nd—yao, from xiphoid process to supraclavicular notch the 3rd–yao,from supraclavicular notch to the tip of the nose the 4th–yao, from the tip of nose to brow the 5th–yao, and from brow to the vertex of the head the top–yao. The upper limb is also divided into three yao,which correspond with those of the lower limb and the head and neck. In this way, the three yao of the lower and upper hexagrams interlock at the chest and abdomen (Fig. 2–17).

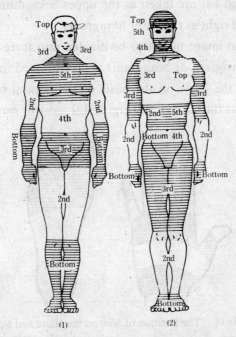

Fig. 2–17   The Position of Yao (Yin and Yang Lines)

This relationship of the yao positions is suitable to both the channel system and the nervous system. The part of the spinal column and waist, for example,is the 4th–yao of the lower hexagram and at the same time the bottom–yao of the upper hexagram; disorders of this part may be manifested by symptoms of the lower limbs. When stagnation of qi and other abnormal conditions occur in one part of the body, imbalance of internal and external qi may be detected at this part or its corresponding region. Furthermore,the yao image of the diagrams is not limited to the division of the six yao positions on the upper and lower part of the body, it can be positioned at the anterior and posterior, and the left and right, of which the posterior and left are taken as the upper hexagrams while the anterior and right as the lower hexagrams.

The yao image may also be divided into three or six yao sections (a trigram or hexagram) and positioned in a specific location of the body on the basis of the natural body partitions, such as the hand, foot (Fig. 2—18), nose or ear, so that

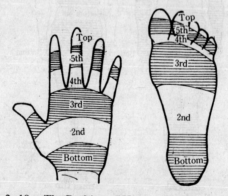

Fig. 2—18   The Position of Yao on the Hand and Foot

the relationship between this specific part and the whole body or even the natural environment can be observed. As the human body is "a small circle of qi" and the epitome of the "large circle of qi" of the universe, the manifestations of the hand,foot,face, ear or nose may provide basis for diagnosis and treatment of diseases and even for perception and prediction of certain future life particulars. All this embodies the doctrine that Heaven, Earth and man are a combination of one and exist in the same world of qi.

Again, Tang Rongchuan stated in *Yiyi Xiang Jie (Detailed explanations of Application of the Book of Changes to Medicine)*, "Taking a herb as an example, the root of the herb is the bottom—yao, the stalk the 2nd—yao, the upper stem the 3rd—yao, the branch the 4th—yao, the leaf the 5th—yao and the flower and fruit the top—yao". So when the plant serves as a medicine, its height of the yao position may manifest its property in terms of ascending, descending, floating and sinking. Take achyranthes root as an example, it corresponds with the bottom—yao, so it can penetrate down to the tibia and foot. In contract, honeysuckle flower and chrysanthemum flower correspond with the top—yao, so they are effective for diseases of the head, eyes, etc.

3. The Yao Image and the Internal Organs

In *Yiyi (Application of the Book of Changes to Medicine)* of *Lei Jing Tu Yi (Illustrated Supplementary to the Classified Canon)* written by Zhang Jiebin, it is stated that "as the images of the zang and fu organs are concerned, the part from the bottom—six, which initiates from Mingmen (Du 4), to the top—six is regarded as yin and related to the zang organs, ... while that from the bottom—nine, which originates from the urinary bladder, to the top—nine is taken as yin and related to the fu—organs. ... Being aware of this, one will be clear about the inner image concerning the yin or yang aspect of zang or fu organs, and the position of them". This indicates that the internal organs (the zang and fu organs) of the human body are, too, conform to the law of the yao image. Relating the yao image with the zang and fu organs, the inner yin and yang nature and the function of the internal organs can be deduced. Speaking in detail, the Kun Diagram is attributed to yin and ascribed to the five zang (solid) organs and Mingmen (Du 4), with its bottom—yao being Mingmen (Du 4), the 2nd—yao the kidney,the 3rd—yao the liver, the 4th—yao the spleen,the 5th—yao the heart, and the top—yao the lung. Qian is attributed to yang and ascribed to the six fu (hollow) organs, with its bottom—yao being the urinary bladder, the 2nd—yao the large intestine, the 3rd—yao the small intestine, the 4th—yao the gallbladder, the 5th—yao the stomach and the top—yao the Sanjiao (the three warmers) (Fig. 2—19).

4. The Appearance of the Diagrams and Diseases

The ancients took the appearance of the diagrams to explain the etiology, the pathology, the clinical manifestations and the principles≡≡of treatment of diseases. The mechanism can be seen from the following examples.

The Tai Diagram : With the Kun trigram expressed by yin lines at the upper and the Qian trigram

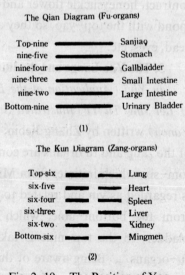

The Qian Diagram (Fu-organs)

Top-nine	Sanjiao
nine-five	Stomach
nine-four	Gallbladder
nine-three	Small Intestine
nine-two	Large Intestine
Bottom-nine	Urinary Bladder

(1)

The Kun Diagram (Zang-organs)

Top-six	Lung
six-five	Heart
six-four	Spleen
six-three	Liver
six-two	Kidney
Bottom-six	Mingmen

(2)

Fig. 2—19   The Position of Yao on the Zang and Fu Organs

expressed by yang lines at the lower and with yang ascending and yin descending and the two coordinative, this hexagram is the symbol of strong and healthy constitution with balanced and coordinative yin and yang. During Qigong practice and outgoing–qi therapy, the Tai Diagram can be obtained by guiding yang–qi down and yin–qi up.

The Pi Diagram ☰☷ : In this hexagram, it can be seen that the Kun trigram is below Qian and yin lines are below yang, meaning yang ascending and yin descending and yin and yang disassociated and incoordinative, which is an evidence of stoppage of life.

The Jiji Diagram ☵☲ : In this hexagram, the Li trigram is below the Kan. Li is referred to as fire and related to the heart; while Kan referred to as water and related to the kidney. With the Kan–water above the Li–fire, which means the descending of water and ascending of fire, it is the symbol of coordination between fire (heart) and water (kidney). The same principle is explained in *Yiyi (Application of the Book of Changes to Medicine)of Lei Jing Tu Yi (Illustrated Supplementary to the Classified Canon)* written by Zhang Jiebin of the Ming Dynasty (1368 – 1644), who held " The Jiji Diagram means the coordination between the heart and the kidney" . During Qigong practice and outgoing–qi therapy, one should guide the heart–fire down to the kidney and the kidney–water up to the heart so as to achieve the state of Jiji Diagram.

The Weiji Diagram ☲☵ : From the hexagram it can be seen that the trigram Kan is below Li and the Li–fire is above the Kan–water, indicating incoordination between water (kidney) and fire (heart) and discordance between yin and yang, which is an evidence of incoordination between the heart and the kidney. The clinical manifestations may include insomnia, vexation,hot sensation in the heart, palms and soles and dreaminess because of hyperactivity of the heart—fire due to insufficiency of the kidney—yin and failure of kidney—water to coordinate with the heart—fire. To correct this, one should nourish the kidney—yin and purge the heart—fire and try to attain the Jiji Diagram mentioned above, which is the symbol of recovery and fitness. In Qigong practice, if the practitioner does not concentrate himself and keep a calm heart, he may fail to guide the heart—fire down to the kidney. As a result, disassociation between yin and yang as manifested by the Pi Diagram other than positive effect of Qigong may occur.

The Daguo Diagram ☰☱ and the Xiaoguo Diagram ☳☶ : The former has the trigram Xun below the Dui while the latter has the Gen below the Zhen, both having yin—yao (negative line) at the top and bottom,with yang lines in between. The two hexagrams symbolize the gradual invasion of yin—cold and failure of yang to extend, which is an indication of stagnation, stasis and abdominal mass. As Zhang Jiebin states in *Yiyi (Application of the Book of Changes to Medicine)* of his work *Lei Jing Tu Yi (Illustrated Supplementary to the Classified Canon),*" The Daguo and Xiaoguo represent the gradual invasion of yin—cold and abdominal mass".

The Zhongfu Diagram ☴☱ and the Yi Diagram ☶☳ : The former has the trigram Dui below the Xun while the latter has the Zhen below the Gen, both with the yang—yao (positive lines) embracing yin—yao in between, which are indicative of gradual waning of yang—qi (positive qi) and tympanites.

The Guan Diagram ☴☷ and the Bo Diagram ☶☷ : The former has the trigram Kun below the Xun, indicating the gradual weakening of yang—qi; the latter has the trigram Kun below the Gen, indicating the gradual collapse of yang—qi. The weakening of yang is often manifested by short breath, perspiration and thready pulse while the collapse of yang by clamminess of the body, weakness of breath and loss of consciousness.

The Twelve Informatory Diagrams

The Twelve Informatory Diagrams (hexagrams) are also termed Twelve Pi diagrams. The doctrine was put forward by Meng Xi of the Han Dynasty (206 B.C. — A.D. 220) who took the Twelve Pi diagrams as the representative of the order of the twelve months of the year. The twelve diagrams consist of seventy—two yao lines, which symbolize seventy—two climatic seasons. As the changes of the seventy—two yao lines, termed hardness and softness (yin and yang), embody the process of waning and waxing of yin and yang, Wei Boyang of the Eastern Han Dynasty (25—220) took them to analogize the extent of small or large circle of qi in practice of training qi, and the physicians of the ancient time then used them to interpret the relationship between nature and growth and development as well as the visce— ra, channels and circulation of qi.

1. The Contents of the Twelve Informatory Diagrams

They refer to the twelve hexagrams of Fu ☲☲ , Lin ☲☲, Tai ☲☲ , Dazhuang ☲☲ , Guai ☲☲ , Qian ☰☰ , Gou ☰☰ , Dun ☰☰ , Pi ☰☷ , Guan ☴☷ , Bo ☶☷ ,and Kun ☷☷ . The first six hexagrams, from the Fu to Qian, indicate the process of gradual waxing of yang—yao and gradual waning of yin—qi; while the other six, from Gou to Kun, represent the process of gradual waxing of yin—yao and the increase of yin—qi. They are given the general term of Twelve Informatory (Waning and Waxing) Diagrams right for the reason that the first six implicate the wax of yang and the wane of yin and the second six implicate the wax of yin and the wane of yang. The Twelve Informatory Diagrams represent the law of the changes of hardness and softness (the domination and yield) and the growth and decline of yin and yang, and explicate the close relationship between the seasons, the time, the zang and fu organs, the channels, and the transformation and circulation of qi. They are taken as the theoretical principle guiding Qigong practice and diagnosis and treatment of diseases with outgoing—qi (Table 2—3).

Table 2—3   The Relationship between the Twelve Informatory Diagrams and Time and the Internal Organs

Diagram	Picture	Month	Season	Time	Earthly Branches	Organs	Pulse	Channels for Qi Flowing
Fu		Nov.	Winter	23—1	Zi	Kidney	Deep	Gallbladder
Lin		Dec.	Winter	1—3	Chou	Sanjiao	Deep	Liver
Tai		Jan.	Spring	3—5	Yin	Liver	Taut	Lung
Dazhuang		Feb.	Spring	5—7	Mao	Gall—bladder	Taut	Large Intestine
Guai		Mar.	Spring	7—9	Chen	Peri—cardium	Taut	Stomach
Qian		Apr.	Summer	9—11	Si	Small Intestine	Full	Spleen
Gou		May	Summer	11—13	Wu	Heart	Full	Heart
Dun		June	Summer	13—15	Wei	Spleen	Full	Small Intestine
Pi		July	Autumn	15—17	Shen	Stomach	Super—ficial	Urinary Bladder
Guan		Aug.	Autumn	17—19	You	Lung	Super—ficial	Kidney
Bo		Sept.	Autumn	19—21	Xu	Large Intestine	Super—ficial	Pericardium
Kun		Oct.	Winter	21—23	Hai	Urinary Bladder	Deep	Sanjiao

2 The Practice of Qigong According to the Twelve Informatory Diagrams

The process of waxing and waning of yin and yang of the human body in all one's life, or a year, a month, and even a day can all be manifested by the Twelve Informatory Diagrams. Take, for example, a year as one week, a month is then one diagram; a month as a week, two and half days are then a diagram; and a day as a week, the one two—hour period is a diagram. Now let us take a month as one week, which has two and half days in one diagram, as an example. The process of fluctuation of yin and yang starts at the beginning of the month when yang—qi begins to grow, which is regarded as the Fu Diagram ䷗ indicative of the generation of vitality, or to put it differently, one yang generates from the Kun Diagram ䷁ , which is of whole yin. Then the yang aspect continues to grow while the yin aspect begins to decline to enter into the state of yin and yang in equilibirium, a state of Tai Diagram ䷊ indicative of coordination between yin and yang, then into the Qian Diagram ䷀ indicative of the period of full bloom of yang, just at a time of the fifteenth day of the month. From the beginning of the next half of the month, yang will wane gradually and yin begins to flourish, entering the state of yang decline expressed by the Gou Diagram ䷫ , then into Pi Diagram ䷋ , which is indicative of incoordination between Heaven and Earth and discordance between yin and yang, a state at which vitality is at its lowest ebb. The same thing happens in a year, a month, a day and during the physiological and pathological processes. The life process from its beginning to its prime, decline and death, is also in accord with this law (Fig.

2-20).

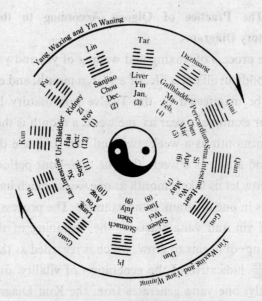

Fig. 2-20 The Twelve Informatory Diagrams
Note: 1. The months are in lunar canlender.

2.The numerals in brakets from (1) to (12) refer respectively to:
the Winter Solstice, Great Cold, Rain Water, the Spring Equinox,
Grain Rain, Grain Full, the Summer Solstice, Great Heat, the Limit
of Heat, the Autumn Equinox, Frost's Descent and Slight Snow.

So long as Qigong practice is concerned, at the stage of the Fu
Diagram☷☳ which means more yin than yang, the practitioner
should regulate himself with the stress put on nourishing yang,
which requires long inhaling and short exhaling. While at the
stage of Gou Diagram ☰ , which represents more yang and
less yin, one should do short inhaling and long exhaling. It is
for this reason that when the time and direction for Qigong
practice and the methods of respiration and mind concentration required are determined properly in accordance with the
Twelve Informatory Diagrams, the result of "turning Pi into

Tai" can be attained and the physiological function of the body can be maintained in a normal state with coordination of yin and yang, which is a state of Tai Diagram.

3. The Twelve Informatory Diagrams and the Physiological Function

Of the Twelve Informatory Diagrams, the Tai ☷ and Pi ☰ represent the best and the worst stages of the physiological function of the human body respectively. The Tai Diagram consists of half Yin and half Yang with the former located above the latter,indicating the descending of yin and ascending of yang, a stage of smooth circulation of qi inside the body,and a stage of physiological equilibrium between yin and yang, the state which, as tradition has, is "the coordination of yin and yang that reveals vigorous life vitality". On the contrary, the Pi Diagram has yang above yin, which indicates the disorderly descend and ascend of yin and yang and the incoordination between them, showing the decline of the physiological function which, as tradition holds, is "the state of separation of yin and yang that indicates the end of life".

The modern biorhythm doctrine has proved that the physiological function of the human body changes in a regular way during a year, a month or even a day. The law of its changes is hereof explained in the light of the ebb and flow of yin and yang of the Twelve Informatory Diagrams, with a year as an example. Of the Twelve Informatory Diagrams, The Tai, Dazhuang and Guai are related to the spring, or the first, second and third months of the lunar year. As this period is the time when yang flows and yin ebbs gradually and the wood—qi or the liver and gallbladder qi is vigorous, the pulse is often felt taut. And because the exuberance of the spring—wood restricts the spleen—earth, diseases due to asthenia of the spleen and stomach occurring at this time may be imputed to the disadvantage of the climate.

If the law of growth and decline of yin and yang included in the Twelve Informatory Diagrams is used to explain the human life, the Kun Diagram then means the period of fetus, Fu refers to the period of newborn and childhood, Tai the puberty, Qian the prime of life or the middle age, Pi the geratic period, and Kun the death. The physiological status of the aged is identical with the Pi diagram, which indicates the waning of yin and decline of yang and incoordination between them, so the aged should practise Qigong against this physiological law to try to gain the state of Tai Diagram back through regulation of posture, respiration and mind concentration to suppress yin and help recuperate yang. Only in this way, they can build up their health and prolong the life.

4. The principle of Qigong Practice During the Zi, Wu, Mao and You Periods

Most of the Qigong practitioners advocate the practice of Qigong during the Zi, Wu, Mao and You periods, which are given the term of "the four principal periods". We here analyse the mechanism of Qigong practice during these periods on the basis of the growth and decline of yin and yang of the Twelve Informatory Diagrams. Traditional Chinese medicine holds that Zi is related to the kidney; the kidney is the source of qi. The kidney—qi is called "ministerial fire of Mingmen (Du 4 or the gate of life)", or "young fire", which is the root of life formed through the supreme combination of the primordial yin and yang and stored seclusively in the kidney–water. The Zi period is in accord with the Fu ䷗ , a diagram with five yin lines at the top and one yang line at the bottom. This is right the period when qi of the natural world and yang–qi (positive energy) in the kidney are in full accord, generating continuously and vibrating vigorously. To practice during this period is highly effective and can get twice the result with half the effort.

Mao is the period when the sun rises and yang progresses.It is in accord with the Dazhuang Diagram ䷡ which has two lines of yin and four lines of yang withthe yang waxing and the yin waning. This is a period during which yang–qi of the human body is in full bloom. So practice at this period helps the vigorous growth of yang.

The Wu period is matched with the diagram Gou ䷫ with five yang lines and one yin line, meaning the exuberance of yang at the top. Wu is regarded asheart–fire. The channel qi of the human body flows right along the Heart Channel. As the heart is considered Taiyang in the yang, the combination of the two yang will naturally result in the flourishing of yang. However, as the one line of yin is the dominating aspect, yang–qi tends to wane other than to grow. And because yin and yang are interdependent, to practice at this period will certainly help the growth of yin–qi and the suppression of the hyperactivity of yang, leading to the tranquilization of the five yang along with the development of one yin to avoid generation of pathogenic dryness.

The You period is matched with the diagram Guan ䷓ , which has four lines of yin and two lines of yang. It is a period when qi of the natural world turns from lucid to turbid, a time when Qigong practice is helpful to the progress of primordial yin and the conservation and nourishment of yang.

To practise Qigong during the Zi, Wu, Mao and You periods is right to facilitate the vigorous growth of the internal qi along with the changes of qi of nature. However, because of the difference of the individuals in health status and constitution, "to practise during the four principal periods" can only be taken as a principle guiding the selection of the time for practice. The actual conditions of the individuals, the number of yin and yang in nature and the fluctuation of yin and yang should also be taken into consideration.

5. The Twelve Informatory Diagrams and the Circulation of Qi

As a law, qi and blood circulate, in terms of time, in the Gallbladder Channel during the Zi period, in the Liver Channel during Chou, in the Lung Channel during Yin, in the Large Intestine Channel during Mao, in the Stomach Channel during Chen, in the Spleen Channel during Si, in the Heart Channel during Wu, in the Small Intestine Channel during Wei, in the Urinary Bladder Channel during Shen, in the Kidney Channel during You, in the Pericardium Channel during Xu and in the Sanjiao Channel during Hai (Fig. 2—21). The Gallbladder Channel belongs to yang, to wood and to the diagram Fu at the Zi period, a time when one yang of nature is beginning to grow and qi and blood of the body circulate in the Gallbladder Channel.So qi of the liver and gallbladder is vigorous at this time. So long as the relationship between gallbladder–wood and the internal organs is concerned, the prosperity of liver / gallbladder—wood restricts the spleen—earth; the lung—metal restrics the gallbladder—wood whilethe flourishing of the gallbladder—wood impairs the lung—metal; kidney—water generates gallbladder—wood and the flourishing of wood results in hyperactivity of water; gallbladder—wood generates

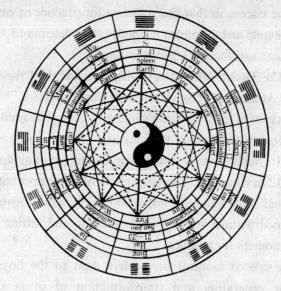

Fig. 2—21 The Twelve Informatory Diagrams and
the Flowing Order of the Channels
Note: The names of the internal organs represent the channels.

heart—fire, but when fire purges wood, the gallbladder will weaken, and when gallbladder—wood is vigorous, the heart—fire is benefited. The relations of generation, restriction, subjugation and reverse restriction between the Five Elements change at different time with the changes of qi of nature and the increase and decrease of qi and blood in the viscera. This relationship can be seen clearly from the illustration of the

Twelve Informatory Diagrams and the circulation of qi and blood along the channels and collaterals. In the practice of Qigong to keep fit or cure diseases and in outgoing—qi treatment of patients, full consideration should be given to the relationship between the time of practice or treatment and the status of the viscera so that the guideline for practice or emission of outgoing—qi and the proper methods can be determined. Only in this way,can satisfactory effect be attained.

6. The Twelve Informatory Diagrams and the Crucial Moment for Attainment of Small or Large Circle of Qi

Circle of qi is divided into small and large. The small circle of qi refers to the level of attainment of transforming essence into qi. Its main characteristic lies in circulation of qi along the Ren and Du Channels. The large circle of qi means a more sophisticated skill. The most important thing is that neither can be attained without a good understanding and seizing of the crucial moment for practice.

The crucial moment here refers right to the favourable turn for generation and transformation of qi in Qigong practice. Taking advantage of this turn, the practitioner can regulate his own posture, respiration and mind concentration according to the law of Qigong practice at will; otherwise, he will loose the favourable opportunity for achivements. To facilitate the understanding and mastery of this doctrine, the ancient Qigong masters explarued the crucial moment for attainment of small or large circle of qi and the changing property of the qi field by way of the Twelve Informatory Diagrams and Yueti Najia (the Moon Embraces the Heavenly Stems).

Take the Twelve Informatory Diagrams as an example. It

is stressed that the practice of the small or large circle of qi should be started at the Zi period when one Yang is beginning to generate. The reason lies in that Zi is the period related to Fu ䷗ of the Twelve Informatory Diagrams, which indicates the generation of one yang. Practising at this period, which is called "the live Zi period" in old times, the internal qi will accumulate continuously and form a flow of energy, bringing about the first phenomenon, among others, of "the impulse of the scrotum". This is right the crucial moment for attainment of circle of qi, at which one should use "wuhuo" or vigorous conscious breathing, mind concentraing and posturing to help the accumulation and circulation of energy in a progressive way to experience the state of the hexagrams of Lin, Tai, Dazhuang, Gui and Qian, a process traditionally called "the progression of yang—fire". But when the yang—fire reaches its climax, it will turn naturally to the yin aspect, which, illustrated on the Twelve Diagrams ䷫ , is the Gou , which indicates the generation of one yin, a moment that requires one to use "wenhuo" or gentle breathing and mind concentrating till the period representative of Kun ䷁ is attained. This is traditionally called "retrogression of yin—symbol".

Yueti Najia (The Moon Embraces the Heavenly Stems)

The doctrine of Yueti Najia is applied to training of active substance inside the body. It is put forward in *Zhouyi Can Tong Qi (Tally to the Book of Changes)* by Wei Boyang of the Eastern Han Dynasty (25 – 220). The doctrine is used to explain the law of growth and decline of qi inside the human body during Qigong practice, in which the crucial moment for Qigong practice changes with the waxing and waning and the position of the moon and, it is for this reason that the poem "When one asks me about my practice of Taoism, I just show him the remote moon in the sky" was prevalent among the alchemists (fangshi).

1. The Contents of Yueti Najia

The Ten Heavenly Stems in the order of Jia, Yi, Bing, Ding, Wu, Ji, Geng, Xin, Ren and Kui represent the positions of the moon. Or to put it differently, Jia—Yi—wood represents east, Bing—Ding—fire south, Geng—Xin—metal west, Ren—Kui— water north and Wu—Ji—earth the centre. On the Congenital Eight Diagrams, the symbols of the trigrams represent the appearance of the moon, the Heavenly Stems represent the positions of the moon. Literally, "Yueti" means "the body of the moon" and "Najia" means "embracing Jia" (one of the Ten Heavenly Stems). Yueti Najia is so termed because everyone of the Eight Diagrams (trigrams) embraces one or two of the Ten Heavenly Stems. And as Jia is the first stem, which is embraced by Qian, the first in the Congenital Eight Diagrams, it is taken as the representative of the other stems. Specifically, Qian ☰ embraces Jia and Ren, Kun ☷ embraces Yi and Kui, Zhen ☳ embraces Geng, Xun ☴ embraces Xin, Gen ☶ embraces Bing, Dui ☱ embraces Ding, Kan ☵ embraces Wu, and Li ☲ embraces Ji. Of the Eight Diagrams, Qian and Kun embrace two of the Ten Heavenly Stems while the others embrace one respectively. This is because Jia and Yi of the ten stems represent the origination of yin and yang while Ren and Kui represent the termination of yin and yang. To match Qian and Kun with Jia, Yi, Ren and Kui indicates yin and yang from beginning to end, as is stated by Wei Boyang of the Eastern Han Dynasty (25 − 220) in his book *Zhouyi Can Tong Qi (Tally to the Book of Changes)* that "Ren and Kui are combined with Jia and Yi, and Qian and Kun comprise the beginning and end". The symbol of the trigrams used in the doctrine of Najia is explained as ☳ indicating the appearance of the moon at the third of the lunar month; ☱ indicating an up−stringed moon at the eighth of the month; ☰ indicating the appearance of a full moon at the fifteen, ☴ indicating the appearance of the moon at the sixteenth; ☶ indicating a downstringed moon at the twenty−third; and ☷ indicating a dark moon at the thirtieth of the month. The appearance of the moon during the first half of the lunar month symbolizes the waxing of yang and waning of yin, while that during the second half symbolizes the waning of yang and waxing of yin. ☵ and ☲ indicate medicaments (the component for training qi, referring to the sun and moon) (Fig. 2−22). In fact, the ancients divided the month into six sections, each being five days. Except that Kan and Li represent medicaments, each of the other six trigrams represents one section. For example, Zhen represents the first five days of a month, with the third day representative of the phase of the moon at this section. The same arrangement is applied to other trigrams.

Why the diagrams are so matched with the Ten Heavenly Stems? The explanation is that at the dask of the third of a lunar month, a new moon appears in the west, which means that

Zhen ☳ contains Geng; at the eighth when an up-stringed moon appears in the south, Dui ☱ contains Ding; at the dask of the fifteenth, a full moon appears in the east, meaning that Qian ☰ contains Jia; at dawn of the sixteenth, the slight dent moon appears in the west, meaning that Xun ☴ contains Xin; at dawn of the twenty-third, a down-stringed moon appears in the south, meaning that Gen ☶ contains Bing; and at dawn of the thirtieth, a dark (Hui) moon appears in the east, meaning Kun ☷ contains Yi.

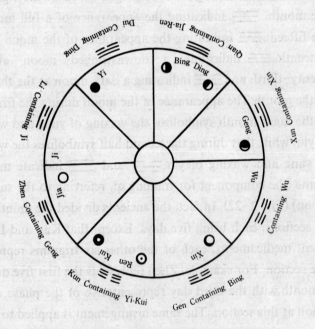

Fig. 2-22 Yueti Najia (The Moon Embraces
the Heavenly Stems)

2. Regulation of Breathing at Fixed Time and Orientation

Now that it is clear that the changes of yin and yang of the four seasons are caused by the waxing and waning of the sun and the moon, Qigong practice and treatment of illnesses should comply with the climatic changes. The time and orientation for Qigong practice and the methods of breathing regulation should be determined in the light of the law of Yueti Najia in order to facilitate the intake of essence of the universe to nourish the body and live one's full span. To explain it,when Zhen ☳ contains Geng which implies two yin and one primarily generating yang, at a time from the first to the fifth of a lunar month when the moon appears in the west at dask with its surface accepting less sunlight, breathing regulation should be carried out with the practitioner facing east and the duration for intake of qi should be longer in order to absorb yang to nourish yin. Dui ☱ containing Ding is from the sixth to the tenth when the moon appears in the south at dask with its shape turning from crescent to half and its surface accepting more sunlight. The practitioner should practise even breathing facing south. Qian ☰ containing Jia is from the eleventh to the fifteenth when the moon is full with its surface accepts sunlight best (called full yang in yin), and at dask a bright moon will appear in the east. This is the time to carry out breathing regulation facing east, and as yin—qi and yang— qi are plentiful at this time, even breathing should be taken. The above mentioned are the regulation methods at the first three periods of a lunar month from the beginning of the month till the moon is full. Xun ☴ containing Xin is from the sixteenth to the twentieth when the sunlight on the moon surface becomes less, yang wanes and yin waxes and the moon appears in the west at dawn. It is a time to face west for regulation.

Gen ☶ containing Bing is from the twenty-first to the twenty-fifth when the moon accepts much less sunlight and appears in the south at dawn, a time for the practitioner to face south for regulation. Kun ☷ containing Yi is from the twenty-sixth to the thirtieth when the moon surface is dark which leads to the period of yin (Kun), and the practitioner should face east for regulation. As yin grows and yang declines from the sixteenth to the end of the month, regulation of breathing at this period should be aimed at replenishing yang to help yin to nourish the yin essence.

3. Tonification of Deficiency and Purgation of Excess

The doctrine of Yueti Najia demonstrates the definite influence of the changes of the position of the earth, sun and moon on man, which can be seen from the changes of the moon. *Ling Shu − Sui Lu Lun (Miraculous Pivot − On the Year)* states, "Man is closely related to the universe and corresponds with the sun and the moon". *Su Wen − Ba Zheng Shen Ming Lun* (a chapter of *Plain Questions*) holds " When the moon begins to wax, qi and blood of man start to be nourished; when it is full, they are substantial; when it wanes, the muscles become thinner and the channels and collaterals deficient" . The ancients came to the conclusion that qi and blood of man are influenced by the turning of the sun and the moon on the basis of their observation of the tide of the sea water, which is influenced by the sun and the moon. They therefore put forward the tonifying and purging principle for qigong practice in terms of "performing no tonification at the fifteenth when the moon is full, no purgation at the thirtieth when the moon is dark, no tonification when qi and blood are sufficient, and no purgation when they are deficient". To provide reference for qigong practice and clinical treatment, the Eight Diagrams, the Ten Heavenly Stems, the appearance of the moon and the tide as well as their relations with the principle of tonification and purgation of qi and blood of man are listed below.

Table 2–4   The Relationship between Yueti Najia and the Principle of Tonification and Purgation

Diagrams & Stems	Date	Appearance of Moon	Position of Moon	Cause of the Moon Appearance	Tide	Qi & Blood	Regulation
Zhen contains Geng	1st	New	West at dask	Moon between th sun and earth	Spring	Turning excessive	No tonification
Dui contains Ding	8th	Up-stringed	South at dask	Moon 90 degrees east of sun	Neap	Deficient	No purgation
Qian contains Jia	15th	Full	East	Moon opposite sun with earth in between	Spring	Excessive	No tonification
Xun contains Xin	16th	Dent	West in the mornngn	Ditto (but to the west)	Medium	Turning deficient	No purgation
Gen contains Bing	23th	Down-stringed	South in the morning	Moon 90 degrees west of sun	Neap	Deficient	No purgation
Kun contains Yi	30th	Dark	East in the morning	Moon between the sun and earth	Medium	Deficient	No purgation

For example, yang–qi of the natural world becomes plentiful gradually from the 11th to the 15th. Influenced by this, spring tide occurs at the 15th when the moon is full, and qi and blood of man will become vigorous, too. This is a good opportunity for qigong practitioners suffering from qi deficiency to replenish qi. However, those with sufficiency of qi should not take the tonifying method lest over—exuberance of qi occur.

The River Chart and the Luo River Graph

The River Chart (Hetu) and the Luo River Graph (Luoshu) are two very old drawings. Legend has it that one day in the reign of King Fu Xi, a dragon horse with a pattern of spots on its back appeared from under the water of a river. The pattern was then given the name "River Chart". King Fu Xi himself drew the Eight Diagrams based on the spots. And when Yu, the reputed founder of the Xia Dynasty (c. 21th — 16th century B.C.) carried out his engineering to regulate rivers and watercourses, an immortal turtle came out of the Luo River, with a graph carved on its shell, which was given the name "Luo River Graph". Yu then drew down the graph and arranged it in nine scopes. So *Zhouyi — Xici* (a chapter of the Book of Changes) says that "The River Chart and the Luo River Graph come from the rivers and are developed by the sages".

1. The Contents of the River Chart and the Luo River Graph
(1) The River Chart
Nan Yi Xun Yuan (Searching for the Source of Difficulty and Simplicity) states, "Heaven—one generates water and results in Earth—six; Earth—two generates fire and results in Heaven—seven; Heaven—three generates wood and results in Earth—Eight; Earth—four generates metal and results in Heaven—nine; and Heaven—five generates earth and results in Earth—ten". *Lei Jing Tu Yi (Illustrated Supplementary to the Classified Canon)* describes, "The numbers one and six are lo—

cated at the bottom, two and seven at the top. three and eight on the left, four and nine on the right, and five and ten in the centre". The two passages introduce in detail the arrangement of the River Chart, in which the yang numbers are odd, representing yang and Heaven, the yin numbers are complex, representing yin and Earth. The numbers in the River Chart are arranged with yin and yang mutually connected and supplemented, an arrangement from which qi of the Five Elements (wood, fire, water, metal and earth) is generated. Yang grows on the basis of yin and vice versa; the extremity of yang results in generation of yin and vice versa. In this way, yin and yang connect with and replace each other to generate qi, or to say, the intercourse between one yin and one yang results in qi.Speaking of the arrangement of the River Chart again, the numbers one and six are in the north and regarded as Ren–Kui–water, two and seven in the south as Bing–Ding–fire, three and eight in the east as Jia–Yi– wood, four and nine in the west as Geng–Xin–metal, and five and ten in the centre as Wu–Ji–earth (Fig. 2–23).

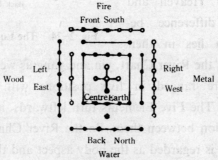

Fig. 2–23 The River Chart

(2) The Luo River Graph

Tan Rongchuan says in his book *Yiyi Tong Shuo (A General Description of Application of the Book of Changes to Medicine)*, "In the centre stands the number five, with the number nine above, one below, three on the left, seven on the right, two and four as its shoulders, six and eight as its feet, yang numbers as Heaven, yin numbers as Earth, yang numbers turning leftward (clockwise), and yin numbers turning rightward (counterclockwise)". This explains the composition of the Luo River Graph. The arrangement is: the number one is in the north, three in the east, nine in the south, seven in the west, the yang numbers going leftwards; the yin going rightwards, two in the southwest, four in the southeast, eight in the northeast, and six in the northwest (Fig. 2-24).

2. The Difference between the River Chart and the Luo River Graph

The River Chart and the Luo River Graph are all composed of yin and yang numbers of Heaven and Earth. The difference between them lies in their

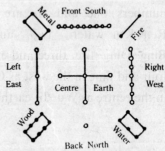

Fig. 2-24   The Luo River Graph

structure. In the River Chart, yin and yang as well as the Five Elements are ranged in five positions with appropriate copulations. The Five Elements turn leftwards, indicating the interpromotion between them. So the River Chart represents Heaven and is regarded as the body aspect and the congenital structure. In the Luo River Graph, yin and yang and the Five

Elements are arranged in nine positions. The yang numbers go leftwards while the yin go rightwards, indicating the evolution and exchanges between them. The Five Elements also turn rightwards, which is indicative of the interrestraint between them. So the Luo River Graph represents Earth, the application aspect and the acquired structure. As stated in *Xuan Zhen Yin—Yang Wuxing Zhuj i (The Foundation of Yin—Yang and the Five Elements by Xuanzhen)*, "The River Chart results from the harmonious copulation of yin and yang while the Luo River Graph from the evolution and exchanges of them; the former is congenital while the latter acquired. The combination of the congenital (as the body aspect) and the acquired (as the application aspect) will bring about growth and development of all things of the universe".

3. The Numbers in the River Chart and the Luo River Graph and Their Relationship with Tonification and Purgation in Qigong

The numbers in the River Chart are congenital which are matched with congenital qi of man, with the generating dominating the resultant. The north kidney—water is copulated with one and six, south heart—fire with two and seven, east liver—wood with three and eight, west lung—metal with four and nine, and centre spleen—earth with five and ten. With one aspect generative and the other resultant in each pair, the generating and restricting functions of the internal organs expressed by the Five Elements are established. Congenital insufficiency will lead to disorder of the internal organs and the Five Elements, which should be regulated with the numbers in the River Chart. For instance, deficiency of kidney—essence and congenital qi should be replenished with the resultant number (six) of north kidney—water first, then with the resultant number (nine) of west lung—metal (to tonify the mother).

The numbers in the Luo River Graph are acquired. The kidney is copulated with north, water, and one; the liver with east, wood and three; the heart with south, fire and nine; the lung with west, metal and seven; and the spleen with centre, earth and five. So pathogenic excess of the lung should be restricted with south—fire—nine.

In the Luo River Graph, the positive (yang) numbers are arranged in an endless cycle from one to three, then to nine, to seven and back to one; the negative (yin) numbers from two to four, to eight, to six and then back to two. To explain it in detail, the negative numbers are the results of multiplication of two by two which equals four, by four which equals eight, by eight which equals sixteen (but ten is not counted), and by six which equals twelve (ten is not counted). The positive numbers are the results of multiplication of three by one which equals three, by three which equals nine, by nine which equals twentyseven (twenty is not counted), and by seven which equals twenty—one (twenty is not counted). The cycling of the negative (yin) and positive (yang) numbers indicates the law of motion of yin and yang in all things. So the principle "to rotate leftwards (clockwise) for tonification" and " to rotate rightwards (counterclockwise) for purgation" is adhered to in Chinese qigong, massage (Tuina) and acupuncture and moxibustion, for it is widely accepted that rotating clockwise means "yang promoting growth", which facilitates the continuous circulation of yang—qi and is helpful to tonification of qi and replenishment of deficiency; while rotating counterclockwise along with yin and against yang means "yin killing evils" , which helps to purgate excess and expel pathogenic evils.

4. The River Chart and Essence, Spirit, Spirit Soul, Material Soul and Intention

Zhang Jiebin stated in *Lei Jing Tu Yi — Yiyi(Illustrated Supplementary to the Classified Canon — Application of the Book of Changes to Medicine)*, "So far as spirit manifestations are concerned, north—water—one is my essence of life, so it is said that the kidney stores essence; south—fire—two is my spirit, so it is said the heart stores spirit; east—wood—three is my spirit soul, so it is said the liver stores spirit soul; west—metal—four is my material soul, so it is said that the lung stores material soul; and centre—earth—fire is my intention, so it is said that the spleen stores intention". This explains the relationship between the generating numbers, the Five Elements as well as the five viscera and essence, spirit, spirit soul, material soul and intention. As the numbers three and two in the River Chart have the same aim for qi, four and one have the same origin of qi and five in the centre governs qi of the four aspects, Zhang Jiebin states in the same book that "spirit and spirit soul are stored in the southeast" , "essence and material soul are stored in the northwest", and as earth governs qi of the four aspects, intention is in the centre coupled with the number five.

Chapter Three   The Points

Other names for the points (Xueqiao) used in qigong include Shuxue, Xuedao, Xuewei, and Qixue. In outgoing—qi therapy, they are habitually termed Qiqiao (qi orifice) or Xueqiao (point and orifice). A point is the locus where qi and blood of the zang (solid) and fu (hollow) organs and the channels and collaterals of the human body comes in and goes out.It interrelates the internal organs and tissues through the channels and collaterals and can manifest the physiological and pathological changes in the organs and tissues. A point can also serve as an exchanger of qi (vital energy) between the human body and the universe. It responds to the stimulations triggered off by needling,moxibustion, massage (Tuina) and electricity and, similarly, to provocation by outgoing—qi. through which it regulates the functions of the inner related zang and fu organs and the channels to cure diseases.

A point plays a special role in Qigong practice. Having undergone the self—training of mind concentration, breathing and posturization, a skilled Qigong practitioner can direct some of his points to "open" or "close". Once the point is opened, the practitioner will be sensitive to qi, able to perceive and differentiate the healthy qi, the pathogenic qi and qi of other types. This function was called "shen" (spirit) by the ancients. Outgoing—qi therapy is right developed from this philosophy. The therapist detects diseases and emits outgoing—qi based on his own sensitivity to qi and the ability of his points to open and close in order to regulate the qi activities of the patient and to expel the pathogenic qi to cure diseases.

Section One   Dantian (Elixir Field) and Sanguan (Three Passes)

1. Dantian (Elixir Field)

(1) Location

Dantian is a collective term for the Upper Dantian, the Middle Dantian and the Lower Dantian. The Lower Dantian is also called Qihai (sea of vital energy), Shenlu (stove of spirit) and Tiangen (root of Heaven), which is located 1.3 cun below the umbilicus and 3 cun inside the lower abdomen. The synonyms for the Middle Dantian are Huangting, Shangjin and Xuanqiao, which is located 3 cun inside the point Shanzhong (Ren 17). The Upper Dantian is otherwise named Qianding, Tiangu, Neiyuan and Niwan (Mud Ball), which is located 3 cun inside Yintang (Extra 1). Dacheng Jieyao (Essentials of Great Achievements) holds that a point is "a void spherical space 1 cun and 2 fen in diameter". Some people consider Dantian to be three areas of the human body, stating that the Lower Dantian spreads between Huiyin (Ren 1) and Qihai (Ren 6), the Middle Dantian between Shenque (Ren 8) and Shanzhong (Ren 17), and the Upper Dantian between the two eyebrows up to the forehead.

(2) Application

Dantian is not only an important point for self applied

Qigong in terms of cultivation and conservation of genuine qi, attainment of small or large circle of qi and the circulation of qi along the Ren Channel, but also an important location toward which the Qigong therapist emit outgoing-qi to activate and regulate the qi activities of the patient.

The Lower Dantian is the priority point for mind concentration and for transformation of essence into qi (the small circle of qi). "Concentrating the mind on the qi point", a popular term in ancient China, refers to concen-tration of the mind on the Lower Dantian for training qi. When regulating the deranged qi of the patient, the therapist must guide qi of the patient to Dantian, which is termed "leading qi back to its origin". Emission of qi toward the Lower Dantian may encourage, facilitate and train the qi activities of the patient to make it easier for the pathogenic qi to be expelled.

The Middle Dantian is the place for transforming qi into spirit. Failure to guide qi in a proper way during Qigong practice or emission of outgoing-qi may lead to adverse flowing of qi to the Middle Dantian, which often condenses there causing stuffiness and pain in the chest and suffocation.

The Upper Dantian is where spirit is trained to achieve the state of "nihility". Concentrating the mind on this point may help improve intelligence and open up the potentials of the human brain. But for those who are not experienced or who are careless with practice, concentration of mind here may cause headache and dizziness. Emitting qi to this point via Yintang (Extra 1) with vibrating and quivering manipulations has the function of inducing sleep, tranquilizing the mind and regulating qi in the Upper-jiao (the Upper Warmer). However, when qi is emitted with the method of making three points linear, the patient may develop the symptoms of dizziness, vertigo or even syncope. This calls for special attention.

2. Sanguan (The Three Passes)

(1) Location

Sanguan refers to the three important places on the Du Channel (the Back Midline Channel), namely, Weiluguan (Coccyx pass) or Luluguan, which is located at the lowerest segment of the spine and posterior to the anus near the point Changqiang (Du 1); Jiajiguan (Spine pass, a pair of points), which are located at the lateral sides of Mingmen (Gate of life, Du 4); and Yuzhenguan (Occiput pass), which is inferior to the occipital bone where the brain originates.

(2) Application

As the three suguan points are the places most difficult for qi to circulate through the Du Channel in practice of the small circle of qi, they are given another name, "Tiebi", meaning "iron wall". Qi may pass through them smoothly or be impeded at any of them. If it is impeded at Weiluguan (Coccyx pass), the practitioner will have aching—pain, heaviness sensation and a sensation of impeded qi in that place. When this happens, he should lead qi to flow upwards with faint will on the one hand, and on the other hand, he may prop the tongue against the palate, inhale deeply and contract the anus to facilitate its passage. Jiajiguan (Spine pass) is usually easier for qi to pass through except that those who have disorders in this location may have aching—pain and a sensation of fracture of waist and spine when qi circulates through there. Impediment of qi is most commonly felt at Yuzhenguan (Occiput pass), manifested as stiffness of the neck and heaviness and aching—pain in the occipital region as if there was something sticking to it which can not be got rid of readily. If this happens, the practitioner may close his eyes and look upward with inward vision, with the head raised slightly, to lead qi to pass by will. When qi is not able to get through Sanguan because of the poor background in Qigong practice, the practitioner should not carelessly guide it to pass by will lest Qigong deviations should occur. If disorders of qi activities and impediment of qi in the Du and Ren Channels develop, outgoing—qi therapy by emitting qi toward the three passes is the method of choice because of its function of facilitating and regulating the qi flow in the Du Channel. So the three passes are also essential for treatment of diseases in the neck and the lumbosacral region.

Section Two   The Points of the Fourteen Channels and the Extrachannel Points Commonly Used in Qigong

Points at the Head and Face

Baihui (Du 20)

Location: Right on the vertex, the midpoint of the line joining the apexes of the ears.

Indication: Headache, dizziness, vertigo, apoplexy, epilepsy, tinnitus, deafness, nasal obstruction, and prolapse of anus or uterus.

Application: Also named Sanyang, Wuhui, Tianman, Weihui and Niwangong (Mud Ball Palace), Baihui is an important point for qigong exercise and outgoing–qi therapy.

(1) The head is the place where all the yang channels converge. As Baihui is located at the top of the head and joints the Three Yang Channels of Hand and the Three Yang Channels of Foot with the Du Channels, it has the function of linking up the channel qi, invigorating the vital function and qi and replenishing and refreshing the mind. Concentrating the mind on Baihui in Qigong practice may help the collapsed yang–qi (positive vital energy) due to dificiency of qi to ascend to cure collapse of uterus, gastroptosia, and collapse of anus and enuresis. When qi flows up to but is not able to pass Yuzhenguan (Occiput pass) during practice of small circle of qi, concentration of the mind on Baihui with the head held up in combination with breathing will facilitate the passage of it.

(2) The line joining Baihui and Huiyin (Du 1) divides the human body vertically into yin and yang.This also stresses the importance of Baihui in Qigong exercise and outgoing–qi therapy.To open through the qi vessels between Baihui and Huiyin (Du 1) or Yongquan (K 1) with a certain qi–emission hand gesture can facilitate qi activities, balancing yin and yang and expel pathogenic factors. And emitting qi to Baihui with vibrating and quivering or pushing and pulling manipulations can help replenish the brain, transquilize the mind, reduce sleep and activate yang.

Tianting (Extra, the Middle Part of the Forehead)

Location: The midpoint of the line joining Yintang (Extra 1) and the front hairline.

Indication: Sticking sensation at the forehead, headache, dizziness, amnesia and palpitation.

—111—

Application: The synonyms of the point are Tianmen (Heavenly Gate), Tianmu (Heavenly Eye), Tiangen and Tianxin. There has been some controversy over its position as to a little higher or lower than the location mentioned above. It is the place where mentality and consciousness store and generate. As the old saying goes, "The success in training of vital essence, qi and spirit brings about light shining over the forehead". Here the forehead refers to Tianting, which, if opened through when qi is sufficient after persistent practice of Qigong, can conduct exchanges with the outside world, view the inner sight of the human body and detect diseases through perspective and remote sensing. Emission of outgoing–qi toward this point with specific manipulations may facilitate qi activities of the qi recipient and induce his specific physiological function, or putting it differently, "open Tianmu (the Heavenly eye)". Carelessness should be avoided when emission ofoutgoing–qi toward it with the qi–guiding method of making three points linear lest disorders of qi activities, syncope and dizziness should occur.

Yintang (Extra 1)

Location: The midpoint between the medial ends of the two eyebrows.

Indication: Headache, dizziness, epilepsy, infantile convulsion, eye congestion with pain, insomnia and vertigo.

Application: As Yintang is located on the Ren Channel, it is the key point for regulating qi in Tianting (Extra), Baihui (Du 20) and the Gallbladder Channel. Qigong deviations such as heavy sensation in the vertex and sticking sensation at the forehead, migraine, dizziness and eye congestion can be well treated by emitting outgoing–qi toward this point as well as Baihui (Du 20) and Taiyang (Extra 2) to make the circulation of qi along the Du Channel, Ren Channel and the Shaoyang Channels facilitated.

Hanyan (GB 4)

Location: Posterosuperior to the hairline of the temporal region. There is a slight movement here during chewing.

Indication: Migraine, vertigo, tinnitus, toothache, epilepsy induced by terror and clonic convulsion.

Application: Digital kneading and flicking manipulations followed by emission of outgoing–qi toward it and guiding of the patient's qi along the Shaoyang Channels with pushing and pulling manipulations can be taken to open the point, dredge the channels to facilitate qi, soothe the liver and suppress the sthenic yang and balance yin and yang between the left and right of the body. In clinical application, the usuage of the point at the two sides is often compatible and the left is usually regulated first in male and the right first in female.

Fengfu (Du 16)

Location: 1 cun superior to the midpoint of the posterior hairline.

Indication: heaviness and pain in the back of the head, apoplexy, hemiparalysis, common cold, headache, neck stiffness, vertigo, sore throat and nausea.

Application: Also called Sheben, Guizhen, Guilin, Caoxi and Xingxing, it is the converging point of the Du Channel and the Yangwei Channel. The point is considered the gate of pathogenic wind invasion. The pathogenic wind may enter Fengfu, spread over the brain and affect the Taiyang and

Shaoyang Channels, causing chills and fever, dizziness, neck stiffness, sore throat and the like. Emission of qi toward this point to open it may facilitate the expelling of the pathogenic wind. In regulation of qi activities, it is often used together with Fengchi (GB 20) and Yanglingquan (GB 34).

Fengchi (GB 20)

Location: Lateral to Fengfu (Du 16), in the triangle depression between the sternocleidomastoid muscle and the trapezius muscle.

Indication: Migraine, occiput pain, vertigo, neck stiffness and pain, apoplexy, exopathy, and pain in the back.

Application: Also called Refu, it is a point of Gallbladder Channel of FootShaoyang and a converging point of the Sanjiao Channel of Hand—Shaoyang, the Gallbladder Channel of Foot—Shaoyang, the Yangwei Channel and the Yangqiao Channel. Located at the back of the head, it is the hub where pathogenic wind often invades into the brain. Emission of outgoing—qi to it followed by guiding qi along the Gallbladder Channel can help dredge the channels and collaterals, regulate qi and blood, expel pathogenic wind from the body surface, dispel wind and remove heat, restore consciousness and reduce resuscitation, and improve visual and auditory acuity.

To treat neck stiffness and pain by expelling pathogenic factors, pushing and pulling are the manipulations of choice for emitting qi toward Fengchi to drive pathogenic factors to go along the Gallbladder Channel and finally out from Yanglingquan (GB 34).

Points at the Chest and Abdomen

Quepen (St 12)

Location: Directly above the nipple, in the middle of the supraclavicular fossa.

Indication: Dyspnea, sore throat and pain in Quepen.

Application: Also called Tiangai and Chigai, it is the place where the channels of Foot−Yangming, Hand−Shaoyang, Hand−Taiyang and Hand−Yangming pass. So emitting qi to it and guiding qi along the channels can help regulate qi circulation in the above−mentioned channels to get qi balanced inside and outside. Emission of qi to it together with guidance of qi to flow along the Stomach Channel and Gallbladder Channel can treat chest stuffiness, cough, hot sensation in the chest and other disorders.

It deserves special attention that during outgoing−qi treatment, the pathogenic qi of the patient may invade via Quepen into the internal organs of the therapist and cause chest distress, chest pain and other symptoms due to stagnation of qi.

Zhongfu (Lu 4)

Location: 6 cun lateral to the thoracic midline, in the interspace of the 1st and 2nd ribs.

Indication: Cough, chest distress and pain in the shoulder and back.

Application: Also called Yingzhongshu, Fuzhongshu and Yingshu and located on the Lung Channel of Hand−Taiyin as a Front−mu point related to the lung, it is the place where qi gathers and stores and where the Channels of Hand–Taiyin and Foot–Taiyin converge. Emission of qi to this point has the function of removing heat from the Upper–jiao (the Upper Warmer), dredging and regulating the lungqi and subduing cough and asthma. Emitting qi toward it together with guiding qi along the Channels of Hand–Taiyin and Foot–Taiyin with pushing and pulling manipulations can help dredge the channel qi and expel the pathogenic qi out of the Taiyin Channels.

Tiantu (Ren 22)

Location: Right at the centre of the suprasternal fossa.

Indication: Cough, difficult expectoration, sore throat, chest distress, nausea and vomiting.

Application: Also called Yuhu and Tianju, it is a point on the Ren Channel and a converging place of the Ren and Du Channels. As the thoracic part controls qi (the vital energy) and Tiantu is located at the top of the chest, emission of outgoing–qi toward this point can ventilate the lung and resolve phlegm, keep the adverse qi flowing downward to relieve asthma, and relieve sore throat to recover voice. Emission of outgoing–qi toward it as well as Fengmen (GB 12) and Feishu (GB 13) can regulate yin–qi (negative energy) and yang–qi (positive energy) between the anterior and posterior.

Xuanji (Ren 21)

Location: In the depression 1.6 cun inferior to Tiantu (Ren 22).

Indication: Sore throat, stuffiness and pain in the chest and hypochondrium, hiccup and adverse rising of lung–qi, cough, dyspnea, pulmonary abscess, etc. *Application*: It is a point of the Ren Channel. Literally, "Xuan" refers to the second star of the

Bid Dipper and "Ji" refers to the third. Xuan and Ji rotate along with the automatic rotation of the Big Dipper. The health preservers take Xuanji as the rotation phenomenon of the laryngeal periosteal bone circle. Therefore, emission of outgoing qi toward this point can promote the dispersing function of qi in the Upper-jiao, remove stagnation and stasis, subduing swelling and pain, moistening the dryness, and check the adverse flowing of qi to allay asthma. Clinically, the point is often used in combination with Qihai (Ren 6) and Dantian for emission of outgoing-qi. As Xuanji is located above Qihai (Ren 6) and Dantian, it is important for clearing heat of lung-qi while Qihai and Dantian are important for supplemen- ting primordial qi.The combination of the three, which are mutual supplementary, is quite effective for regulating qi activities of the zang-organs and fuorgans, clearing and regulating the lung, and improving inspiration to relieve asthma. In the case of Qigong deviations manifested as chest and hypochondriac pain, the therapist should first emit qi toward Xuanji to get the patient's qi circulation smooth, and then guide qi with pushing and leading manipulations to flow back to its origin.

Huagai (Ren 20)

Location: 1.6 cun inferior to Xuanji (Ren 21).

Indication: Dyspnea, cough, and fullness and pain in the chest and hypochondrium.

Application: Huagai is a point of the Ren Channel. Inside this point lies the lung, where all the vessels converge and normal gas exchanges take place, a time when yang-qi is in exuberance. So emitting qi toward this point can soothe the chest oppression and regulate qi. The point at the same level of it, which belongs to the Kidney Channel, is Yuzhong (K 26), a point having the function of suppressing the kidney—water and nourishing the lung—metal. So Huagai is often used together with Yuzhong (K 26) to attain the effect of mutual promotion of the lung and the kidney and curing the mother (lung) and child (kidney) simultaneously (the lung and the kidney are of mother—child relationship). When emitting qi to Zhongwan (Ren 12) and Qihai (Ren 6) to expel pathogenic factors, it is advisable no to forget emission of qi toward Huagai, Xuanji (Ren 21) and Yuzhong (K 26) so as to avoid the upward rushing of turbid qi.

Yuzhong (K 26)

Location: 2 cun lateral to Huagai (Ren 20).

Indication: Cough, chest distress, phlegm accumulation, distending pain in the chest and hypochondrium and loss of appetite.

Application: Emission of qi toward this point may clear the lung and regulate qi, check the upward adverse flow of qi and resolve phlegm and regulate qi activities. Clinically, it is often applied in combination with Shanzhong (Ren 17), Huagai (Ren 20) and Xuanji (Ren 21) so as to prevent stagnation of pathogenic factors and adverse rising of qi of the Chong Channel to the chest.

Shanzhong (Ren 17)

Location: At the midpoint between the breasts.

Indication: Chest distress, dyspnea, cough, chest pain, hypogalactia after delivery, mammary abscess, and pain in the back.

Application: Also called Yuanwu, Yuanjian, the Upper Qihai and the Middle Dantian, it serves as the sourse of qi of the Ren Channel, the sea of pectoral qi and the converging place of general qi. Emission of outgoing–qi toward this point can therefore regulate qi and check its upward adverse flow, clear away heat from the lung and resolve phlegm, and soothe the chest and regulate qi. Emission of qi toward it in combination with Neiguan (P 6) can regulate qi of the chest, heart and stomach as a whole, which is applied specially to soothe the chestand regulate regulate qi of the chest, heart and stomach as a whole, which is applied specially to soothe the chest and regulate qi, invigorate the heart and tranquilize the mind and activate the collaterals to relieve pain. As Shanzhong is located between the Upper and Lower Dantian, stagnation of qi of the three elixir fields (Dantian) should all be treated by emitting qi toward Shanzhong to dredge the channels and facilitate qi back to its origin. Emission of qi to it in combina– tion with Feishu (U B 13) has the function of regulating qi activities of the Upper–jiao (lung) and the Upper Dantian, and that of balancing yin and yang in the anterior and posterior to activate qi all over the body.

Zhongwan (Ren 12)

Location: 4 cun superior to the umbilicus.

Indication: Stomachache, abdominal distention, acid regurgitation, vomiting, diarrhoea, dysentery, jaundice and asthenia of the spleen and stomach.

Application: Its synonyms are Taicang, Weiwan, and Zhongji. As a point of the Ren Channel, it serves as a converging place of the Ren Channel and the Channels of

Hand—Taiyang, Hand—Shaoyang, and Foot—Yangming, as a Front—mu point related to the stomach and as the converging point of the fu—organs. With the help of outgoing—qi, this point has the virtue of calming the nerves, checking the ascending and discending of qi, soothing the stomach—qi, regulating the Middle—jiao, resolving dampness accumulation and removing phlegm stagnation. Clinically, emitting qi toward it together with Fenglong (St 40) can resolve dampness accumulation and remove phlegm stagnation; with Zusanli (St 36) can strengthen the spleen and soothe the stomach; with Pishu (U B 20) can regulate the spleen—qi and stomach—qi as well as yin—qi and yang—qi at the anterior and posterior. Because it locates between the Lower and Middle Dantian, it is of utmost important for regulating qi of the two elixir fields with outgoing—qi. Emitting qi toward Zhongwan with vibrating and quivering manipulations has the function of inducing sleep and tranquilizing the nerves.

Lanmen (Extra, Ileocecal Junction)

Location: 1.5 cun superior to the umbilicus.

Indication: Abdominal distention and pain, diarrhoea, constipation, vomiting, and stagnation of qi between the upper and the lower.

Application: Lanmen is located on the Ren Channel, joining the stomach and the small intestines. Emitting outgoing—qi toward it can correct the disorder of qi, regulate the stomach and the small intestines and facilitate qi of the Middle—jiao.In clinical treatment of diseases of the zang—organs and fu—organs with emission of outgoing—qi, qi of this point should be the first to be facilitated, then the other points in combination. Emitting qi toward Lanmen together with Zhongwan (Ren 12) may regulate qi of the Middle—jiao; with Qihai (Ren 6) may regulate qi of the Lower—jiao and can guide qi back to its origin; and with Shanzhong (Ren 17) may regulate qi of the Upper—jiao.

Shenque (Ren 8)

Location: Right in the middle of the umbilicus.

Indication: Abdominal pain, diarrhoea, stagnation of qi and congenital and acquired insufficiency.

Application: Also termed Qishe, Mingdi, Qizhong and Weihui, the point is both the house of acquired qi and the reservoir of congenital qi. Emitting qi toward this point and guiding qi here can facilitate the congenital and acquired qi, culture the primordial qi to consolidate the origin, recuperate depleted yang and rescue the patient from collapse, and diagnose diseases. Guiding qi to rotate round Shenque by will is termed attaining the "circle of qi" or "automatic circular rotation of qi", which is quite effective for regulating qi activities of all the channels and for treatment of diseases of the digestive, cardiovascular and other systems.

Qihai (Ren 6)

Location: 1.5 cun inferior to the umbilicus.

Indication: Abdominal pain and distention, dysmenorrhea, amenorrhea,disorder of qi activities, and failure of qi to flow back to its origin.

Application: Also called Boying, Xiahuang and Dantian, Qihai is the origin of qi of the Ren Channel and the source of qi of the male, the returning place of primordial qi and the fundamental point for abdominal inspiration. Emitting qi to it can activate and mobilize the primordial qi, invigorate the kidney—qi, warm the Lower—jiao, dispel the pathogenic cold and dampness and replenish the kidney qi to relieve asthenia type asthma. Qihai is very important for training qi, guiding qi and emitting outgoing—qi. Abdominal respiration depends whollyon the oscillation of qi in Qihai. In clinical application, qi is often emitted to it in combination with Shanzhong (Ren 17) and Xuanji (Ren 21) for mutual assistance. Purgation manipulation on Qihai or guiding the pathogenic qi out from this point should be avoided lest the vital qi (vital energy) be impaired.

Guanyuan (Ren 4)

Location: 3 cun inferior to the umbilicus.

Indication: Deficiency of vital—qi, abdominal pain, dysmenorrhea, amenorrhea, enuresis, diabetes and vertigo.

Application: With many synonyms such as Dantian, Dahai, Jinglu, Liji, Dazhongji and Huangzhiyuan, Guanyuan is a point of the Ren Channel, a Front—mu point related to the small intestine, a converging point of the Three Yin Channels of Foot and the Ren Channel, and a place where qi of Sanjiao (three warmers) generates. Qihai is considered as the reservoir of essence of the male and of blood of the female, a hub of life, a storehouse of genuine qi and a place where the kidney—yin and kidney—yang meet. So emitting outgoing—qi to this point can invigorate the kidney to consolidate the fundamental essence, nourish and replenish the primordial qi, supplement the brain and the spinal cord, facilitate qi activities, check the mental activity, strengthen the waist and knee, warm yang and help the transformation of qi and promote diuresis and remove dampness. In clinical treatment, emitting qi to Guanyuan in combination with Shenshu (U B 23) can replenish qi, nourish yin and keep qi in the Lower—jiao, which in turn can help replenish the congenital and acquired qi and facilitate inspiration to relieve asthma. Emitting qi in combination with Mingmen (Du 4) can invigorate qi, strengthen yang and activate qi activities, which ususlly induces spontaneous movements of the patient. Qi may be better activated if Dazhui (Du 14) and Feishu (U B 13) are added for outgoing—qi emission. So Guanyuan is the main point for training qi, guiding qi and emitting qi.

Huiyin (Ren 1)

Location: In the centre of the perineum, between the anus and the scrota in the male or the posterior labial commissure in the female.

Indication: Disorder of qi in the Ren Channel and Du Channel, deranged qi activities, seminal emission, impotency, prospermia, irregular menstruation, headache, epilepsy induced by terror and syncope.

Application: Also called Haidi, Xiajidihu, Digen and Yinqiaoku (yinqiao storehouse), Huiyin is the originating point of the Ren Channel, Du Channel and Chong Channel, and a collateral point (point where the collaterals originate) of the Ren Channel. During Qigong practice, the accumulation and circulation of qi often makes this point throb, a phenomenon indicative of the activation and mobilization of qi of the Ren, Du and Chong Channels. So emitting outgoing qi toward Huiyin can regulate qi of the Ren, Du and Chong Channels in overall. And as Huiyin joints Baihui (Du 20) forming a line of demarcation of yin and yang inside the body, emitting qi toward these two points can facilitate the exchange of qi inside and outside the body. This is a favourable opportunity for training and regulating qi and for facilitating qi activities of the whole body to balanced yin and yang and circulate qi smoothly, and by this way, the purpose of diagnosis and treatment of diseases can be achieved.

Zhangmen (Liv 13)

Location: On the free end of the 11th rib.

Indication: Distending pain in the costal region, abdominal distention, borborygmus, mass in the abdomen, vomiting, vertigo, insomnia, and vexation.

Application: Also named Zhoujian, Changping and Xieliao, Zhangmen is the Front—mu point related to the spleen, a converging point of the zang—organs and a meeting place of the Channels of Foot—Shaoyang and Foot—Jueyin. Emitting outgoing—qi toward it can facilitate and regulate the qi activities of the Liver Channel and the Gallbladder Channel, so it is often applied to soothe the liver and regulate qi, promote blood circulation to remove stasis and to disintegrate masses. Emitting outgoing—qi to open qi in Zhangmen and the Inner Laogong (P 8), which are mutually promotive, is very effective for guiding the pathogenic fire to descend, clearing away the heart—fire and liver—fire and soothing the liver and regulating the stomach.

Daimai (GB 26)

Location: Directly inferior to the free end of the 11th rib, level with the umbilicus.

Indication: Disorder of qi of the Dai Channel and the Gallbladder Channel, abdominal pain, amenorrhea, leukorrhea with reddish discharge, hernia, and pain in the lumbocostal region and the lower extremities.

Application: Daimai is a converging point of the Dai Channel and the Channels of Foot—Shaoyang. Literally, "Dai" means "belt", so the Dai Channel is regarded as "the waist belt", which joints all the vertically lying channels of the body. Qigong masters attach great importance to the smooth circulation of qi along this channel. Emitting outgoing—qi toward Daimai may activate and regulate all the vertically lying channels. When Daimai is opened through, qi of the three elixir fields (the three Dantian) will be easy to communicate. If this point is kept tense, there will be stagnation of qi activities of the Dai Channel, leading to disorder of qi flow in the Ren, Du and Chong Channels and all the other channels of the body.

Guilai (St 29)

Location: 4 cun inferior and 2 cun lateral to the umbilicus.

Indication: Pain in the abdomen and the lumbosacral region, asthenia of the lower extremities accompanied with pain, amenorrhea, irregular menstruation, leukorrhea, coldness, swelling and pain in the genitals, prolapse of uterus, impotency and prospermia.

Application: Another name for Guilai is xigu. The point is important for lowering the abdominal qi along with exhaling to get qi to its origin during Qigong exercise. Emitting outgoing—qi toward it may help activate qi in Dantian, lower qi to the Lower Dantian along with exhaling, and warm the channels to expel cold and replenish Chong and Ren Channels.

Qichong (St 30)

Location: 5 cun inferior and 2 cun lateral to the umbilicus.

Indication: Stagnation of qi in the Chong and Ren Channels, abdominal distention and pain, borborygmus, hernia, swelling of the genitals, impotency and irregular menstruation.

Application: Also called Qijie, it is the originating point of the Chong Channel, a channel that receives qi and blood of all the Twelve Regular Channels. When inhaling, the abdominal qi will rush upward from this point and join with qi of the Middle—jiao; when exhaling, the abdominal qi will descend from Guilai (St 29). So Qichong and Guilai (St 29) work together as "a qi pump" for training qi in Dantian. Emitting outgoing—qi toward Qichong has the function of regulating and facilitating the qi activities of the Ren Channel, Chong Channel and the Stamoch Channel, promoting circulation of qi and blood, and dispelling cold and dampness.

Points at the Back and Waist

Jianjing (GB 21)

Location: At the midpoint of the line joining the inferior aspect of the 7th cervical vertebral process and the acromion.

Indication: Stiffness and pain in the neck, pain in the shoulder and back, inability to raise the arm, and mammary abscess.

Application: It is a converging point of the Channels of Hand—Shaoyang, Foot—Shaoyang and Foot—Yangming and the Yangwei Channel, and a place for the Gallbladder Channel to join with all the Yang Channels when it passes through the shoulder. So emitting outgoing—qi toward Jianjing can regulate qi activities all over and dredge qi of all the Yang Channels. It also serves as a point for the overall regulation of qi after clinical treatment.

Dazhui (Du 14)

Location: Between the spinous processes of the 7th cervical vertebra and the 1st thoracic vertebra.

Indication: Stagnation of qi in the Du Channel, occiput pain due to qi stagnation, rush of qi into Baihui (Du 20), dysfunction of yang—qi (positive energy), vertex pain, fibrile diseases, epilepsy, hectic fever due to yin— deficiency, night sweat, and visual and auditory hallucination.

Application: The synonyms are Bailao and Shangshu. The Du Channel is the back midline throughfare of the small circle of qi. The point Dazhui is referred to as the yang aspect of yang, a crux for regulating and replenishing yang—qi, and a place where the Du Channel meets the Channels of Hand—Taiyang, Hand—Yangming and Hand—Shaoyang. So it is often used to regulate yin or yang when they interclock or when either of them is over exuberant. Before emitting and guiding qi to regulate the Du Channel and the Urinary Bladder Channel of Foot—Taiyang, the point Dazhui should be first regulated together with some adjunct points because it is most helpful to excitation and activation of yang—qi. Emitting outgoing—qi to Dazhui and its adjunct points Mingmen (Du 4) and Weiluguan (Coccyx pass) tends to induce the dynamic phenomenon (spontenous movement) of the patient. However it may also cause the phenomenon of syncope in some patients. This calls for special attention of the therapist in clinical treatment.

Mingmen (Du 4)

Location: Inferior to the lower border of the spinous process of the 2nd lumbar vertebra.

Indication: Asthenia of yang—qi (positive energy), insufficiency of kidney—yang, coldness and pain in the waist and knee, soreness of the waist and back, rigidity and pain, impotency, seminal emission, diarrhoea and leukorrhea.

Application: Also named Jinggong and Zhuzhang, it is located between the two kidneys. As the storage of essence, the kidney is the root of life, the origin of innateness, and the crux thoroughfare of qi flowing along the Du Channel. So emitting outgoing—qi to Mingmen can regulate the Du Channel in general, excite yang—qi, strengthen yang and replenish the kidney, and facilitate qi to go through the three passes to reach the desired points. Emission of outgoing—qi to it together with its adjunct points Weiluguan (Coccyx pass), Dazhui (Du 14) and Yuzhenguan (occiput pass) has the function of regulating the Du Channel and exciting yang—qi to open through the small circle of qi.

Feishu (UB 13)

Location: 1.5 cun lateral to the lower border of the spinous process of the 3rd thoracic vertebra.

Indication: Cough, dyspnea, hemoptysis, hectic fever due to yin—deficiency, chest distress, hypochondriac pain and rigidity and pain in the back.

Application: As the lung lies inside it, Feishu is a place where the lung carries out exchanges of qi, serving as an important point for treatment of the lung diseases. Emitting outgoing—qi toward it for conduction of qi may help dredge and regulate the channel qi, nourish yin and clear away heat from the lung,and replenish qi to subdue asthma. By opening through Feishu with outgoing qi together with exciting its adjunct point Xinshu (UB 15) to achieve the result of will following the circulation of qi, the effect of dynamic phenomenon of the patient can be most easily induced. Emitting qi toward Feishu and its adjunct point Zhongfu (Lu 1), one in the anterior and the other posterior, has the function of regulating the lung—qi and keeping the lung—qi downwards.

Xinshu (UB 15)

Location: 1.5 cun lateral to the lower border of the spinous process of the 5th thoracic vertebra.

Indication: Precordial pain, insomnia, vexation, palpitation due to fright, amnesia, epilepsy and hysteria.

Application: As a key point for treatment of heart diseases, it is a place for transformation and exchange of the heart—qi at the back. Emitting outgoing qi to it can help nourish the heart—qi and regulate the heart and kidney. Emitting qi to it together with its adjunct points Shanzhong (Ren 17) and Juque (Ren 14) and guiding qi between the anterior and posterior can balance yin and yang of the above two aspects.

Ganshu (UB 18)

Location: 1.5 cun lateral to the lower border of the spinous process of the 9th thoracic vertebra.

Indication: Chest and hypochondriac pain, margins of eyelids, dizziness, depressive psychosis, epilepsy.

Application: It is internally related to the liver, serving as the location for the liver—qi to transport and exchange at the back and a point for treatment of the liver diseases. Emitting outgoing—qi toward it together with guiding qi can help regulate the circulation of qi along the Liver Channel, calm the liver to stop pathogenic wind, and improve the visual acuity and check the exuberance of yang. Clinically, it is often used with Zhangmen (Liv 13) and Qimen (Liv 14) as the adjunct points.

Pishu (UB 20)

Location: 1.5 cun lateral to the lower border of the spinous process of the 11th thoracic vertebra.

Indication: Vomiting, abdominal distention, diarrhoea, dysentery, edema, pain in the waist and back and lassitude of the extremities.

Application: It is internally related to the spleen and serve as a location for the spleen—qi to transport and exchange at the back and a key point for treating diseases of the spleen and stomach. Emiting outgoing qi toward this point can activate qi of the Spleen Channel, reinforce the spleen to remove dampness, and replenish qi and regulate blood circulation. Emiting qi toward it with Dantian as the adjunct point can help activate and regulate both the congenital and acquired qi.

Shenshu (UB 23)

Location: 1.5 cun lateral to the lower border of the spinous process of the 2nd lumbar vertebra.

Indication: Pain in the loins and legs, enuresis, seminal emission, impotency, irregular menstruation, vertigo, tinnitus and deafness.

Application: It is internally related to the kidney, serving as a place for the kidney—qi to transport and exchange at the back and a key point for treating diseases of the kidney. Emitting qi toward it together with conducting qi has the function of supplementing the congenital qi, tonifying the kidney to arrest spontaneous emission and removing dampness to relieve edema. And with Dantian as its adjunct point for emittng and guiding qi, the effect of facilitating the congenital qi and guiding qi back to its origin can be achieved.

Points at the Upper Limbs

Jiquan (H 1)

Location: At the centre of the axilla, on the medial side of the axillary artery.

Indication: Precordial pain, pain and fullness in the hypochondrium and pain in the arm.

Application: The point is where the transformation of heart—yang into yin takes place. It is internally related to the heart, joins the lung and has its outer opening at the axilla. Emitting outgoing qi to this point has the function of general regulation of qi of the Lung Channel of Hand—Taiyin and the Heart Channel of Hand—Shaoyin, the function of promoting circulation of qi and blood and that of regulating the blood vessels. Emitting outgoing—qi to it and Xiaohai (SI 8), Hegu (LI 4) and Quchi (LI 11) with rotating manipulation can help activate, check and promote the qi flow in the upper limb.

Shaohai (H 3)

Location: In the depression at the ulnar end of the transversal cubital crease which appears when the elbow is bent.

Indication: Precordial pain, pain in the axillary and hypochondriac region, epilepsy and scrofula.

Application: Shaohai is the He (Sea) point, or the converging point of the Channels of Hand—Shaoyin. Emitting outgoing—qi toward it together with guiding qi can help dredge the channels and collaterals, regulate the blood vessels and resolve phlegm to calm the heart. Clinically it is often applied together with Jiquan (H 1), Quchi (LI 11) and Hegu (LI 4).

Quchi (L I 11)

Location: In the depression at the radial end of the transverse cubital crease when the elbow is flexed.

Indication: Vertigo, common cold, sore throat, gingivitis, dryness in the throat, thirst, manic—depressive psychosis, abdominal pain, vomiting and diarrhoea, pain in the shoulder, arm and elbow, and flaccidity of the upper limb.

Application: Quchi is also termed Guichen and Yangze. It is the place where qi of the Large Intestine Channel of Hand—Yangming enters. Emitting outgoing—qi toward this point together with guiding qi can help dispel pathogenic wind from the body surface, regulate the stomach and intestines, resolve stasis and swelling, and relax the muscles and tendons to lubricate the joints. As Quchi is in charge of desending and Zhongchong (P 9) in charge of ascending, the combination of the two for emission and guidance of qi may achieve harmony of qi descending and ascending, making the heart, lung and the large intestine pure and clear, the stomach regulated with adversely—rising qi checked, vomiting relieved and vertigo improved.

Hegu (L I 4)

Location: Between the 1st and 2nd metacarpal bones, approximately level with the midpoint of the 2nd metacarpal bone.

Indication: Headache, toothache, conjunctival congestion and pain, deafness, sore throat, deviation of the eye and mouth, syncope, manic–depressive psychosis and epilepsy.

Application: Also termed Hukou, Hankou and Hegu, it is a source point (the point where the primordial qi of the viscera flows and stays) of the Large Intestine Channel of Hand–Yangming. Emitting qi toward it together with guiding qi can clear and activate the channels and collaterals, promote circulation of qi to induce resuscitation, dispel pathogenic wind from the body surface, and relieve muscular spasm and tranquilize the mind. When it is applied in combination with Taichong(Liv 3) for emission of qi, satisfactory effect is often attained in the treatment of joint pain, syncope, epilepsy, and the like. Patients who are sensitive to outgoing–qi can readily feel the effect of qi or feel the vibration of qi when the therapist emits it toward his Hegu point.

Inner Laogong (P 8)

Location: In the middle of the palm, between the 3rd and 4th metacarpal bones.

Indication: Manic–depressive psychosis, epilepsy, hysteria, vomiting, halitosis and aphthae.

Application: Also named Guilu, Yinggong, Wuli and Zhangzhong, it is a point of and representative of the Pericardium Channel of Hand–Taiyin, the place where qi of this channel passes, a spring point (one of the five shu points), and a point of great importance for emission and guidance of qi. A well versed Qigong practitioner can get this point open and emit qi out of his body. When the therapist emits outgoing–qi toward the Inner Laogong of the patient, the pa-

tient, if sensitive to outgoing—qi, can feel qi apparently. Emitting outgoing—qi toward this point may help clear away the
heart—fire, tranquilize the mind, remove dampness—heat, dissipate stasis and disperse the accumulation of pathogen, lower
the adversely ascending qi to soothe the stomach and remove
heat from the blood to stop pathogenic wind.

Point at the Lower Limbs

Yanglingquan (GB 34)

Location: In the depression anterior and inferior to the
small head of the fibula.

Indication: Pain in the knee, paralysis, hemiplegia, eye disease, bitterness in the mouth and dryness of the throat, dizziness, vertigo, hypochondriac pain, pain in the shoulder joint
and sciatica.

Application: Also named Jinhui and Yangling, the point
belongs to the Gallbladder Channel of Foot—Shaoyang, serving as the entrance of qi of this channel. Emitting qi toward
this point together with guiding qi can help relax the muscles
and tendons and activate the flow of qi and blood in the channels and collaterals, relieve spasm and pain, clear away dampness—heat, treat shaoyang disease, and disperse the stagnated
liver—qi and gallbladder—qi. Emitting qi to Yanglingquan in
combination with Zhigou (S J 6), with one in the upper and the
other in the lower, can ensure a smooth flow of qi in the two
channels (the Gallbladder Channel and the Sanjiao Channel),
facilitate qi in Sanjiao (three warmers) and resolve stagnation
and masses.

Zusanli (St 36)

Location: 3 cun inferior to the lateral depression of the knee.

Indication: Stomachache, abdominal distention, vomiting, dysphagia, edema, constipation, and pain in the waist, knee and leg.

Application: Also called Xialing and Guixie, it belongs to the Stomach Channel of Foot—Yangming, serving as a converging point at the lower part of the channel. Emitting qi to this point together with guiding qi can help regulate the stomach and intestines, facilitate qi to relieve distention, dissipate stagnation and obstruction, promote the circulation of qi to allay pain, alleviate water retention to subdue swelling, and activate the flow of qi and blood in the channels and collaterals. Emitting qi toward it in combination with Quchi (LI 11) has the functions of general regulation of qi of the yang channels, regulation of the spleen, stomach and intestines and of general health care.

Weizhong (UB 40)

Location: Exact the midpoint of the popliteal transverse crease.

Indication: Lumbago, flaccidity of the lower limbs, abdominal pain accompanied with vomiting and diarrhoea, and swelling and pain in the neck.

Application: Weizhong belongs to the Urinary Bladder Channel of Foot—Taiyang as a converging point at its lower part. Emitting outgoing—qi toward it to guide qi can relax the muscles and tendons and activate the flow of qi and blood in the channels and collaterals, reinforce the waist and knee and cool the blood to stop bleeding.

Yongquan (K 1)

Location: In the depression when the toes are plantar flexed.

Indication: Vertex pain, dizziness, vertigo, infantile convulsion, depressive psychosis, sore throat, aphonia, and hot sensation in the sole.

Application: The synonyms are Diheng, Dichong, and Juexin. It belongs to the Kidney Channel of Foot−Shaoyin, serving as an exit of the channel qi. Emitting qi toward it can help restore consciousness and reduce resuscitation, tranquilize the mind, clear away heat and purge pathogenic fire and calm the liver to stop the pathogenic wind. Yongquan is a point connected with the Earth− qi. Emitting qi toward it in combination with Laogong (P 8) can facilitate the coordination of qi inside and outside the body and regulate the internal qi.

Other Points

Besides the above−mentioned commonly used points, there are some other regular points and extrachannel points used as adjuncts in outgoing−qi therapy, which are listed in brief below.

Table 3−1   List of Other Commonly−used Points

Channel: The Lung Channel of Hand−Taiyin
Yunmen (LU 2)

Location: 6 cun lateral to the thoracic midline, inferior to the lateral end of the clavicle, 1 cun above Zhongfu (LU 1).

Indication: Cough, dyspnea, pain in the chest, shoulder and back, and hot sensation in the cheSt

Chize (LU 5)

Location: In the middle of the cubital crease, at the radial side of the tendon of brachial biceps.

Indication: Contracting pain in the elbow and arm, cough with dyspnea, fullness in the chest and hypochondrium and infantile convulsion.

Lieque (LU 7)

Location: Superior to the styloid process of radius, 1.5 cun above the transverse crease of wrist

Indication: Cough, sore throat, hemiplegia, stiffness of the neck with pain, headache, facial paralysis and toothache.

Yuji (LU 10)

Location: On the palmar surface, in the middle of the first metacarpal bone at the junction of the "white and red" skin.

Indication: Pain in the chest and back, headache, vertigo, sore throat, fever and aversion to cold.

Shaoshang (Lu 11)

Location: On the radial side of the thumb, about 0.1 cun posterior to the corner of nail.

Indication: Apoplectic coma, contracture of the fingers with pain and infantile convulsion.

Channel: The Large Intestine Channel of Hand—Yangming

Yangxi (LI 5)

Location: On the radial side of the back of the wrist, in the hollow between the tendons of m. extensor pollicis longus and brevis.

Indication: Headache, tinnitus, toothache, soreness and

pain in the arm, sore throat and edema.

Shousanli (LI 10)

Location: 2 cun direct below the point Quchi (LI 11).

Indication: Spasm of elbow with difficulty in extension and flexion and numbness and aching—pain in the arms.

Jianyu (LI 15)

Location: In the depression of the acromion when the arm is raised.

Indication: Pain in the shoulder and arm, dysfunction of the shoulder joints and hemiplegia.

Yingxiang (LI 20)

Location: 0.5 cun lateral to the nasal ala, in the naso—labial groove.

Indication: Rhinitis, stuffy nose and facial paralysis.

Channel: The Stomach Channel of Foot—Yamgming

Sibai (St 2)

Location: In the depression at the infra—orbital foramen, directly below the pupil when one is looking straight ahead.

Indication: Facial paralysis and conjunctival congestion with pain and itching.

Dicang (St 4)

Location: 0.4 cun lateral to the corner of mouth.

Indication: Slobbering and facial hemiparalysis.

Daying: (St 5)

Location: In the depression at the lower border of m. masseter, 1.3 cun anterior to the angle of jaw.

Indication: Lockjaw and toothache.

Jiache (St 6)

Location: In the depression one finger width superior to

the angle of jaw, at the prominence of the masseter muscle when the jaw is shut tight.

Indication: Facial paralysis, toothache and swelling of cheek.

Xiaguan (St 7)

Location: In the depression at the lower border of the zygomatic arch, at the prominence of the masseter muscle when the jaw is shut tight.

Indication: Facial paralysis and toothache.

Touwei (St 8)

Location: 0.5 cun directly above the midpoint of the frontal hairline.

Indication: Headache and vertigo.

Renying (St 9)

Location: 1.5 cun lateral to the thyroid cartilage.

Indication: Sore throat, asthma and shortness of breath.

Shuitu (St 10)

Location: On the anterior border of m. sternocleidomastoideus, 1 cun inferior to Renying (St 9).

Indication: Fullness in the chest, cough with dyspnea, stiffness of the neck and sore throat.

Tianshu (St 25)

Location: 2 cun lateral to the umbilicus.

Indication: Diarrhoea, constipation, abdominal pain and irregular menstruation.

Biguan (St 31)

Location: On the line between the anterior—superior iliac spine and the lateral border of the patella, at the level of the gluteal groove.

Indication: Pain in the waist and legs, numbness and flaccidity of the lower limbs with contracture and spasm of muscles with stiffness and difficulty in extension and flexion.

Futu (St 32)

Location: 6 cun above the superolateral border of the patella.

Indication: Cold and numbness of the knee with pain; lower limbparalysis.

Liangqiu (St 34)

Location: 2 cun above the superolateral border of the patella.

Indication: Pain, cold and numbness in the knee.

Waixiyan (Dubi, St 35)

Location: At the lower border of the patella, in the depression lateral to the patellar ligament.

Indication: Aching pain in the knee with difficulty in movement.

Shangjuxu (St 37)

Location: 3 cun inferior to the point Zusanli (St 36).

Indication: Pain around the navel, diarrhoea, lower limb paralysis.

Jiexi (St 41)

Location: On the midpoint of the dorsum of foot at the transverse malleolus crease, between the tendons of m. extensor digitorum longus and hallucis longus.

Indication: Sprain of the ankle and numbness of the foot.

Channel: The Spleen Channel of Foot–Taiyin

Sanyinjiao (Sp 6)

Location: 3 cun above the tip of the medial malleolus, on

the posterior border of the medial aspect of the tibia.

Indication: Insomnia, abdominal distention, indigestion, enuresis and irregular menstruation.

Yinlingquan (Sp 9)

Location: In the depression on the inferior border of the medial condyle of tibia.

Indication: Soreness of the knee joint and pain in the knee.

Xuehai (Sp 10)

Location: 2 cun superior to the medial border of the patella.

Indication: Irregular menstruation and pain in the knee.

Daheng (Sp 15)

Location: 4 cun lateral to the navel.

Indication: Diarrhoea of deficiency—cold type, constipation and pain in the lower abdomen.

Channel: The Heart Channel of Hand—Shaoyin

Jiquan (H 1)

Location: At the centre of the axilla.

Indication: Stuffiness in the chest, hypochondriac pain and coldness and numbness of the arm and elbow.

Shaohai (H 3)

Location: In the depression at the ulnar end of the transversal cubital crease which appears when the elbow is flexed.

Indication: Numbness and pain in the arm and elbow.

Shenmen (H 7)

Location: On the transversal crease of wrist, at the radial side of the tendon of m. flexor carpi ulnaris.

Indication: Palpitation due to fright, severe palpitation, insomnia and amnesia.

Channel: The Small Intestine Channel of Hand−Taiyang

Shaoze (SI 1)

Location: At the ulnar side of the little finger, about 0.1 cun posterior to the corner of nail.

Indication: Fever, apoplectic coma, hypogalactia and sore throat.

Xiaohai (SI 8)

Location: In the depression between the olecranon of the ulna and the tip of the medial epicondyle of the humerus when the elbow is flexed.

Indication: Toothache, pain in the neck and soreness and pain in the upper extremities.

Bingfeng (SI 12)

Location: In the centre of the superior fossa of spinascapula, directly above Tianzong (SI 11).

Indication: Pain in the scapular area, difficulty in raising the arm and soreness and numbness of the upper arm.

Jianwaishu (SI 14)

Location: 3 cun lateral to the lower border of the spinous process of the 1st thoracic vertebra.

Indication: Pain in the shoulder and back, stiffness of the neck and coldness and pain in the upper limb.

Jianzhongshu (SI 15)

Location: 2 cun lateral to the point Dazhui (Du 14).

Indication: Cough, shortness of breath, pain in the shoulder and back and blurred vision.

Jianzhen (SI 9)

Location: 1 cun superior to the posterior axillary fold.

Indication: Soreness and pain in the shoulder joint with difficulty in movement, and upper limb paralysis.

Tianzong (SI 11)

Location: In the centre of the superior fossa of spinascapula.

Indication: Soreness and pain in the shoulder and back, dysfunction of the shoulder joint and upper lim paralysis.

Quanliao (SI 18)

Location: Directly below the outer canthus, in the depression below the lower border of the zygomatic bone.

Indication: Facial hemiparalysis.

Channel: The Urinary Bladder Channel of Foot–Taiyang

Jingming (UB 1)

Location: 0.1 cun lateral to the inner canthus.

Indication: Diseases of the eye.

Zanzhu (UB 2)

Location: In the depression proximal to the medial end of the eyebrow.

Indication: Headache, insomnia, pain in the supra–orbital bone, conjunctival congestion and pain.

Tianzhu (UB 10)

Location: 1.3 cun lateral to the point Yamen (Du 15), in the depression at the external border of the trapezius muscle.

Indication: Headache, rigidity in the neck, stuffy nose, pain in the shoulder and back.

Dashu (UB 11)

Location: 1.5 cun lateral to the lower border of the spinous process of the 1st thoracic vertebra.

Indication: Fever, cough, rigidity in the neck and pain in the shoulder and back.

Fengmen (UB 12)

Location: 1.5 cun lateral to the lower border of the spinous process of the 2nd thoracic vertebra.

Indication: Cold, cough, rigidity in the neck and pain in the shoulder and back.

Weishu (UB 21)

Location: 1.5 cun lateral to the lower border of the spinous process of the 12th thoracic vertebra.

Indication: Gastric diseases, vomiting of milk in infants, and indigestion.

Sanjiaoshu (UB 22)

Location: 1.5 cun lateral to the lower border of the spinous process of the 1st lumbar vertebra.

Indication: Intestinal gargling and distention, vomiting, rigidity and pain in the waist and back.

Qihaishu (UB 24)

Location: 1.5 cun lateral to the lower border of the spinous process of the 3rd lumbar vertebra.

Indication: Pain in the waist and lower limbs.

Dachangshu (UB 25)

Location: 1.5 cun lateral to the lower border of the spinous process of the 4th lumbar vertebra.

Indication: Pain in the waist and lower limbs, lumbar muscle strain and enteritis.

Guanyuanshu (UB 26)

Location: 1.5 cun lateral to the lower border of the spinous process of the 5th lumbar vertebra.

Indication: Pain in the waist and lower limbs and

diarrhoea.

Baliao (the Eight Liao)

Location: A collective term for Shangliao (UB 31), Ciliao (UB 32), Zhongliao (UB 33) and Xialiao (UB 34), located in the 1st, 2nd, 3rd and 4th posterior sacral foramen respectively.

Indication: Pain in the waist and lower limbs and diseases of the urogenital system.

Zhibian (UB 54)

Location: 3 cun lateral to the lower border of the 4th sacral process.

Indication: Pain in the waist and lower limb, flaccidity of the lower extremities, difficulty in micturition, and constipation.

Yinmen (UB 37)

Location: 6 cun inferior to the midpoint of the gluteal fold.

Indication: Sciatica, paralysis of the lower extremities, pain in the waist and back.

Chengshan (UB 57)

Location: At the top of the depression between the two gastrocnemius muscles. *Indication*: Pain in the waist and legs and systremma.

Kunlun (UB 60)

Location: In the depression between the posterior border of the lateral malleolus and the medial aspect of the tendo calcaneus.

Indication: Headache, stiff neck, lumbago and sprain of ankle.

Channel: The Kidney Channel of Foot—Shaoyin

Taixi (K 3)

Location: In the depression between the tip of medial malleolus and tendo calcaneus.

Indication: Sore throat, insomnia, toothache, impotency and irregular menstruation.

Shuiquan (K 5)

Location: 1 cun directly inferior to Taixi (K 3).

Indication: Irregular menstruation, dysmenorrhea, difficulty in micturition, dizziness and blurred vision.

Zhaohai (K 6)

Location: In the depression on the inferior of the medial malleolus.

Indication: Irregular menstruation.

Channel: The Pericardium Channel of Hand—Jueyin

Quze (P 3)

Location: In the middle of the transverse cubital crease, at the ulnar side of tendon of m. biceps brachii.

Indication: Aching—pain in and trembling of the upper limbs.

Neiguan (P 6)

Location: 2 cun above the transverse carpal crease, between the tendon palmaris and the mediocarpal tendon.

Indication: Stomachache, vomiting, palpitatiom and mental disorders.

Daling (P 7)

Location: At the midpoint of the transverse crease of wrist, between the tendon palmaris and the mediocarpal tendon.

Indication: Pain in the costal region, palpitation, stomachache, vomiting and pain in the chest and hypochondrium.

Channel: The Sanjiao Channel of Hand—Shaoyang

Zhongzhu (SJ 3)

Location: On the dorsum of the hand, between the small ends of the 4th and 5th metacarpal bones, in the depression posterior to the metacarpophalangeal joint when the hand corms a fiSt

Indication: Migraine, pain in the palm and fingers or in the elbow and arm.

Waiguan (SJ 15)

Location: 2 cun above the transverse crease of dorsum of wrist, between the radius the ulna.

Indication: Headache, pain in the wrist or fingers with difficulty in stretching and flexing.

Yangchi (SJ 4)

Location: On the dorsum of wrist, in the depression lateral to the medial border of m. extensor digitorum.

Indication: Pain in the shoulder and arm or wrist, diabetes, deafness.

Jianliao (SJ 4)

Location: Lateral and inferior to the acromoin, in the depression about 1 cun posterior to the point Jianyu (L I 15).

Indication: Aching—pain in the shoulder and arm and difficulty in shoulder joint movement.

Channel: The Gallbladder Channel of Foot—Shaoyang

Tongziliao (GB 1)

Location: Lateral to the outer canthus, in the depression at the lateral border of the orbital bone.

Indication: Headache, conjunctival congestion, irritated epiphora.

Yangbai (GB 14)

Location: 1 cun superior to the midpoint of the eyebrow.

Indication: Headache, vertigo and pain in the eye.

Juliao (GB 29)

Location: At the midpoint of the line between the anterosuperior iliac spine and the highest point of the greater trochanter femur.

Indication: Pain in the loins and legs, soreness and pain in the hip joint and sacro—iliilis.

Huantiao (GB 30)

Location: At the junction of the external one third and the internal two thirds of the distance between the highest point of the greater trochanter of femur and the hiatus of sacrum.

Indication: Pain in the loins and legs, sciatica, hemiparalysis and flaccidity of the lower extremities.

Fengshi (GB 31)

Location: On the lateral midline of the thigh, 7 cun superior to the popliteral transverse crease.

Indication: Hemiplegia, flaccidity and numbness of the lower extremities and aching—pain in the knee joint.

Guangming (GB 37)

Location: 5 cun above the tip of external malleolus, close to the anterior border of fibula.

Indication: Pain in the knee, flaccidity of the lower limb, pain in the eye and distention of the breaSt

Xuanzhong (GB 39)

Location: 3 cun above the tip of external mallelus, close to the anterior border of fibula.

Indication: Headache, rigidity in the neck and soreness and pain in the lower limbs.

Qiuxu (GB 40)

Location: Anterior and inferior to the external malleolus, in the depression on the lateral side of the tendon of the m. extensor digitorum longus.

Indication: Pain in the knee joint, chest and hypochondrium.

Channel: The Liver Channel of Foot—Jueyin

Taichong(Liv 3)

Location: On the dorsum, in the depression distal to the articulation of the 1st and 2nd metatarsals.

Indication: Headache, dizziness, hypertension and infantile convulsion.

Zhongdu(Liv 6)

Location: 7 cun superior to the tip of the malleolus, on the posterior border of tibia.

Indication: Abdominal pain, diarrhoea, hernia, metrorrhagia and metrostaxis, and lochiorrhea.

Qimen(Liv 14)

Location: Directly below the nipple, in the intercostal space between the 6th and 7th ribs.

Indication: Pain in the chest and hypochondrium, vomiting, abdominal distension and diarrhoea.

Channel: The Ren Channel

Shimen (Ren 5)

Location: 2 cun inferior to the umbilicus.

Indication: Abdominal pain, irregular menstruation, fullness in the epigastric region, amenorrhea and dysmenorrhea.

Juque (Ren 14)

Location: 6 cun superior to the umbilicus.

Indication: Precordial pain, gastric regurgitation, manic-depressive psychosis and painful syndromes.

Jiuwei (Ren 15)

Location: 7 cun superior to the umbilicus and inferior to the sternum. *Indication*: Precordial pain, gastric regurgitation, gastric diseases and pain and fullness in the cheSt

Channel: The Du Channel

Changqiang (Du 1)

Location: 0.5 cun inferior to the tip of the coccyx.

Indication: Diahorrea, constipation and prolapse of anus.

Yaoyangguan (Du 3)

Location: Inferior to the spinous process of the 4th lumbar vertebra.

Indication: Pain in the waist and back, flaccidity of the lower limbs and irregular menstruation.

Jizhong (Du 6)

Location: Inferior to the spinous process of the 11th thoracic vertebra.

Indication: Rigidity and pain in the waist and along the spine, diarrhoea, and prolapse of anus.

Taodao (Du 13)

Location: In the depression inferior to the spinous process of the 1st lumbar vertebra.

Indication: Headache, rigidity in the neck, aversion to cold, fever, cough with pain in the chest and soreness and pain in the back and along the spine.

Renzhong (Du 28)

Location: At the junction of the upper one-third and lower two-thirds of the midline of the nasolabial groove.

Indication: Infantile convulsion, facial hemiparalysis, coma and dizziness.**Extrachannel Points**

Yuyao (Extra)

Location: In the middle of the eyebrow.

Indication: Congestion of the eye with pain, blepharoptosis and facial hemiparalysis.

Anmian (Extra)

Location: On the midpoint of the line joining Fengchi (G B 20) and Yiming (Extra).

Indication: Insomnia, headache, vertigo, palpitation, deafness and hypertension.

Weishang (Extra)

Location: 4 cun lateral and 2 cun superior to the umbilicus.

Indication: Gastroptosia, stomachache and abdominal distention.

Dingchuan (Extra)

Location: 0.5 cun lateral to the midpoint of the lower border of the spinous process of the 7th cervical vertebra.

Indication: Cough with dyspnea, pain in the shoulder and back, stiffneck and pain in the the upper limbs with difficulty in raising the arm.

Jiaji (Extra, a group of points)

Location: 0.5 cun lateral to the lower borders of the spinous processes from the 1st thoracic vertebra to the 5th lumbar vertebra.

Indication: Rigidity and pain in the spinal collumn and diseases of the extremities and the viscera.

Shiqizhui (Extra)

Location: At the lower border of the spinous process of the

5th lumbar vertebra.

Indication: Pain in the waist and legs, dysmenorrhea and pain in the lumbo- sacral portion.

Shixuan (Extra)

Location: At the tips of the ten fingers, 0.1 cun from the nails.

Indication: Syncope, sore throat and infantile convulsion.

Jianneiling (Extra)

Location: At the midpoint of the line connecting the upper end of the anterior axillary fold and the point Jianyu (L I 15).

Indication: Soreness and pain in the shoulder joint with dysfunction of shoulder movements.

Sifeng (Extra)

Location: On the palmar surface in the tranverse crease of the proximal interphalangleal joint of the index, middle, ring and small fingers of both hands, 8 points in all.

Indication: Infantile malnutrition, pertusis and infantile diarrhoea.

Qiaogong (Extra)

Location: The line posterior to the ear connecting Yifeng (SJ 17) and Quepen (St 12).

Indication: Headache, dizziness and hypertension.

Taiyang (Extra 2)

Location: In the depression about 1 cun lateral to the line connecting the lateral end of the eyebrow and the outer canthus.

Indication: Migraine headache and conjunctival congestion.

Chapter Four   The Training of Qi

Training of qi is the basic step of guiding and emitting qi. A qigong therapist usually has to undergo long–term painstaking dynamic (physical) and static (internal) exercise before his functional activities of qi can be voluntarily regulated, replenished and circulated down to Dantian, and his qi can flow freely all over the body through the channels. Wherever his mind is concentrated, there is qi; and wherever there is qi, there is strength. This is the foundation for qigong therapists to guide qi and emit waiqi (outgoing–qi). Training of qi is achieved mainly through static exercises, dynamic exercises and Daoyin selfmassage, or in a general term, qigong dirigation.

Section One   The Essentials of the Training of Qi

1. Being Both Dynamic and Static

Qigong exercise calls for selection of methods which suit the health status of the individuals. The practice of static qigong is aimed at training and accumulating qi to get the functional qi substantial in Dantian, and with more practice, to get qi circulating through the Ren and Du Channels and all the other channels, or further, to open the large and small circule of qi. On the other hand, static qigong is aimed at promoting the functional activities of qi to guarantee the free pass of it through all the channels of the human body, which in turn may facilitate the static training of qi. The two methods are supplementary to each other provided they are combined as one.

No matter which of the two is practised, the principle "quiescence in motion and motion in quiescence" should be adhered to. When dynamic qigong is practised, while keeping physical movements going on, one needs to keep the mind concentrated on the effectiveness of limb movements and the circulation of qi along the channels and collaterals. When static qigong is practised,the more serene and relaxed one is, the more one can feel the effectiveness of the circulating qi along the channels and collaterals. A correct realization of the reffectiveness of motion can help one to concentrate himself , expell distracting thoughts and raise the quality of exercise.

2. Being Relaxed and Tranquil Naturally

Relaxation, a principle in qigong exercise, means both physical and mental, for only when one is relaxed mentally can he be so physically. However, relaxation here does not mean slackness or inattentiveness,but means relaxation with attentiveness, relaxation with tension and tension without rigidity, dominated by the conscious mind.

" Tranquil" here means to keep a serene mind during qigong exercise. Tranquillity is relative, there exists no absolute tranquillity. The so called "falling into quiescense" in qigong is different from natural sleep and general rest. It implies a special tranquil state with consciousness, or in other words, a special conscious state with tranquillity.

Relaxation and tranquillity are mutually promotive; proper relaxation often results in tranquillity and tranquillity can facilitate good relaxation.

Both the relaxation and tranquillity mentioned above should be achieved naturally,so should the regulation of posture, breathing and mind concentration.

3. Coordinating Will and Qi (Vital Energy)

The coordination of will and qi, as the term implies, means that in qigong exercise, will should follow qi and vice versa. The practitioner should not put undue emphasis on exerting will to guide qi, which usually leads to forced "gentle, fine, even and long" breathing other than that acquired naturally through correct practice; nor should he force unnecessarily abdominal respiration which leads him to buldge his belly and throw out his chest on purpose,losing naturalness. Another deviation can be seen in the fact that when the motion of qi is felt inside the body, the practitioner forces it by will to flow in a definite direction.This is also against the principle which needs the function to be formed naturally through practice.Xue Yanggui of the Qing Dynasty (1644 − 1911) wrote in his book *Mei Hua Wen Da Pian (Questions and Answers of Meihua)* that " the tranquillity of the mind regulates the breathing naturally and in turn regulated breathing brings on concentration of the mind naturally; this is what is said that mind and breathing are interdependent and regulated respiration produces serene mind".

It is not advisable to put undue emphasis on realization of the flow of qi either. The cold, hot, tingling, distending, itching, light, heavy, floating, deep or warm sensation experienced during qigong exercising will go along a certain route. It is improper to pursue such kind of sensation intentionally or to exaggerate it, or force oneself to gain it.

4. Combining Active Exercise with Inner Health Cultivation

"Active exercise" means a series of procedures controlled by consciousness during qigong exercise in terms of determination of a proper posture, adjustment of the body, achievement of internal and external relaxation, regulation of respiration, as well as the elimination of distracting thoughts. The saying that "active exercise is vigorous breathing (wu huo)", means to conduct breathing training under strong domination of consciousness. "Inner health cultivation" refers to the static state one falls into after active exercise, in which one carries out "wen huo" breathing (gentle breathing), feeling relaxed and comfortable, with his will and respiration feeble and faint.

In qigong practice, active exercise and inner health cultivation are done alternately and the two are interpromotive. For instance, one may have static inner cultivation after active exercise has been practised or vice versa to achieve the effectiveness of "active exercise in static cultivation" or "static cultivation in active exercise", or we can say, "a combination of the two", to raise the quality of qigong exercise.

5. Proceeding in an Orderly Way and Step by Step

qigong exercise needs to be proceeded in an orderly way and step by step. Be aware of the old saying "Haste makes waste". In qigong outgoing–qi therapy, the basis for guiding and emitting qi is, firstly, the hard practice of static and dynamic exercises which is required to get the internal qi substantial and all the channels and collaterals unobstructed; secondly, the training of guidance of qi, which is the skill to make the internal qi circulate with the changes of posture, respiration and mind activities; and lastly, the practice of emitting outgoing—qi, which needs the practitioner to grasp the hand manipulations and to improve the hand sensitivity , the qi—emitting technique and the skills for eliminating pathogenic , filthy qi. Only in this way, can one learn the correct methods of treating diseases with outgoing—qi. Inconstancy in practice should be avoided. Negligence of one's own advantages and disadvantages to pursue merely "super skill" and "emission of outgoing qi" will lead only to the opposite.

Section Two   Essential Factors in Training Qi

1. Posture

Posture in qigong is also called regulation of the body or adjustment of posture. It is especially important for the beginners of static or dynamic qigong to have a good command of proper posturization.

Four postures may be assumed in qigong exercise——sitting, lying, standing and walking. Static qigong usually requires a sitting, lying or standing posture while dynamic qigong often needs the standing and walking. The formal training of outgoing qi therapy often needs a strict posture; however, the skill can also be trained during walking, standing, sitting and lying in daily life.

(1) The Sitting Posture

1) Upright Sitting

Sit upright on a large, even square stool. Ground the feet apart at shoulder width. Bend the knees to form an angle of 90 degrees. Keep the trunk erect, the angle between the trunk and the thigh being 90 degrees. Rest the palms gently on the thighs with the arms bent at the elbows naturally, look straight forward, draw in the chin a little, let down the shoulders and draw the chest slightly inwards to keep the back straight, close the eyes and mouth gently and apply the tongue against the palate (Fig. 4—1).

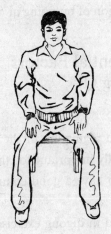 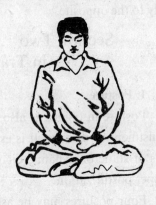

Fig. 4—1 The Upright Sitting   Fig. 4—2 The Cross—legged Zi—
Posture   Wu Sitting Posture

2) Sitting Cross—legged

Sit cross—legged on bed steadily with the two feet under the legs. Cushion the hips to raise them a little, with the body leaning slightly forwards. overlap the hands before the abdomen with the left above the right and the thumb of the right hand pressing Ziwen (the crease joining the palm and the ring finger) of the left hand and the thumb and the middle finger of the left hand jointing together to form a Zi—Wu Jue Shi (a cross—legged Zi—Wu sitting posture) (Fig. 4—2). Or close the two palms in front of the chest to form a Fo Zhang Shi (a cross-legged Buddha-greeting sitting posture) (Fig. 4-3). Or put the two hands on the two knees naturally to form a Jin Gang Shi (a crossed-legged Buddha's-warrior-attendant sitting posture) (Fig. 4-4).

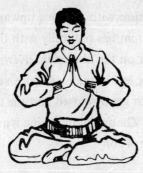 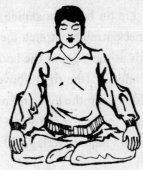

Fig. 4-3 The Crossed-legged Buddhist-Greeting Sitting Posture

Fig. 4-4 The Cross-legged Buddha's-Worrior-Attendant Sitting Posture

(2) The Lying Posture

1) Lateral Recumbent Posture

Lie on bed in lateral recumbent posture (usually on the right side but either side will do), the trunk being kept slightly bent. Rest the head on a pillow and lean it towards the chest a bit. Keep the eyes and mouth slightly closed and the tongue against the palate. Put the hand of the lying side comfortably on the pillow with the palm upwards, and place the other palm on it, the tips of the little, ring, middle and index fingers of the upper hand on the metacarpophalangeal creases of the corresponding four fingers of the lower hand, the thumb of the upper hand resting on the outside part between the thumb and the index finger of the lower hand. Or place the upper arm of the above side naturally on the same side of the body (Fig. 4−5). Stretch the leg of the lying side naturally, with the above bent and resting naturally on it.

2) Supine Posture

Lie on bed in a supine posture with the face upward and the neck straight, stretch the extremities naturally with the two hands at the sides of the body or on the abdomen, overlapping one another (the right above the left in male and vice versa in female), keep the eyes and mouth gently closed and the tongue against the palate to form a Die Zhang Shi (a supine lying posture with hands overlapped) (Fig. 4−6).

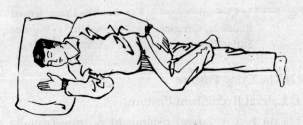

Fig. 4−5 The Lying Posture

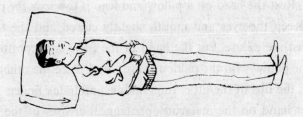

Fig. 4−6 The Lying Supine Posture with Hands Overlapped

(3) The Standing Posture

Stand with feet apart as wide as the shoulders. Keep the

head straight, the trunk erect, the chest slightly inward,the knees at ease and the arms raised and bent a little. Keep the fingers apart naturally, and hold the two hands close to the chest or the lower abdomen as if holding a ball (a ball–holding standing posture) (Fig. 4–7); or close the two palms in a way as if doing Buddhist greeting (a Buddha's greeting standing posture), or press the palms downwards (a palm–pressing standing posture)(Fig. 4–8); or get the right (left) hand upwards with the left (right) palm held erect with the root of the palm pointing at the midpoint of the medial side of the root of the right (left) palm to form a Zhan Zhuang Fang Yuan Shi (a square–round standing posture) (Fig. 4–9). The two hands can also be overlapped against the lower abdomen. The mouth and eyes should be closed gently and the tongue should be propped against the palate during practice.

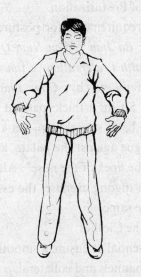

Fig. 4–7 The Ball–holding Standing Posture

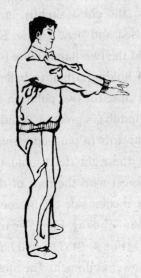 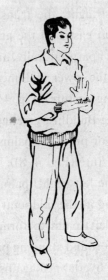

Fig. 4—8   The Palm—pressing   Fig.4—9   The Square—round
         Standing Posture   Standing Posture

(4) Essentials of Posturization

So far as the requirements for posture in qigong are concerned, *Zun Sheng Ba Jian — Yan Nian Que Bing Jian (Eight Annotations on Health Preservation — Annotations on Longevity and Disease Prevention)* by *Gao Lian* (Ming Dynasty, 1368—1644) says, "Sit on a thick—padded cushion, loosen the clothing, keep the back straight up, get the lips close to the teeth, stick the tongue against the palate, keep the eyes slightly open and stare at the apex of the nose". Although there is a variety of postures in qigong exercise, the essential requirements for them remain the same.

1) Loosening the Clothes

This step is essential to ensure a smooth flow of qi through the unobstructed channels and collaterals.

2) Picturing Supporting an Object on the Head

Also called "Suspending the Crown of the Head", it is neccessary to prop the head upward gently, pull in the chin slightly and lift the neck a little to get it straight and relaxed.

3) Relaxing the Shoulders and Dropping the Elbows

This should be done with ease; avoid stiffness of the elbows.

4) Drawing in the Chest and Straightening the Back

The practitioner should not ease his back at will or lean it against anything. Instead, he should keep it erect, and on this basis, draw in his chest a little.

5) Keeping the Waist and the Abdomen Relaxed

The waist and abdomen are two important parts in training and guiding qi. The abdomen is usually taken as the furnace for refining qi and the waist, as the residence of the kidneys, the gate of life and the important pass of qi and blood circulation. Relaxation of the waist and abdomen without slackness is helpful to the training and circulation of qi.

6) Contracting the Buttocks and Relaxing the Knees

Contracting the hips a little helps to straighten the spinal column; relaxing the knees permits free flow of qi through the Three Yang and Three Yin Channels of Foot.

7) Keeping the Toes Clutching the Ground

When the standing posture is taken, stretch the feet and let the five toes of each foot clutch the ground to keep the body as firm as Mount Tai (as stable as possible).

8) Curtain—falling and Inward Vision

It refers to dropping the eyelids to create inward vision on the spot where qi is trained or circulates. *Yin Fu Jing* claims that "the functional activities of qi are determined by the eyes";

Ling Shu — Da Huo Lun (Miraculous Pivot — on Elusiveness) holds that "the eyes are the messengers of the mind, and the mind is the home of vitality". Eyes are of great importance in qigong exercise. Curtain–falling and inward vision can keep mentality undisturbed, turning off hallucination as well as sunlight. The eyes should neither be tightly closed nor left wide open; in the former, drowsiness may occur because of darkness and in the latter, vitality may be deranged because of too much light.

9) Closing the Mouth and "Stopping the Ears"

Laozi (Laotzi) once said "Close the mouth to shut the gate". Shutting the gate here refers to closing the mouth slightly without clenching the teeth or tightening the lips, while stopping the ears means to focus one's hearing to oneself so as to be free from outside interference (inward–hearing).

10) Sticking the Tongue against the Palate

Traditionally called "propping the palate with the tongue tip" or "tongue propping",it means to apply the tongue against the palate naturally and gently to join the Ren and Du Channels. In the course of practice, the strength of the tongue sticking against the palate will increase automatically and the tongue substance will be gradually pulled backward in accord. This is a phenomenon occurring in the course of qigong practice and should not be pursued intentionally.

2. Respiration

Respiration is also called regulation of breathing, breathing method, or venting and taking in (tu na). It is an important link in qigong exercise. The ancients attached great importance to breathing exercises. A great many terms about breathing exercises can be found in books written in ancient times, such as fuqi (inhaling qi), shiqi (eating qi),jinqi (entering qi),yanqi (swallowing qi),xingqi (circulating qi) and caiqi (taking in qi); as for breathing methods, there are terms such as shangxi (upper breathing), xiaxi (lower breathing), manxi (full breathing), chongxi (blurted breathing), chixi (lasted breathing), changxi (long breathing) and shenxi (deep breathing). The following breathing methods as required for training of qi are usually used.

(1) Natural Respiration

Natural respiration is the ordinary breathing under normal physiological condition.Because of the difference in physiology between male and female and in the breathing habits of individuals,natural respiration can be further divided into natural thoracic respiration, natural abdominal respiration and the combination of the two. Any of the above should be dominated by certain consciousness, performed naturally, and taken as the usual way of breathing in qigong exercise.

(2) Orthodromic Abdominal Respiration It refers to trained natural orthodromic abdominal breathing formed gradually through practice of natural respiration under guidance of will. To train orthodromic abdominal respiration, one employs a little consciousness to relax the abdominal muscles during inhaling to make the abdomen bulged naturally, and during exhaling , uses some consciousness to get the abdominal muscles contracted. The contraction and relaxation of the abdominal muscles are intensified gradually and naturally through a certain period of practice. Forced exertion must be avoided. The orthodromic abdominal respiration tends to appear when one concentrates his mind on the navel.

(3) Antidromic Abdominal Respiration

Antidromic abdominal respiration is the main breathing method used in training qi, guiding qi and in emitting outgoing—qi.To get it, one uses will to guide the abdominal muscles to contract and make the abdomen sunken during inhaling and , during exhaling , relaxes the abdominal muscles gradually to get the abdomen bulged. Training in this way for a certain period of time will make antidromic abdominal respiration a natural one in qigong exercise.

When antidromic abdominal respiration becomes more or less natural, it can be done in cooperation with contraction of the anus, which means to contract the anus and pudendum slightly during inhaling and relax them during exhaling.

(4) Latent and Embryo Breath

Latent breath may occur when respiration of the practitioner is in an extremely gentle state which is built up through long—term qigong exercise. Embryo breath is a kind of abdominal respiration much more gentle than the latent breath, with which there is almost no movement of the abdominal muscles and the practitioner can only feel respiratory rhythm at the navel. The method is considered somewhat mysterious and miraculous in ancient literatures. They may be achieved when the training of qi has reached the peak period. One should not try to get it by importunity.

(5) Other Breathing Methods

Apart from the above—mentioned main breathing methods, others that can be trained may include long inhaling and short exhaling, short exhaling and long inhaling, nasal exhaling and inhaling, nasal inhaling and oral exhaling and respiratory pause after exhaling or inhaling. The selection of the breathing methods is based on the methods of qigong exercise and the stage in practice.

(6) Essentials of Respiration Training

1) It is preferable to train mainly posturization first when one starts practising dynamic or static qigong. Training of respiration should begin when one is skilled and natural in posturization. Otherwise adverse effects such as respiratory distress, emotional upset, chest stuffiness and headache may occur.

2) The final goal of respiration training is to achieve deep, long, even and fine respiration. This is the result gained from long term practice; forced lengthened breathing or oppressed breathing should be guarded against.

3) The ancients laid much stress on the manner of breathing in their practice of regulation of respiration, stating four phases (xiang) of respiration: wind phase (feng xiang), gasp phase (chuan xiang), air phase (qi xiang) and rest phase (xi xiang). With the wind phase, one can hear the rough sound of his own breath; with the gasp phase, though he may hear no sound of his breath, he may feel stagnated and obstructed ventilation of air; with air phase, he may neither hear the rough sound of breath nor feel the stagnated and obstructed ventilation of air yet his breath is not even; and with the rest phase, which is a state of extreme quietness, he may achieve deep, long and even respiration. It was believed in ancient times that "concentrating on the wind phase may derange the mentality, on the gasp phase may cause knotted mentality, on the air phase may strain the mentality, and only on the rest phase can the mentality be set peaceful".

4) Before starting respiration training,it is desirable to open the mouth to exhale, imagining that the obstructed parts

of all the vessels are dredged and the turbid qi is expelled from the body along with exhaling; then to close the mouth to take in the fresh. The above inhaling and exhaling should be carried out three times and then natural breathing should be taken, which should be further adjusted by will to be one desired for training.

3. Mind Concentration

Mind concentration is also known as will control or regulation of the mental activities. The training of mind concentration is an important link in training qi. *She Sheng San Yao (The Three Gists of Regime)* says, "Preservation of essence of life rests with cultivation of vital energy (qi) which in turn rests with mental focalization. Mental focalization is to vital energy as mother is to child. So concentration of the mind would have vital energy consolidated while distraction of the mind would have it dispersed. He who only tries to save essence of life but neglects mental concentration knows the how but does not know the why". Here the relationship between essence of life, vital energy and mental concentration needed in qigong exercise is stressed and importance is attached to mental activities.

An essential thing in training of qi is the training of mind concentration. This is especially true of guiding qi and emitting outgoing–qi.

(1) Localized Mind Concentration

During qigong exercise, concentration of the mind on a certain part or a point of the body such as the Upper Dantian, Lower Dantian and Middle Dantian, Yongquan (K 1), the Inner Laogong (P 8), the fingertips or palms, or on something or a spot fixed outside the body is known as localized mind concentration.

(2) Directive Mind Concentration

It refers to mind concentration following the circulation of qi along the channels when qigong exercise is practised or when qi is emitted; or the sensation obtained when the mind is concentrated on the two hands or on a certain part of the body.

(3) Rhythmical Mind Concentration

It occurs repeatedly or vibrates rhythmically or moves subtly with normal respiratory cycles during qigong exercise or emission of qi, like the vibration produced by driving a pile and the quivering of the hand in emission of outgoing-qi.

(4) Power-strengthening Mind Concentration

During qigong exercise or emission of qi, one may think that he had as much strength as he could imagine. For example, he may imagine that he is strong enough to push down a hill, to hold up the sky or to pull nine oxen back by the tails. This kind of mind concentration is named power-strengthening mind concentration.

(5) Suggestive Mind Concentration

It refers to training of the thought during qigong exercise and emission of qi, by which the movements are induced in coordination with language, e.g., saying some words silently or meditating the results one wishes to achieve by exercise.

(6) Representative Mind Concentration

While practising qigong exercises, one may perform some imaginary movements and get qi response in the long run. For instance, he may imagine he is stroking a ball, pressing qi, instilling qi and expelling unhealthy qi, and he may feel qi as hot as fire, as cold as ice, as sharp as a sword, or as soft as cotton.

(7) Essentials of Training Mind Concentration

1) Mental activities should be coordinated naturally with

respiration and posture. For example, in dynamic qigong exercises or Daoyin, mental activities must be adapted to the posture and the lifting, lowering, opening and closing manipulations of the hand.

2) Mental activities should be carried out naturally in a composed state of mind. The mind should be kept clear and the distracting thought should be expelled. While one should not forget mind concentration, one should not force himself to get it.

3) Training of mind concentration cannot go without "confidence". No matter what kind of mental activity one is training, one should be confident that he can realize the goal, though he should not expect unpractical quick results.

4) Do not be overjoyed or frightened if something unexpected happens or something is perceived by consciousness during exercise. Do not worry or talk about it. Take advantage of this good effect to keep the mind concentrated and qi consolidated.

Section Three   The Time and Direction for Training Qi and The Points for Attention

The Time for Training Qi

The training of qi should be adapted to nature. The qigong exercises to be practised should be selected according to the season or even to the month or the date, and to the physical conditions of the individuals. The time of exercise is determined on the basis of the time of advance and retreat of yin and yang. *Su Wen − Si Qi Tiao Shen Da Lun (Plain Questions − Treatise on Regulation of Vitality in Four Seasons)* emphasizes the principle of "nourishing yang in spring and summer and replenishing yin in autumn and winter". In one day, the first six of the 12 two-hour periods (the twelve Earthly Branches by which the 24-hour day is divided), i.e., Zi (11 pm − 1 am), Chou (1 − 3 am), Yin (3 − 5 am), Mao (5 − 7 am), Chen (7 − 9 am) and Si (9 − 11 am) are called the sixyang periods, while the second six, i.e., Wu (11 am − 1 p m) , Wei (1 − 3 pm), Shen (3 − 5 pm), You (5 − 7 pm), Xu (7 − 9 pm) and Hai (9 − 11 pm), are called the six yin periods. The antients believed that during the six yang periods of the day the external world is filled with active force (the force promoting growth and development) while during the six yin periods the external world is enveloped in stagnant force. So it is advisable to train qi during the six yang periods.

The beginners can practise training of qi mainly in the morning and evening based on their own conditions of constitution and their working habit, and can practise some more flexibly at the free hours. When one's qi activities inside the body are vigorous, his vital energy is replenished and he can realize that there is a kind of vital qi enveloping him or enveloping around him, he can begin to practice during the Zi, Wu, Mao and You periods, or during the period when he is most sensitive to qi or his qi activity is most vigorous, to achieve twice the result with half the effort.

A master qigong practitioner usually practises qigong exercises during the Zi, Wu, Mao and You periods when he has gained certain experiences. In the concrete, training of qi is performed during the Zi and Wu periods, and nourishing of qi (muyu) during the Mao and You periods. And because the Zi, Wu Mao and You periods represent the fluctuation of yin and yang in terms of its advance and retreat in winter, summer, spring and autumn respectively (there are one yang and five yin during the Zi period, one yin and five yang during the Wu period, four yang and two yin during the Mao period and four yin and two yang during the You period), the number and advance and retreat of yin and yang during the four periods are geometrically symmetric and balanced, which can keep the practitioner's yin and yang in equilibrium and is helpful to and ideal for the training of qi.

Because of the difference between people in physique, such as shaoyang physique, taiyang physique, shaoyin physique, taiyin physique and yin−yang− balanced physique, the time for practice should be determined according to one's own conditions and to the fluctuation of yin and yang in a whole day. Those with yang deficiency should do some practice during the six yang periods to replenish yang−qi; while those deficient in yin should practise more during the six yin periods to get the kidney−yin (kidney essence) sufficient, which in turn may facilitate the preservation of yang qi.

For a patient, the time for practice should be selected in line with the philosophy of yin, yang, the Five Elements, the time of circulation of qi and blood along the course of the channel as well as the severity of illness. For instance, the Hai and Zi periods are good for regulating the function of the kidney, the Yin and Mao periods for the liver, the Si and Wu periods for the heart, the Shen and You periods for the lung, the Zi period for the Gallbladder Channel, the Chou period for the Liver Channel, the Yin period for the Lung Channel, the Mao period for the Large Intestine Channel, and the Chen, Xu, Chou and Wei periods for the Spleen Channel.

The Direction for Training Qi

Su Wen — Ci Fa Lun (Plain Questions — On Acupuncture) states that " Those with lingering kidney disorder can face south during the Yin period quietly with no distractions". Because the Yin period pertains to the spring—wood and relates to the liver, training of qi during this period, i.e., "the early spring" period when the Shaoyang Channels are vigorous, will render the exuberant wood (liver) to control earth (spleen) to prevent earth from inter— restraining water (kidney), which "enables water (kidney) to develop and become healthy",just as the saying goes, "Kidney diseases heal in spring (Yin period)". On the other hand, the intrinsic qi is in the Lung Channel in the Yin period, and because the lung—metal can generate kidney—water, " the kidney deficiency can be cured by reinforcing its mother" (the kidney and the lung are in child—mother relationship). It is generally believed that practising qigong facing south and east is helpful to yang, while facing west and north helpful to yin.

The majority of qigong schools in ancient times attached emphasis on practice of qigong in certain directions. The reason for that is just because the directions——east, west, south and north, as well as the sun, moon and stars of the universe have direct influence on the human body.

Generally speaking, beginners may practise qigong facing east or southeast, or in the day time facing the sun and in the evening facing the moon. As the purpose of qigong practice is to train yang—qi inside the body to make genuine qi (pure yang—qi) accumulated and activated to link up with qi of the universe, the direction of yang (positive aspect) should be taken as the main direction for qigong practice so as to take qi from Heaven and Earth to nourish the human body. However, when one has practised qigong to a certain extent with his vital energy rendered sufficient, his qi circulation active and his perception to qi sensitive, he can choose the place and direction all by himself according to his own experiences and understandings. This will be more efficient. The method of direction selection is, when a proper place is determined, the practitioner may assume a suitable posture and get into "quiescence", a state in which he may feel qi clearly and his qi activity is vigorous, then try attentively to perceive at which direction, say east, west, south or north, his body is most stable and his qi is most active. This direction is therefore the optimal one for training qi. For example, the practitioner is standing or sitting facing south and feels that his body is enveloped with qi but he is being turned by a force toward southeast and can not stand or sit stably, then he can change his direction to southeast, and the like. The desired place and direction are those in which the practitioner can stand or sit as stable as Mount Taishan. Some beginners may feel no qi around though he may feel turning of the body. This is mostly caused by improper mind concentration and posturization, and the practitioner should correct it through regulation of mental activities and posture so that good effect can be attained rather than being misled by the suspicion that he himself has attained real perception of qi, lest qigong deviations occur.

Points for Attention in Training Qi

1. Have a good understanding of training qi and study carefully the essentials of it and adhere to its principles. Pay attention both to the teacher's instructions and to one's own initiatives. Be confident and do the exercises in sequence and step by step.

2. Once a method of practice is determined, one should be constant and persevere with it. Do not waste the time on changing the practice methods.

3. The frequency and duration of training—qi practice should be determined flexibly in line with the physique and health status of the individuals and their skill in qigong. It is advisable to increase the practice frequency and duration gradually.

4. It should be taken as a principle that the practitioner should choose a quiet environment with fresh air for practice. Better results can be achieved if the dynamic exercise is done in the open or in a place with flowers, grass and trees. Practice in the hot sun or against cold, strong wind and rain with thunders and lightening, or in a place near old, withered trees or near old graves should be avoided.

5. The training of qi should be combined with cultivation of one's moral character. *Qian Jin Yao Fang* (*Valuable Prescriptions*) written by Sun Simiao (Tang Dynasty, the middle of 7th century) says, "The way to keep in good health is to avoid long—time sole walking, standing, sitting, lying, looking and listening." and "He who is good at health preservation is who knows the twelve mottos or the twelve lesses——less thinking, longing, desire, meddling, talking, laughing, anxiety, amusement, joy, anger, readiness and wickedness". Practice under overfatigue, starvation and overeating should be avoided. The practitioner should keep a light heart and lead a regular life.

6. To be ready for the practice, go defecate, loose the

clothes and wear soft flat—sole shoes.

7. Adhere to the principle of the three steadiness——steady starting, steady performance and steady closing of the exercise.

8. Do not premeditate qigong effect, e.g., to force yourself to experience hot sensation in the lower abdomen or a certain sensation of qi. If qi effects occur during practice, do not try to identify it or to be overjoyed or frightened. Just let it take its own course.

9. Attention should be paid to avoid sudden panic. If one is suddenly frightened during exercise, one should not be panic—striken. The proper way is to find out the cause of the panic and to guide qi to its origin (the Lower Dantian), then continue or terminate the exercise.

Section Four   Static Qigong for Training Qi

The Three Regulations

1. Posture

Sitting, standing or lying posture may be selected for the training of qi. One may select the standing, upright sitting or the cross—legged sitting that is most suitable for him as the main posture and take the other postures as the supplementary ones so that he can take the advantage of any opportunities to practise.

2. Respiration

Antidromic abdominal respiration is mainly adopted. The beginners may practice natural and then orthodromic abdominal respiration at the first stage and, when used to it, shift to antidromic respiration. The purpose for such respiration training is to get the breath deep, long, fine and even. The training of respiration should be guided by consciousness at the beginning. After some practice, it can be done with neither negligence nor forcibility.

3. Mind Concentration

Setting the mind on the Lower Dantian is the main method of mental concentration in training qi in static qigong. The method is literally called "concentration on the qi point", which is practised to gain substantialness of qi in Dantian and to open "Zhou Tian" (the circule of qi) when one can guide qi to flow inside the body by consciousness on the requirements for training qi.

Methods of Practice of Static Qigong

1. Be in a proper posture, relax all over and get rid of distractions. Imagine that the turbid qi within the body is expelled through the mouth,nose and pores all over the body along with exhaling.After three times' exhaling,get the upper and lower teeth tapping each other 36 times, then move the tongue within the mouth and swallow the saliva three times, imagining that the clear qi of Heaven and Earth comes together with the saliva down to Dantian to nourish the whole body.

2. Regulate the breath to get it even and smooth, expel distractions, concentrate the mind on the Lower Dantian, close the mouth and focus the hearing to the Lower Dantian, and close the eyes gently to look inwardly at the Lower Dantian. All these should be carried out naturally and lively. Voluntary stop of respiration and rigid mind concentration should be avoided. While one should not forget qi, one should not speed up its circulation but simply follow it naturally as it progresses.

3. Training of qi should be combined with nourishing of qi. Conditions permit— ting, it is better to do qi training sometime in the period from 11:00 pm to 1:00 am (Zi period) and from 11:00 a.m. to 1:00 pm (Wu period). During the other periods, inner cultivation of qi should be mainly carried out. It goes without saying that in any episodes of training, neither of the two aspects (training qi and inner cultivation of qi) should be neglected. During the exercise, when one has entered "quiescence" by practising antidromic abdominal respiration and mind concentration on Dantian, the soft, even and fine breathing can be achieved.

4. This step can be called "qi generating in Dantian and circulating all over". After a certain period of practice, qi will be substantial in Dantian during exercise, and one may have a feeling of substantialness, warmth, or movement of qi cluster or other strange but comfortable feeling. This sensation of qi will become stronger and stronger as time goes by. When one has entered "quiescence", he may feel hot in Dantian and a stream of warm air (qi) rushing from Dantian towards the coccyx area, which makes him relaxed and comfortable all over. Sometimes the point Huiyin (Ren 1) will throb first. Under this circumstance, one should guide the genuine qi to circulate along the Du Channel towards the two qigong passes—— Jiajiguan (spine pass) and Yuzhenguan (occiput pass) and further, through Baihui (Du 20) and go along the Ren Channel down back to Dantian. In this aspect, the principle of "focusing attention merely when qi has not started to move and leading qi to circulate when it is about to move" should be adhered to. Then it is the time to guide the genuine qi to flow in the Ren and Du Channels, with mind concentration carried out in cooperation with breathing. Inhaling, conduct qi to flow along the Du Channel to the Upper Dantian; exhaling, conduct it down along the Ren Channel to the Lower Dantian. This is traditionally called "small circle of qi" (Xiao Zhou Tian). As the time passes, qi gathered in Dantian will not disperse; it will circulate naturally along the Ren and Du Channels without the guidance by will and the help of breathing.

5. Carry out the closing process seriously after each exercise session. This is the skill with which one may shift the attention slowly off the point he has been concentrating on, lead qi to the Lower Dantian, relax all over, open the eyes slowly, and do some self-massage.

Self-massage include rubbing the hands, bathing the face (rubbing the face with the palms), combing the hair with the fingertips and dredging the Twelve Regular Channels. Rub from the chest to the hands to dredge the Three Yang Channels of Hand, and from the hands, the shoulders and the lateral sides of the head down to the chest and abdomen to dredge the Three Yin Channels of Hand. Rub from the waist and hips to the feet to dredge the Three Yang Channels of Foot, from the feet to the abdomen to dredge the Three Yin Channels of Foot. The above procedures should be performed 7 times each followed by limbering oneself up to end the exercise.

Section Five   Dynamic Exercise for Training Qi

The Twelve–Form Sinew–Transforming Exercise (Yijin Jing)

Sinew–transforming exercise (Yijin Jing) is one of the set of dynamic qigong exercises. Here it is taken as the foundamental exercise for guiding and emitting qi in outgoing–qi therapy. Literally, "yi" means "transform", "jin" means "sinew" and "jing" means " method". As the term implies, "sinew– transforming exercise" is the method to train the tendons and muscles. The exercise is designed according to the course and the characteristics of qi circulation in the Twelve Regular Channels and the Du and Ren Channels. It has been passed from generation to generation without recession at any times. Qigong emphasizes coordinative practice of dynamic exercise and static exercise so that qi activities of the channels and the extremities can be kept smooth. During practice of sinew–transforming exercise, qi and blood usually circulates appropriately with proper speed and no sluggishness or stagnation. The exercise is a highly salubrious one of its kind.

1. Form One   Wei Duo Presenting the Pestle

Pithy Formula

Keep erect when standing,

Hold the hands before the chest as if praying.

Set the breath even and keep the mind calm,

With the heart clear, soft and warm.

Posture and Essentials

First, step out with the left foot to set the feet apart at shoulder—width, hands hanging naturally, head and neck upright, eyes slightly open and looking straight ahead, tongue stuck against the palate, shoulders relaxed with elbows dropping, chest drawn in and back straightened, abdomen contracted and buttocks relaxed, knees at ease and slightly bent, and feet set steadily on the ground. Relax all over.

Second, turn hands into yin palms (palms facing the ground) and lift them slowly to shoulder—level. Turn hands into yin—yang palms (palms facing each other) and draw them towards each other and close them before the chest. Bend the elbows slowly to get the fingertips pointing upward, the point Shaoshang (Lu 11) on the two thumbs touching each other gently. Relax the shoulders and drop the elbows (Fig. 4—10).

Respiration and Mind Concentration

Take natural respiration when performing the first step, with the mind clear and calm and concentrated. Take abdominal respiration during the second step, with qi guided down to Dantian. When you feel the flow of qi, have your mind follow the flow of qi and, during inhaling, guide qi to flow out of the fingertips, enter the nostrils and go down to Dantian. During ex-

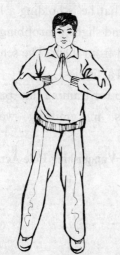

Fig. 4—10 Wei Duo

Presenting the Pestle

—181—

haling, guide qi from Dantian to the chest and then to the palms along the Three Yin Channels of Hand to fill the fingertips. Do the exercise for 6 or 12 respiratory cycles.

Eff ect

The Lung Channel of Hand—Taiyin is 3 chi and 5 cun (about 117 cm) long, along which qi circulates from the chest to the hand. The qi activities induced during the practice of this form can be felt most apparently in this channel, then it diffuses gradually to the Channels of Hand—Jueyin and Hand—Shaoyin. At the first stage of practice, the practitioner may have a slightly tingling sensation along the medial side of the arm, and an itching and worm—crawling one along the external side, indicating that qi has been activated. After long term practice, the effect that the lung governs qi, connects all the vessels and can spread qi to various parts of the body can be realized. The practitioner may feel that he is holding a hot inflated ball, his ten fingers distending and slightly throbbing as if something thready was being released from them. The sensation is usually accompanied with mental activities.

This form is the foundamental step for training flat—palm pushing and pulling manipulations in emitting waiqi (outgoing—qi).

2. Form Two   Carrying A Monster—Vanquishing Pole Across on the Shoulders

Pithy Formula

Stand on tiptoe upright,

Stretch the two arms wide,

Set the mind quiet,

    the breath even,

And the eyes and mouth widely open
   as if stunned.

Posture and Essentials

Proceed from the last stance. Turn both palms slowly into yin palms (palms facing the ground) and move them sideways respectively to form a straight parallel line. Simultaneously, lift the heels slightly to stand on tiptoe (when skilled one may touch the ground with only the big toes). Concentrate the mind and look fixedly ahead, with the chest drawn in and the back straightened, abdomen contracted and buttocks relaxed, and tongue stuck against the palate (Fig. 4–11). Do it for 9 or 18 respiratory cycles.

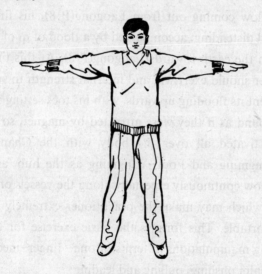

Fig. 4–11   Carrying a Monster–Vanquishing
Pole Across on the Shoulders

Respiration and Mind Concentration

Breathe naturally, concentrate the mind on Laogong (P 8)

—183—

and on the toes. Turn natural respiration into abdominal when one gets familiar with the exercise; concentrate the mind on Laogong (P 8) when inhaling, and when exhaling, guide qi along the Channel of Hand—Yangming to the Channel of Foot—Yangming then to the big toes, on which the mind is then concentrated.

Effect

The Large Intestine Channel of Hand—Yangming originates from the head. It is identical with the Stomach Channel of Foot—Yangming in the nature of qi. At the beginning of practice, the practitioner may feel heaviness in the two shoulders and hotness in the palms. When he is well versed he may feel a qi flow coming out from Laogong(P 8), his fingertips itching and distending, accompanied by a flood of qi of yin—essence from the earth towards Laogong(P 8). At this time, the practitioner should exert will and internal strength to suppress qi to prevent its flooding upwards, with his toes setting steadily on the ground as if they were attracted by magnet, so that qi can be activated all over the body with the Channels of Hand—Yangming and Foot—Yangming as the hub, and rendered to flow continously especially along the vessels of the extremities, which may make the practitioner extremely ralaxed and comfortable. This form is the basic exercise for training qi—emitting manipulations in terms of one— finger—meditation and flat—palm pushing, pulling and leading.

3. Form Three Holding the Heavenly Gate with the Palms

Pithy Formula

Hold the heavenly gate with the palms and look inwardly up,

Stand on front sole and upright.
The whole body is planted as a sturdy pine,
And the teeth are clentched tight.
Saliva gushes as the tongue is pressed against the palate,
With nasal breathing the mind is set quiet.
As the two fists are slowly lowered,
Strength is exerted as if pulling a heavy weight.

Posture and Essentials

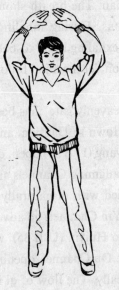

Fig. 4–12   Holding the Heavenly
Gate with Hands

Proceed from the last stance. Raise the hands (in yin palms) slowly from their respective side in an arch till they are above the head. Turn the yin palms into yang (palms facing upwards),with fingers of the two hands pointing each other and the back of the hands toward Tianmen (2 cun above the front hairine), as if holding the heavenly gate. Lift the heels simultaneously to stand on tiptoe, the heels inclining slightly outwards to set the "Yinqiao Storehouse" (the point Huiyin, Ren 1) closed, at the same time set the point Huiyang (UB 35, 5 fen lateral to the coccyx, a point of the Urinary Bladder Channel) open. Clench the teeth and rest the tongue against the palate. Apply inward–vision to stare through Tianmen (Heavenly Gate) at the space between the two hands (Fig. 4—12). The procedure may last for 14 or 28 respiratory cycles.

Make fists, the arms falling slowly along the original arc until they are in the stance "Carrying a Monster—vanquishing Pole Across on the Shoulders".

Respiration and Mind Concentration

Take nasal inhaling and oral exhaling first. When the posture of the form is assumed, turn both inhaling and exhaling into nasal and guide qi down to Dantian. The breath should be fine, even, long, slow and continuous. During inhaling, the mind is set on Dantian and, during exhaling,lifted to between the two palms. When qi is in circulation, let the mind follow qi.

Effect

After the posture "holding the heavenly gate" has been assumed with the breath even, qi sent down to Dantian, and the point Huiyin (Ren 1) closed and Huiyang (U B 35) open, qi will be activated along and around the Yangming Channels and all the qi vessels of the body will be filled with qi naturally. The practitioner may feel qi of the Three Yin Channels go adversely up along the Three Yang Channels to Huiyin (U B 35), where it continues to flow upward along the Du Channel, opening up Sanguan (the three passes) automatically. The flow of qi is felt most apparently when it goes along the Stomach Channel, the Liver Channel, the Gallbladder Channel and the Large Intestine Channel. Sometimes qi is still active and in circulation after exercise. When staring at Tianmen (Extra), the beginners of the exercise may feel a force of attraction between the two palms while the experienced may feel that there is white cloud floating between the two palms, a lingering charm that gives one an extremely graceful feeling. When the teeth are clenched, quivering of the root of the ears may occur and the quivering will spread to the temples. The mouth will be full of saliva which should be swallowed and sent mentally down to Dantian.

This form is essential for exerting "internal strength" and guiding qi in emission of qi with manipulations with pushing, pulling and leading and hand gestures of one—finger—meditation, flat—palm and sword—fingers.

4. Form Four   Plucking and Resetting the Stars

Pithy Formula

Over the head hold the sky with one palm,

Stare at Inner Laogong in calm.

Inhale by nose and exhale by mouth,

Attentively   shift   the
eyesight to another palm.

Posture and Essentials

Proceed   from   the   last
stance. Lift the right hand slowly
in an arc to about one fist off the
forehead. Lower the left hand
simultaneously and rest the back
of it on the left side of the small
of the back (Yaoyan, Extra).
Concentrate the sight on Inner
Laogong (P 8) of the right palm
(Fig. 4—13).

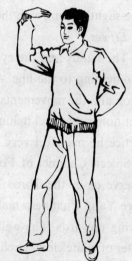

Fig. 4—13 Plucking and
Resetting the Stars

Lift the left hand to about
one fist off the forehead and lower the right one and rest its

back on the right side of the small of the back. Concentrate the sight inwardly on Laogong (P 8) of the left palm. Exchange hands and do the same. Practise for 11 or 22 respiratory cycles.

Respiration and Mind Concentration

Take nasal inhaling and mouth exhaling and make the breathing even. While concentrating the mind on Laogong (P 8) of the raised hand, make the Inner Laogong (P 8) of the raised hand, the two eyes and the Outer Laogong (P 8) at the back of another hand linear, and as one exhales and inhales, the point Yaoyan (Extra, the small of the back) will fluctuates. Concentrate the attention on the Inner Laogong (P 8) of the raised hand when exhaling and on the Outer Laogong (P 8) of the lower hand when inhaling. The mind, the Inner Laogong (P 8), the eyes and Yaoyan (Extra, the small of the back) should move slightly along with the fluctuation.

Eff ect

The hands and the eyes are linear as if they are attracted by something to the line. Along with breathing, mind concentration and the movements of the eyes and Yaoyan (Extra), the practitioner may feel itching of the eyes at first, but after some practice he may feel very comfortable. This form emphasizes the Spleen Channel of Foot—Taiyin. It may help collect and preserve qi of the Three Yin Channels and convey it to the Three Yang Channels, making qi in the Three Yang Channels flowing upwards. The well versed practitioner may perceive a cluster of white cloud circling around Laogong (P 8).

The form is foundamental for training qi—emitting manipulations of pushing, pulling and leading with spreading—claw, dragon—mouth and flat—palm hand gestures.

5. Form Five   Pulling Nine Oxen by Tails

Pithy Formula

The front leg is a bow and the back an arrow;

The lower abdomen is filled with qi as if hollow.

The strength is directed to the two arms,

As if seizing something with the palms,

And the eyes look inwardly at the hand they follow.

Posture and Essentials

Proceed from the last stance. Take the right hand off the right Yaoyan (Extra), drop it slightly, turn it naturally into yin palm and thrust it forward until it is up to shoulder level. Then bring the fingers together to form a spreading—claw gesture with the wrist bent a little, the fingers pointing inwardly to the right and the strength focused on the inner side of the wrist. Along with the above movements, the right leg takes a big step forward and bends, the left leg stretches straight to form a forward lunge (the front leg is like a bow and the back an arrow as in martiar arts or gymnastics).At the same time, drop the left hand and thrust it backwards to the left with the fingers close to each other, the tips pointing upwards and outwards and the wrist and arms bent a little. The right hand is held at the level of the forehead, and the left completes an angle of 15 degrees with the straightened left leg (Fig. 4—14).

Change the last stance, getting the left leg bent, the right straight and the left hand up and the right down in ´the same way as required in the first procedure. Perform each procedure 6 or 12 respiratory cycles.

Respiration and Mind Concentration

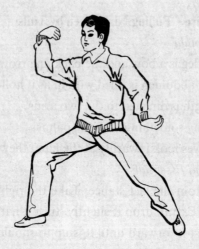

Fig. 4—14 Pulling Nine Oxen by the Tails

This form needs also nasal inhaling and mouth exhaling. Imagine that your hands are in a line as if pulling the tail of an ox. When inhaling, look at the front hand with inward—vision and pull it; when exhaling, look at the hand with inward—vision and lean the body forward a little as if to seize the tail, The forward and backward movement of the body should be in coordination with the fluctuation of qi in Dantian at the lower abdomen. The legs, waist, back, shoulders and the elbows, too, move or vibrate correspondingly with the forward—seizing and backward—pulling movement.

6. Form Six　Stretching Paws and Spreading Wings

Pithy Formula

Stand erect and stare glaringly,

Push the window open to look at the moon steadily.

Topple the mountain and return the tide,

With respiration in guide,

And do it seven rounds straightly.

Posture and Essentials

Proceed from the last stance. Take the advantage of the "backward—pulling", get the bent leg back to stand with heels closed. Draw back the hands and hold them at the hypochondria, fingers straight upward and palms facing the front, to form "mountain—toppling palms".

Then push the "mountain—toppling palms" slowly forward.The forward pushing is very gentle as if pushing a window open. Stop the pushing when the shoulders, elbows and wrists are at the same level, then separate the fingers forcefully, keep the body straight, hold the breath, open the eyes widely, look straight ahead without any movement of the eyeballs or even a blink, and concentrate the mind on the palms (Fig. 4—15).

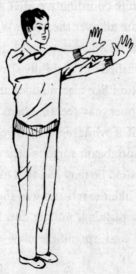

Fig. 4—15 Stretching Paws and Spreading Wings

Finally draw the "mountain—toppling palms" back slowly until they touch the hypochondria. Do the pushing and withdrawing for 9 or 18 respiratory cycles.

Respiration and Mind Concentration

Take nasal inhaling and mouth exhaling. Exhale when pushing gently forward, but hold breath somewhat when the arms are straight and begin to push with force to stretch the arms as much as possible as if gathering all the strength to topple a mountain. Exhale when drawing the palms back. Concentrate the attention on the two palms.

Effect

This form is designed mainly for training qi of the Channels of Hand—Taiyang and Foot—Taiyang. When respiration and movements are quite coordinative after a certain period of practice, qi will circulate all over the body. With the help of the movements and breathing, the palms and fingers are full of energy. When they are pushed out and fully stretched, the practitioner can get a sensation like electric discharge at Laogong (P 8). The versed practitioner may feel that he is enjoying the sight of a bright moon as if a white light revolves around the two palms or the bright moonbeam spreads all over the sky. When the hands are drawn back, he may feel that qi is returning from the palms to the body like the returning of the tide. The form is important for training pushing, pulling and leading manipulations with flat—palm and spreading—claw hand gestures in outgoing—qi therapy.

7. Form Seven Nine Ghosts Pulling Out Sabres

Pithy Formula

Turn the head and bend the elbow,

Hold the head and pull the ear,
Keep the right armpit open and the left closed,
Vibrate Kunlun with the right hand,
And touch the interscapular region with the left.

Change hands and repeat the same with the body
stretched and erect.

Posture and Essentials

Proceed from the last stance.
Stretch the arms sideways with the
palms downwards. Raise the right
arm towards the back of the head
and apply the palm to
Yuzhenguan(the occiput pass).
Press and pull the tip of the left ear
(point Tiancheng, G B 9) with the
index, middle and ring fingers, and
keep the shoulder and the elbow
parallel and the right armpit open.
The left hand draws the half circle

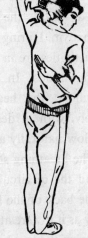

Fig. 4—16   Nine Ghosts
Pulling Out Sabres

leftwards until the back of the palm touches the interscapular
region. Keep the left armpit closed tightly (Fig. 4—16).

Then stretch the arms sideways again. Exchange the
movements of the hands and do the same procedure mentioned
above. Perform the two procedures alternately for 14 or 28
respiratory cycles.

Respiration and Mind Concentration

This form needs nasal inhaling and mouth exhaling. When
inhaling, concentrate on the tip of the lifted elbow, which is
pulled upward a little, and move the head and neck in

coordination with the manipulation of the hand. When exhaling, concentrate on the Outer Laogong (P 8) of the hand set at the interscapular area, and move qi down to Dantian.

Effect

The practice of this form activates qi of the Channels of Hand—Taiyang and Foot—Taiyang to make the two channels connected with the channels of Hand—Shaoyin and Foot—Shaoyin. During practice, the posture, breathing and the mental activities are in perfect harmony and the circulation of qi is continuous. In cooperation with breathing and the hand—pulling, the head and the elbows tense and relax alternately, with qi descending slowly down to Dantian. Qi should flow naturally and should not be guided to go up and down. The breathing should be gentle, the body should be relaxed and the qi circulation should be particularly slow and deep. The back of the hand is rested on the back of the body naturally as if it were attracted by the back, and it is as ifthat is a line joining the two hands through the ear. The form is essential for training pushing, pulling and leading manipulations with one— finger—meditation, sword—fingers and flat—palm hand gestures.

8. Form Eight   Three Dishes Falling to the Ground

Pithy Formula

The tongue is rested on the hard palate,

The eyes are open and the teeth gnashed,

The legs are bent in a horse stance,

And the hands are pressing and holding;

The palms are turned and raised upwards,

As if a great amount of weight is added;

With oral exhaling and nasal inhaling,

The feet are set firm and the body straight.

Posture and Essentials

Proceed from the last stance. Raise and stretch out the arms to both sides to form a straight line at shoulder level, with the palms facing floor. At the same time, the left foot takes a big step to the left to keep about 0.7–1.7m between the two feet (the distance can be altered according to the height of the individual practitioners).

Then bend the knees and squat down slowly to form a horse stance, with the chest drawn in, the back straightened, the angle between the thigh and shank being 90 degrees. Simultaneously, press the two yin palms downwards until they are at the knee level. The movement should be slow, and the strength exerted steadily, with tongue pressed against the palate and eyes wide open (Fig. 4–17).

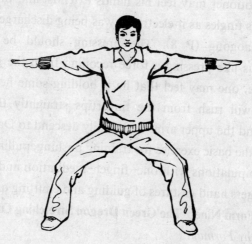

Fig. 4–17   Three Dishes Falling to the Ground

Finally turn palms up into yang palms. Picturing holding

something, move the palms upwards along the straightening movement of the legs until they are at chest level. Do the exercise for 3 − 5 respiratory cycles repeatedly at the first stage of practice, and up to 11 when one is experienced.

Respiration and Mind Concentration

Exhale by mouth when squatting down and let qi down to Dantian. Concentrate the mind on the two palms as if pressing an elastic thing. Inhale by nose at rise and concentrate the mind also on the palms as if holding a heavy thing.

Effect

During the practice of this form with yin and yang corresponding with each other, qi will move in endless circles along the Channels of Hand−Shaoyin, Foot− Shaoyin, HandTaiyang and Foot−Taiyang. When the hands are pressed downwards, the practitioner may feel his hands extends, and the centre of his palms tingles as if electricity was being discharged from the point Laogong (P 8). The pressing should be slow and continous like pressing a force recoiling from the ground. At this time, one may feel that he is holding some heavy things, and qi will rush from the fingertips straightly through the palms and the upper arms and finally descend to Dantian. This form is the basic exercise for training pushing, pulling and leading manipulations with one−finger−meditation and five−thunder−fingers hand gestures of guiding and emitting qi.

9. Form Nine   The Green Dragon Stretching Out Paws

Pithy Formula

The green dragon stretches its paws,

  With the left one following the right.

The paws roll and tumble along the hypochondrium,

The right braves the wind forward,
And the left "cloud gate" is exposed.
Qi is fixed in the shoulders and back,
And the waist and abdomen twist.
While uttering "xu" gently,
The breath is regulated
And the movements of dragon and tiger are imitated.

Posture and Essentials

Proceed from the last stance. Withdraw the left foot back to stand with feet shoulder—width apart. Turn the left palm to face floor to form a "dragon paw" (the joints of the fingers bent, the centre of the palm "empty" and round). By force of the waist, draw the left hand backwards with the elbow tip in the lead; at the same time turn the right palm to face floor and into "dragon paw". Take advantage of the backward drawing of the left hand, stretch the right hand leftwards as if to brave the wind and the wave, to open left the Qimen (Liv 14) and Yunmen (Lu 4) points and close the right ones closed. As the left hand draws and the right stretches, turn the waist and abdomen correspondingly and relax them as much as possible, by which the Dai Channel (Belt Channel) can be trained to be as flexible as silk and its tightness moderate (Fig.4—18).

Then withdraw the right hand and stretch the left rightwards in the same way mentioned above. Whichever hand is being stretched forward, one should utter "xu" in cooperation and should turn the head and neck along with the movements of the hands. Do the exercise for 6 or 12 respiratory cycles.

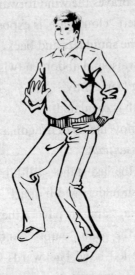

Fig. 4–18 The Green Dragon Stretching Out Paws

Respiration and Mind Concentration

The exercise needs nasal inhaling and mouth exhaling . Inhale during the process of withdrawing the left hand and stretching the right and vice versa and send qi slowly down to Dantian; exhale when the withdrawing and stretching are done to the utmost, while uttering "xu", scratching gently for once with the third segments of the ten fingers and concentrating the mind on the two palms.

Effect

This form is for training qi in Sanjiao (three warmers). Qi activities are most sensible in the Lung Channel, Gallbladder Channel, Liver Channel and Dai Channel (Belt Channel). Qi falls down into Dantian during inhaling, and during exhaling when "xu" is uttered and the scratching movements are carried out, the practitioner may feel that qi rises vividly to his palms, giving the point Laogong (P 8) and the fingertips an electricity—discharging sensation. One may feel that all his channels are governed by the Dai Channel, and the waist and abdomen are circled by something as soft as silk. This kind of feeling is beyond description but can be perceived automatically through long—term practice.

The form is essential for training, guiding and emitting qi with pushing, pulling, rotating and leading manipulations and spread—claw and flat—palm hand gestures.

10. Form Ten   The Hungery Tiger Pouncing on Its Prey

Pithy Formula

Squat with feet apart to incline forward,

Make the right leg an arrow and the left a bow.

Hold up the head and chest to prostrate forward,

Raise the hips towards the sky up and down.

Inhale and exhale the breath is evenly regulated,

Touch the ground by fingertips in support.

Lower the waist and back to flutuate,

And withdraw the legs to resume upright standing.

Posture and Essentials

Proceeding from the last stance. Shift the body weight to the right leg, lean the left knee against the right and place the arms sideways. Make a step forward to the left with the left leg to make a forward lunge. Simultaneously stretch the hands forward to set the fingers on the ground, with the palms suspended (beginners may set the palms on the ground instead) and head raised slightly [Fig. 4—19(1)].

Withdraw the left foot and rest its back against the right heel [Fig.4—19(2)]. Do a push—up first and then lower the body and withdraw the buttocks slowly, with the eyes looking straight ahead, the waist relaxed and the arms stretched like a tiger ready to pounce on its prey [Fig. 4—19(3)].

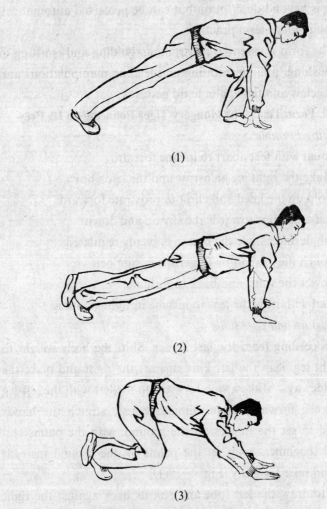

(1)

(2)

(3)

Fig. 4—19 The Hungery Tiger Pouncing on Its Prey

Hold up the head, prostrate the chest to about 4 cun from the ground and get the head, waist, buttocks and extremities moving forward up and down like waves. Assuming a tiger ready to pounce on its prey, get the two eyes looking ahead. Throw out the chest a little when the arms are straight and withdraw it when the arms are bent. Do this repeatedly 8 or 16 times (beginners may do it 1 − 3 times) and return to the left forward lunge.

Draw the right foot back to stand upright. The left foot takes a step forward to the left to make a left forward lunge. Do right the same mentioned above. Return to the posture of the left forward lunge and then to the standing posture with feet shoulder−width apart.

Respiration and Mind Concentration

The exercise requires nasal inhaling and mouth exhaling . When the two palms are rested on the floor in a forward lunge, regulate the breath evenly When doing the push−up, inhale when the body is raised and exhale when it is lowered. And inhale when withdrawing the body and contracting the abdomen with eyes looking forward as if going to pounce on something. Qi is sent along the Ren Channel down to Dantian. Exhale when the body is sent forward to get qi to rise along the Du Channel.

Effect

This form is, in a low position of the body, to facilitate q circulation along the Ren and Du Channels as well as the Twelve Regular Channels. Long−term practice of it may result in maximum activation of qi in all the channels and collaterals, or in other words, a climax of qi circulation that should be acquired in the practice of Sinew—transforming Exerccise. At this stage, the practitioner may firstly feel qi in Dantian substantial and the back and shoulders hot. Then he may feel qi circulating all over the body. Following various movements and the inhaling and exhaling, qi circulates with Ren and Du Channels as the hub throughout the whole body, making the practitioner sweat slightly and feel indescribably comfortable and relaxed.

This form is very important for training the skill of pushing, pulling, rotating and leading manipulations needed in flat—palm, spreading—claw, one— finger—meditation, dragon— mouth and sword—fingers hand gestures.

11. Form Eleven　Bending the Waist and Striking the Drum

Pithy Formula

Hold the hind head with the palms and bend the waist low,

Bring the head between the legs with teeth clenched and mouth closed;

Rest the tongue gently on the palate and bend the elbows,

Cover the ears to strike the heavenly drums,

As if an orchestra plays the eight tones.

Posture and Essentials

First, proceed from the last stance. Stand upright with feet apart as wide as the shoulders.

Second, clasp the head with both hands,palms covering the ears,the two middle fingers against Yuzhenguan (occiput pass) with the tips touching each other gently. The elbows are bent and raised to shoulder level [Fig.4—20(1)]. Strike with the two middle fingers on Yuzhenguan repeatedly to give rub—a—dub in the ears. This is called " striking the heavenly drum".

Then, after striking, with hands still holding the head, bend slowly down as much as possible to get the head between the legs, with the legs straightened, the waist and buttocks relaxed, the tongue rested on the palate and the teeth clenched. Take a view of the horizon for a moment through the interspace between the legs [Fig. 4−20(2)].

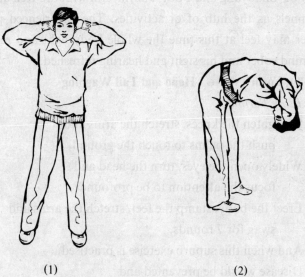

(1)　　　　　　　　　　　(2)

Fig. 4−20 Bending the Waist and Striking the Drum

Finally, rise to get the body upright and beat the "heavenlydrum" again. Do this 14 times. Then return to the upright standing posture.

Respiration and Mind Concentration

Do nasal respiration during the exercise. Hold breath slightly when bending down and rising (the breath can be held completely on rising after a certain period of practice). Concentrate the mind on Dantian when bending down and on the two palms when rising.

Eff ect

This form is the transition to the ending of the whole series of Sinewtransforming Exercise. So far qi has circulated all through the Fourteen Channels (the Twelve Regular Channels plus the Ren and Du Channels) and finally runs to the channels of Foot—Shaoyang and Foot—Jueyin, still with the Ren and Du Channels as the hub of qi activities. The experienced practitioner may feel at this time the whole body light and relaxed, his mind sober and his sight and hearing refreshed.

14. Form Twelve   Head and Tail Wagging

Pithy Formula

Straighten the knees, stretch the arms and
    push the palms to touch the ground,
Widely open the eyes, turn the head and
    focus the attention to be profound,
Erect the body, stamp the feet, stretch the arms and
    swag for 7 rounds,
And when this supurb exercise is practised,
Disease would be prevented and
    life would be prolonged.

Posture and Essentials

Proceed from the last stance. Push the hands forward from the back of the head. Keep the arms stretched at shoulder level.

Then cross the ten fingers with palms facing floor. Withdraw the palms slowly towards the chest until they are two fists away from the chest, then push them downwards till the palms reach the floor, with legs straightened. Push towards the middle, the left and the right once each, with the head nodding accordingly (Fig. 4—21).

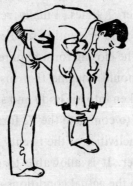

Fig. 4—21 Head and Tail Wagging

Finally straighten the waist slowly to lift the palms. Let go the crossed fingers.

Respiration and Mind Concentration

Do natural respiration during practice. Keep the mind on the centre of the palms while pushing the palms to the ground, and on the tip of the nose while standing straight.

Effect

This is the last and ending step of Sinew—transforming Exercise. The methods of it seem simple, however, it can regulate qi activities of the total of twenty channels of the body. The practitioner may feel extremely relaxed and comfortable after practice.

15. The Closing Form

Proceeding from the last stance, push the hands (palms facing each other) forward and lift the heels slightly to stand on sole. When the arms are straight, abduct the palms slowly and then separate the arms to draw an arch toward the armpit. Set the palms upwards, fall the heels simultaneously and lift the toes. Then push the hands forward again to repeat the procedures for altogether 7 times. Finally resume the posture in Form One——Wei Duo Presenting the Pestle, to end the whole series of exercise. The closing form requires natural respiration. The practitioner should imagine that his qi is now separated from nature and taken into his body and stored in Dantian.

It is advisable to complete the 12 forms step by step in sequence to keep qi activities of the twenty channels of the body coordinated all over. It is allowable to select one or several forms, according to the actual conditions of the individuals, for practice. If the whole series are practised successively, the beginners of the exercise may perform 3 − 7 respiratory cycles (times) for each form and increase the times gradually to the number required.

Double—Nine Yang Exercise

This exercise is often practised on the basis of Sinew—transforming Exercise. The practitioner shakes his body in a spring vibration (like a pile being struck down) in a certain posture and with proper breathing and mind concentration to make qi in Dantian rippling and get it to circulate throughout the body. The exercise is to build up the physique and to activate the vitality of qi. It is the foundamental skill for outgoing—qi therapy with vibrating, quivering and fixing manipulations and other qi guiding and emitting methods.

1. Preparatory Methods
(1) Basic Posture

Take a standing–vibrating posture.

Stand relaxed and quiet, with feet apart as wide as shoulders, toes clutching at the ground, hands falling naturally, head picturing supporting an object on its top, eyes looking straight ahead but seeing nothing, tongue stuck against the palate, chest slightly out, buttocks slightly in, knees relaxed and bent somewhat, mind concentrated, and breath natural.

After adjustment of the posture, expel the turbid qi three times along with exhaling as done in static qigong. Then bend and stretch the knees alternately to cause Dantian and even the whole body to quiver and vibrate. The amplitude of vibration may be too large and unnatural at first. After some practice, however, the vibration will become easy and will converge towards Dantian, and eventually, occur with Dantian as the centre. With Dantian vibrating, qi will diffuse rhythmically throughout the whole body.

(2) Massaging the Dai Channel

Proceed from the last stance. Put the palms on the Dai Channel and massage it in cooperation with antidromic abdominal respiration. During inhaling, take advantage of the vibrating force to push qi of the Dai Channel with the palms (the right is preceded by the left) to flow leftwards, mind following palms to try to sense qi, with the

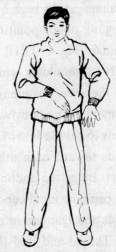

Fig. 4–22 Softening the
Dai Channel

—207—

eyes slightly closed to get inward-vision on the Dai Channel (Fig. 4-22). During exhaling, push qi of the Dai Channel rightwards with the left palm preceded by the right in the same way mentioned above. Repeat the sequence for 9 respiratory cycles. Carry out the same but with palms rightwards when inhaling and leftwards when exhaling for another 9 respiratory cycles.

Breathing, posture and mind concentration should be well coordinated during practice. The waist should be relaxed at the utmost. Turn the waist in small amplitude along with hand manipulations. One may feel the waist as soft as silk, the Dai Channel warm, qi flowing round the waist and circulating freely and vigorously all over the body.

(3) Opening and Closing of the Three Dantian

Take the standing pile-driving vibrating posture. When inhaling, get the back of the palms facing each other (the Outer Laogong points pointing at each other) in front of the Lower Dantian [Fig. 4-23(1)]. Move the hands sidewards to get them apart at shoulders width. Meanwhile contract the abdomen and the anus, imagining that Dantian is open and voluminous qi enters the body by way of Dantian. When exhaling, turn the palms to get the Inner Laogong (P 8) facing Dantian. Draw the hands toward each other [Fig. 4-23(2)] till they are one fist apart. Bulge the abdomen and relax the anus simultaneously, and combine mind concentration, the vibrating movement, the hands and Dantian in one. Gather the qi that has been sensed into Datian and lead the qi breathed in from the mouth and nose down to Dantian too. Repeat the above process for 9 respiratory cycles.

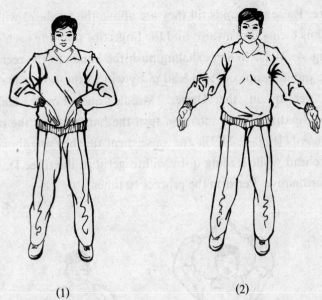

(1)   (2)

Fig. 4–23 Opening and Closing the Three Dantian

Next, move the hands up to the level of the Middle Dantian (around Shanzhong, Ren 17) and do the same hand movements for 9 respiratory cycles, lifting qi to the Middle Dantian while inhaling and sending the genuine qi down to the Lower Dantian while exhaling.

The next step is to open and close the Upper Dantian. Move the hands up to the Upper Dantian (around Yintang, Extra 1) and do the same hand movements for 9 respiratory cycles. However, qi may only be lifted up to the Middle Dantian at the first stage of practice. It can be conducted to the Upper Dantian gradually as the practice is carried on for a longer period of time. Guide qi down to the Lower Dantian during exhaling.

Continue to do the exercise in a standing–vibrating posture. Raise the hands till they are above the forehead with the palms facing downwards and the fingertips pointing each other [Fig. 4—24(1)]. When exhaling push the hands to the region of the pubic symphysis and lead qi by will to the Lower Dantian to get qi in the Upper, Middle and Lower Dantian coordinative. When inhaling, turn the hands to get the palms upwards [Fig. 4—24(2)], and raise them till they are above the forehead while leading qi by will to get it in the three Dantian coordinative. Perform the process 10 times.

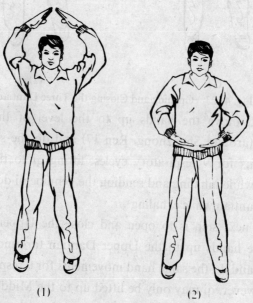

(1)   (2)

Fig. 4—24 Opening Through the Three Dantian

NOTE: The preparatory methods (massaging the Dai Channel and opening and closing the three Dantian) should be practised 55 times in order to mactch with the number of yin and yang of the universe (Heaven and Earth or Qian and Kun).

Qi activities is vigorous throughout the body, fills the three Dantian, and further is made mixed with qi of the universe. Qi inside and outside the body interflows and resonates continuously, making Heaven, Earth and the body a whole to lay solid foundation for training qi and guiding the vibrating qi to the palms and fingertips in various postures. To this stage, qi (vital energy) and strength (force) can be coincident with each other when other exercises are practised, and the practitioner can guide qi by will and facilitate strength with qi at high proficiency.

2. Posture Training

Posture training is done on the basis of practice of the preparatory methods. Qi is made vibrating with Dantian as the centre and circulating along with the vibration, controlled by will. Posture training needs also the standing vibrating posture as its basis, but one must combine the vibrating and the changing of posture in one to get qi to flow following the changes of the posture.

(1)Form One   The Immortals Pointing Out the Way

First,contract the abdomen and anus during inhaling and lift qi from the Lower Dantian up to the Middle Dantian, the two hands moving upwards simultaneously, palms facing upwards and elbows bent backward , to the sides of the waist.

Second, exhaling, gather the genuine qi into Dantian and, with it vibrating in Dantian, guide it by will and in turn get will following it to spread it to the right upper arm, with the four fingers of the hand close together,the thumb stretched, and the joint of the wrist bent up a little. By guiding qi, direct internal strength to the arm, push the hand (palm erect) forward, and gather strength in the thenar eminence minor of the hand (Fig. 4–25).

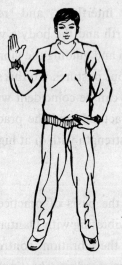

Fig. 4–25   The Immortals
Pointing Out the Way

Finally, inhaling, make fist and draw it back to the chest. Turn fist into palm facing downwards and press down. Turn the left palm up and lift it to hold qi up to the Middle Dantian. Exhaling, push the left hand forward in the same method as described for the right hand. Repeat the process for 9 respiratory cycles for each hand.Finally place the hands back in front of the chest and hold qi up to the Middle Dantian. Then get the palms facing each other to get prepared for the next step.

NOTE: This form is used to train qi of the Shaoyin, Taiyang, Taiyin and Shaoyang Channels. During exhaling, by means of the strength produced by arm–pushing, guide qi in the Middle Dantian, which has been lifted from the Lower, to flow to the arms, the thenar eminence minor and the small finger, and to flow along the Shaoyang and Taiyang Channels. During inhaling,return qi to the Middle Dantian along the Taiyin and Yangming Channels to join with qi rising from the Lower Dantian. Qi flows rhythmically along with the vibration of Dantian and the whole body, coming out from the Lower

Dantian continuously and going back into it continuously like a chain of rolling pearls. This form is basic for emission of qi with pushing, pulling and leading manipulations.

(2) Form Two   Pushing Eight Horses Forward

Proceed from the last stance. Exhaling, direct qi to the Middle Dantian and then to the shoulders and arms. With the two palms facing each other, the thumbs stretched and the four fingers of each hand close to each other, push the hands out slowly till the elbows, palms and shoulders are at the same level. Bend the thumbs backwards hard and lower the palms with strength to make qi fill the tips of the four fingers of both hands [Fig. 4—26(1)].

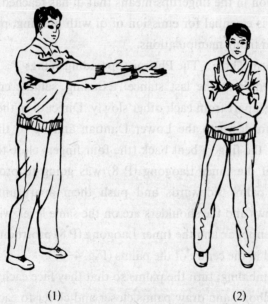

(1)   (2)

Fig. 4—26   Pushing Eight Horses Forward

Then inhaling, relax the four fingers. Bend the thumbs

back and pull the elbows gently, and draw the hands back to the hypochondria. At the same time make qi from the Lower Dantian and that returning from the hands converge in the Middle Dantian. Repeat the above two steps for 9 respiratory cycles. Finally draw the palms back and cross them in front of the chest [Fig. 4—26(2)].

NOTE: This form is to train the Three Yin Channels and the Three Yang Channels of Hand and the energy in the fingertips. Qi is directed mainly through the Channels of Hand—Taiyin and Hand—Yangming to the palms and the fingertips, and then back by way of the Three Yang Channels of Hand and the Channel of Hand—Taiyin. The distending or hot sensation in the fingertips means that qi has reached there. This form is essential for emission of qi with pushing, pulling, leading and fixing manipulations.

(3) Form Three   The Phoenix Spreading Wings

Proceed from the last stance. Exhaling, set the crossed, erect palms apart from each other slowly. Direct qi in the Middle Dantian down to the Lower Dantian and up to the two arms, with the fingers bent back (the four fingers close to each other) as if the Inner Laogong (P 8) was going to protrude. Turn the palms sidewards and push them apart until the hands, elbows and the shoulders are on the same level, with fingers still bent back and the Inner Laogong (P 8) protruding and qi gathered in the centre of the palms (Fig. 4—27).

Then inhaling, turn the palms so that they face each other, bend the elbows and draw palms closer and closer to each other and finally get them crossed in front of the chest. Repeat the procedure for 9 respiratory cycles. Then get the hands to the sides of the chest to be prepared for the next step.

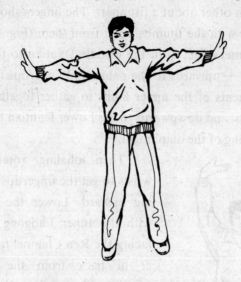

Fig. 4-27   The Phoenix Spreading Wings

NOTE: This form is aimed at training of the Channels of Hand-Jueyin and Hand-Shaoyang. Qi is accumulated in the Inner Laogong (P 8) when the hands are pushed out, in the Outer Laogong and then is sent back to Dantian when the hands are drawn back. As a result of persistent training of this form, the line of qi will always be kept round the palms, the centre of it is between the Inner and Outer Laogong. It is the basic step for traing emission of outgoing-qi with pushing, pulling, quivering and fixing manipulations.

(4) Form Four   Holding the Sky with the Hands

Proceed from the last stance.

Exhaling, lift the palms slowly. When they get to the point Lianquan (Ren 23), abduct them slowly as if to hold something. Continue to lift them until they are above the head, with the arms stretched and the fingertips of the two hands pointing at each other about a fist apart. The fingers should be closed together with the thumbs apart from them (Fig. 4—28). At the same time, direct qi in the Middle Dantian to flow in two directions——upwards to the palms and fingertips following the movements of the upper limbs to gather together between the hands, and downwards to the Lower Dantian following the discending of the diaphragm.

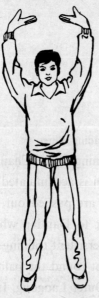

Then inhaling, rotate the wrists to get the fingertips pointing upward. Lower the hands with the Inner Laogong (P 8) facing the Ren Channel to gather qi back from the Inner Laogong (P 8) and up from the Lower Dantian. Repeat the steps for 9 respiratory cycles. Put the hands in front of the chest with palms facing upward in preparation for the next step.

NOTE: This form is aimed at training qi of Sanjiao (three warmers) and the Shaoyang, Taiyang and Shaoyin Channels

Fig. 4—28 Holding the Sky
with the Hands

to make qi of the Yin Channels flow via the Yang Channels upwards to the palms, then via the Yang Channels downwards to Dantian then to the toes. This form is essential for training the emission of qi with pushing, pulling, leading and quivering manipulations.

(5) Form Five   Scooping the Moon from Water

Proceed from the last stance.

Exhaling, get hands apart sidewards. Bend forward and hang down the arms, and draw hands towards each other between the feet with fingertips pointing at each other. Draw hands towards each other until they are one fist apart. Accumulate energy at the fingertips as if holding a bulky weight (Fig. 4—29). Meanwhile, direct qi in the Middle Dantian in two directions——downwards to the Lower Dantian and upwards to between the two hands.

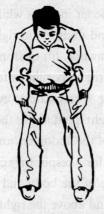

Fig. 4—29   Scooping the Moon from Water

Then inhaling, straighten the waist naturally to hold the "moon" up to the chest and direct qi to Dantian. Repeat the above process for 9 respiratory cycles. Place the two palms upwards at the chest for the next step.

NOTE: When bending forward, one should keep lithe and slow movement of the waist. The eyes are closed appropriately to look at the "moon" (a round object or a light mass or a tiny glittering spot that can be taken as the moon) between the legs, and the hands groping, trying to catch the "moon" and then hold it up to Dantian. The exercise is good for nourishing Dantian and reinforcing the kidneys and can regulate both the Ren Channel and the Du Channel. It is essential for training emission of qi with pushing, pulling and quivering manipulations.

(6) Form Six Holding the Ball and Stroking It Three Times

Proceed from the last stance.

Exhaling, move the hands to the right side of the body with the palms facing each other, the left below the right, as if holding a ball. Inhaling, pull the palms a little farther away from each other as if the ball were being inflated (Fig. 4—30). Then adduct the left palm and abduct the right while pulling them to make qi rotate between the palms and direct qi in the Middle Dantian down to the Lower Dantian and up to the hands. Press the ball as if to compress the air inside it while exhaling and then adduct the left palm and abduct the right to make qi rotate between the palms. Meanwhile, lift qi from the Lower Dantian and draw it back from the upper limbs to the Middle Dantian. Repeat the above for 3 respiratory cycles. While the palms are rotated, bring the right hand above the left to turn the "ball" upside down in front of the abdomen, and do the same "inflating" and "compressing" for 3 respiratory cycles there. Finally shift hands to the left side of the body and turn the "ball" upside down to get the left hand above the right,and do the "inflating" and "compressing" 3 respiratory cycles. Let the hands stay at the left side for the next step.

NOTE: This form is practised for directing qi of the Three Yang and Three Yin Channels of Hand and Foot to the palms. Yin—qi and yang—qi will circulate between the hands like the rotation of a ball. The inflation and deflation of the ball is coordinative with mind concentration. Yin is interlocked with yang. Qi flows endlessly. This form is the art to train emission of qi with pushing, pulling, rotating and quivering manipulations.

(7) Form Seven   Moving the Palms As If Setting Tiles on the Roof

Proceed from the last pose. Exhaling, stretch the left hand forward to send out qi of the Three Yin Channels and pull back the right hand to draw the qi of Three Yang Channels back (Fig. 4–31). Inhaling, stretch out the right hand and pull back the left to get qi of the Three Yin Channels out and that of the Three Yang Channels back. Along with the stretching out and pulling back of the hands, qi of the Three Yin and Three Yang Channels of Hand begins to circulate. Perform the process for 9 respiratory cycles. Place the hands at the sides of the chest, palms upwards, to be prepared for the next step.

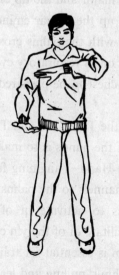
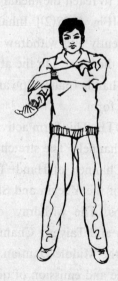
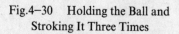

Fig.4–30   Holding the Ball and   Fig.4–31   Moving the Palms As
        Stroking It Three Times   If Setting Tiles on the Roof

NOTE: This form is aimed at guiding qi of the Three Yin and Three Yang Channels of Hand out to the palms and back to Dantian, with yin and yang interlocked and qi circulating endlessly. It is essential for emission of outgoing-qi with pushing, pulling, leading and quivering manipulations.

(8) Form Eight   The Wind Swaying the Lotus Leaf

Proceed from the last stance. Exhaling, cross the palms with the left above the right and both facing upwards. Stretch them out slowly to get the palms and the elbows at shoulder level [Fig. 4-32(1)]. Simultaneously direct qi in the Middle Dantian down to the Lower Dantian and up to the palms to connect qi of the Yin Channels of Hand with that of the Yang. Then separate the arms sidewards and press them down gently to get qi to reach the thenar eminence major and the tip of the thumbs [Fig. 4-32(2)]. Inhaling, stick up the thenar eminence minor gently and withdraw the arms, with the palms crossed, back to the chest. Do the above for 9 or 18 respiratory cycles. Put the hands (palms upward) at the chest to be prepared for the next form.

NOTE: This form activates qi of the Three Yin and Three Yang Channels. The stretching out of the hands is to make qi of the Channels of Hand-Taiyin and Hand-Yangming facilitate qi of the Yueyin and Shaoyin Channels to the palms and fingertips. The withdraw of them is to activate qi of the Shaoyin and Taiyang Channels to facilitate qi of the yin channels to the Middle Dantian. This form is essential for training guidance and emission of qi with pushing, pulling and leading manipulations.

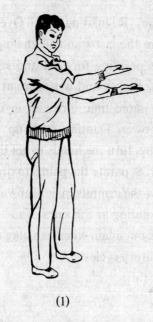

(1)

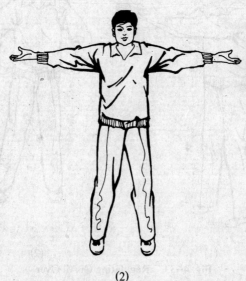

(2)

Fig. 4–32   The Wind Swaying the Lotus Leaf

(9)Form Nine   Regulating Qi All Over

Proceed from the last stance. Exhaling, turn the palms to get the fingertips pointing forward and stretch the palms out till the shoulders, elbows and wrists are at the same level [Fig. 4–33(1)]. At the same time direct qi in the Middle Dantian down to the Lower Dantian and up to the palms and fingertips. Inhaling, turn the hands to get the back of the palms facing each other. Separate the palms to draw an arc with them till they are below the armpits, palms upwards and fingertips of the two hands pointing at the sides of the chest [Fig. 4–33(2)]. Stretch the palms out again when exhaling to repeat the process for 9 or 18 respiratory cycles.

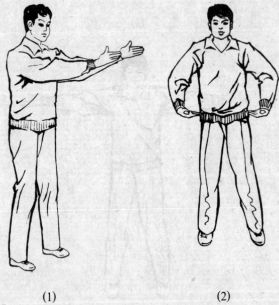

(1)   (2)

Fig. 4–33   Regulating Qi All Over

NOTE: This form is to combine the heavenly, earthly and

human qi in one and to regulate qi of the whole body to get prepared for the closing of the exercise.

(10)Closing Form of Double—Nine Yang Exercise

Overlap the two hands with the right over the left (vice versa in female) and apply them to the Lower Dantian. Stop vibrating gradually and gather qi into Dantian. Breathe naturally and concentrate on Dantian for a while. Rub the hands and face and move freely to end the exercise.

Massaging the Abdomen to Strengthen the Active Substance in the Body

The exercise is an auxiliary to static and dynamic qigong in training qi. The practice of it in combination with static and dynamic exercises can stren— then the internal organs, reinforce intrinsic qi, accumulate qi without leaking, multiply the strength, and open and close the points sensitively so that any risk of deviations can be avoided. This is especially important for those who carry out treatment of patients by emitting outgoing—qi because though they may be able to open the small or large circle of qi and can direct qi to the extremeties at will, they can not ensure his internal qi substantial all the time. If they do not practise the exercise Massaging the Abdomen to Strengthen the Active Substance in the Body but treat patients, they may become insufficient in active substance, deficient in qi and weak in strength. If they emit outgoing—qi to treat patients, their health will be impaired easily by pathogenic qi because they are not strong enough internally, their points are easy to open as soon as qi reaches them and their resistance to external pathogenic factors is weak. This can cause local discomfort or morbid physical state which leads to a general disorder of qi activities, resulting in collapse of the achievements gained through long–term practice. So Massaging the Abdomen to Strengthen the Active Substance in the Body is not only an auxiliary exercise for strengthening the intrinsic qi, but also an indispensable exercise for those who treat patients with outgoing–qi.

1. Methods

(1) Lie supine on bed with both legs stretched naturally, hands at the sides of the body, the whole body (especially the viscera) relaxed, distracting thoughts expelled, breath natural, tongue pressed against the palate, belt released and the region to be massaged exposed.

(2) Apply the right palm (left palm for a female) to the abdomen under the xiphoid process and rotate the palm to knead the upper abdomen clockwise (for a female massaging with the left palm counterclockwise to coincide with yin is tonifying, as it is so for a male to massage with the right palm clockwise to coincide with yang). Do not exert force intentionally lest the hand become stiff. The correct manipulation should be natural and gentle, which gives a soft sensation under the palm inside the upper abdomen. Avoid distractions. Keep inward–vision attentively and concentrate the mind on the Middle Dantian. One should neither forget the flowing of qi, nor should he speed up its flow; just let it progress naturally. Maintain natural breath with a calm mind and try to get the pleasant feeling of warm, gentle and continuous flowing qi under the palm. Each session of practice needs 15 – 30 minutes; the time can be

increased gradually to one hour but overfatigue of the arm should be avoided. Carry out the kneading three times a day: in the morning, at noon and in the evening; or twice a day: in the morning and in the evening.

(3) After about a month's practice and as qi accumulates gradually, one may feel that his stomach—qi is consolidated and his appetite and sleep improved, and he may have "the feeling of qi" in the mid—upper abdomen when it is pressed. The straight muscles of the abdomen may have become more solid or bulged gradually, which may appear more apparently when one directs qi or exerts strength to it. At this stage, the midline from the xiphoid process to the navel may be still soft and dented, indicating that qi in the Ren Channel (the Front Midline Channel) is still not substantial. To improve it, massage the midline with the palmroot and strike along it gently with a "hollow" fist. The dent will disappear then, and qi in the Ren Channel is now rendered substantial. This usually takes one a hundred days to attain.

(4) As a following step, conduct massage on the right side of the abdomen with the right palm first, in a way of spiral kneading from under the ribs down to the groin, 12 times. Do the same with the left palm to the left abdomen counterclockwise 12 times. Then massage with the right palm the lower abdomen where the Lower Dantian is located circularly for 15 — 30 minutes, with the same method of respiration and mind concentration. Pat the same site with a "hollow fist" for some time after the massage. By so doing, Dantian and even the whole abdomen will become substantial with qi and will be strong and solid in about a hundred days.

(5) The next step is to strike with a "hollow fist" on the midline of the chest and the right and left sides of it, followed by massaging the Lower Dantian in the way mentioned in step (4). Long—term practice will make both the chest and the abdomen substantial with qi, indicating that both the Ren and Chong Channels are full of qi.

(6) At this stage, one can direct qi into the Du Channel (the Back Midline Channel). Then, use a ready—made mulberry club or a wooden hammer to carry out self—patting, or ask someone to pat with a hollow fist along the Du Channel and along the first and second collaterals of the Urinary Bladder Channel, up and down and vice versa alternately. Ask him to rub these places with his palm root in order to make qi even and full. In this way, the Du Channel will be substantial with qi in about a hundred days.

(7) When the Ren and Du Channels are filled with consolidated qi, one can carry out self—patting or ask someone to pat with a hollow fist or a readymade tool on the upper and lower extremities from above to below, with emphasis on the regions where there are flably muscles.

The patting or striking of the above—mentioned parts can also be done with a specially made tool.

With about one year's practice of the exercise, one may feel that he is full of substantial and vigorous qi all over. His resistance to external pathogenic factors will be strong, his points will be highly sensitive in opening and closing and will not be affected by turbid qi. On this basis, he can take some time every day to massage the abdomen and pat the extremities as a routine.

The Exercise of Heaven—Earth Rotation
(Qian Kun Yun Zhuan Gong)

The exercise is aimed at facilitating the qi activities of yin and yang of the whole body by means of hand manipulation at the upper and lower, left and right and anterior and posterior parts of the body so as to make yin—qi and yang—qi reach the hands and circulate there alternately to refine qi activities and improve the sensitivity of the hands to qi. It is the essential exercise for guiding and emitting qi.

1. Preparation

Either a standing or sitting posture can be taken. The standing posture is hereof taken as an example.

Stand quiet and relaxed, with the feet at shoulder width, the whole body relaxed, respiration natural, distractions expelled, eyes slightly closed, tongue rested against the palate and hands in front of the chest in a pose of Buddhist greeting.

2. Holding and Rotating the Ball with Hands at Its Upper and Lower Sides

Set the hands naturally in front of the chest and the abdomen respectively as if holding a ball (the left hand above the right in male and vice versa in female), the thumb of the upper hand toward the point Shanzhong (Ren 17), the thenar eminence minor of the lower hand toward the navel, and the Inner Laogong (P 8) of the two hands pointing at each other. Breathe naturally and imagine holding a ball (Yin—Yang Taiji Ball) and yin—qi and yang—qi circulating between the two hands. Firstly, inhale to send qi to Dantian by will and exhale to direct qi from Dantian to between the palms, followed by pushing and pulling

—227—

the hands with internal strength several times. When a sensation of attraction or congestion has been obtained, push and rotate the "inflated" ball with the left hand turning leftwards and the right rightwards as if rubbing the ball, 25 times (the Heaven number). Then exchange the hands and push and rotate the ball in the opposite direction 30 times (the Earth number) (Fig. 4—34). With natural respiration, concentrate the mind on the palms and hold the ball quietly for a moment.

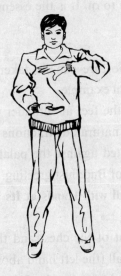 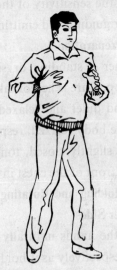

Fig. 4—34 Turning the Ball Up and Down   Fig. 4—35 Turning the Ball Left and Right

3. Holding and Rotating the Ball with Hands at Its Left and Right Sides

Set the hands at the two sides of the hypochondria respectively as if holding a ball, with the point Laogong (P 8) of the two hands pointing at each other and the two thumbs leveling Shanzhong (Ren 17). Inhaling, send qi to Dantian and exhaling direct it to the space between the palms, followed by pushing and pulling the hands with internal strength several times. When the sensation of attraction or congestion is obtained, rotate the "inflated" ball with the palms, the left hand turning leftwards and the right rightwards, 25 times (the Heaven number). Then rotate the ball in the oppisite direction 30 times (the Earth number)(Fig. 4–35). With natural respiration, concentrate the mind on the palms and hold the ball quietly for a moment.

4. Rotating the Sun and Moon in Turn

Set the left hand at the level of the point Tiantu (Ren 22) and the right hand at the level of Shenque (Ren 8), with the centre of the two palms facing each other as if holding something in the arms. Firstly take a breath and send qi down to Dantian, then exhale to guide qi to the space between the palms. Pull the hands toward each other and pull them in the opposite directions alternately with internal strength several times. When the feeling of qi has been attained, turn the hands and the forearms clockwise and

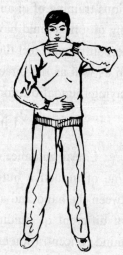

Fig. 4–36   Rotating the Sun and Moon Alternately

counter– clockwise alternately 25 times (the Heaven number). Then turn the hands and forearms counterclockwise and clockwise alternately 30 times (the Earth number)(Fig. 4–36). Close the two palms in front of the chest like a Buddhist greeting to end the exercise.

Chapter Five   The Guidance of Qi

Guiding qi, or directing qi, means to guide intrinsic qi to a certain part (a hand, a point, etc.) where outgoing–qi (waiqi) is emitted. This is usually made only when one has undergone serious training of qi and qi–guiding exercises for long. On guiding qi, one should have qi follow the mind and should be able to control and feel the pattern, nature and amount of intrinsic qi as well as the direction it flows in. The exercise is aimed at laying foundations for hand–emission of outgoing–qi (waiqi).

Linear Guidance of Qi

Linear guidance of qi refers to the formation of a straight line of inductive outgoing–qi between the two hands or between the hand and a certain point outside the body by means of different qi–guiding methods such as hand manipulation, mind concentration and breathing. Its characteristic is that qi is kept still in a line when the practitioner keeps himself in a static state and moves to and fro when he is in a dynamic state. It is the main qi–guiding method of outgoing–qi therapy.

1. One–finger–Meditation to Guide Qi

(1) Posture

Take the standing–vibrating posture, with the left hand lifted to the shoulder level, the wrist bent, the index finger straight and the rest curved, the tips of the thumb and the middle finger touching each other to form a ring; the right hand (in the same gesture as the left) at the right side of the abdomen; the index fingers of the two hands pointing at each other to form a straight line (Fig. 5–1).

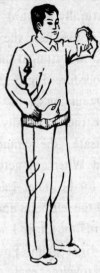

Fig. 5–1   Guiding Qi with One–finger–meditation

(2) Guiding Qi

Breathe naturally and concentrate the attention on Dantian. As soon as qi in Dantian is activated, begin to breathe slowly to direct qi to the tip of the right index finger, and when one feels that qi has reached there (one will feel his fingertip hot and distending as if something is being released from it), direct qi from Dantian to the tip of the index finger of the left hand. As one feels that there is an attractive force between the tips of the two fingers caused by qi, start to rap with the tip of the left index finger on the qi column being emitted from the right; one will get strong feeling of qi at the two hands. Then direct qi to the left index finger to emit it to the right hand, driving the top of the qi column to beat the tip of the right index finger; one will also get a strong feeling of qi. Then change the posture and position of the two hands to train qi.

(3) Time

Do the exercise once or twice a day, 5 – 30 minutes each

time.

2. Palm-pushing and Plam-pulling to Guide Qi

(1) Posture

Take the standing-vibrating posture. Relax the fingers of both hands. Stretch the right hand naturally forward to the right and bent the left to get it in front of the chest, the centre of the two palms facing each other to form a straight line. Exchange hands and carry out the same procedure (Fig. 5-2).

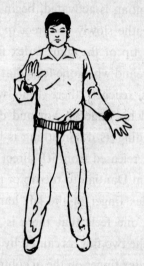

Fig. 5-2　Guiding Qi by Pushing-Pulling the Hands

(2) Guiding Qi

Breathe naturally and concentrate the mind on Dantian. When qi is activated, lead it to the Inner Laogong (P 8) of the left palm and emit it towards the Inner Laogong of the right palm. Push the palms toward each other while emitting qi Holding qi between the palms, draw the palms back to the original position. One will get strong feeling of qi when doing that. Exchange hands and carry out the same procedure.

(3) Do the exercise once or twice a day, 5 - 30 minutes each time.

3. Making Three Points Linear to Guide Qi

(1) Posture

Light a stick of sanitary incense. Put the incense burner on a table or one can take a similar object as a point. Take the standing—vibrating posture, the right palm stretched naturally in front of the incense, the burning tip of the incense pointing at the Inner Laogong (P 8); the left palm, in the one—finger—meditation or sword—fingers or flat—palm gesture, is put at the back of the tip of the burning incense, the fingertip pointing at the incense tip. The three points——the tip of the left index finger, the tip of the burning incense and the Inner Laogong (P 8) of the right palm are thus made linear (Fig. 5—3).

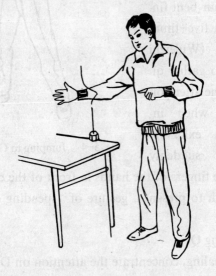

Fig. 5—3   Making Three Point Linear to Guide Qi

(2) Guiding Qi

Proceed from the last stance. Breathe naturally and concentrate the attention on Dantian. Divert the attention onto the tip of the incense and concentrate there. Continue to emit qi and send it farther on. One will have strong feeling of qi in the Inner Laogong (P 8) of the right hand.

—233—

(3) Time

Do the exercise once or twice a day, 5 − 30 minutes each time.

4. Jumping to Guide Qi in Burst

(1) Posture

Stand with feet apart at shoulders width and bend the knees slowly. Rest the thumb on the back of the four bent fingers to form a five−thunder−fingers (Wuleizhi Shi) gesture to gather qi. Concentrate the attention on Dantian when inhaling; when exhaling, jump and suddenly

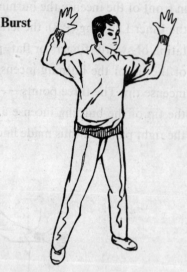

Fig. 5−4   Jumping to Guide Qi in Burst

stretch out the fingers of the hands in front of the chest, palms facing forward, to present a gesture of "speading claw" (Fig. 5−4).

(2) Guiding Qi

When inhaling, concentrate the attention on Dantian. Lift qi to the chest and gather it in the palms. When exhaling, concentrate the attention on the centre of the palms with qi bursting out from the Inner Laogong (P 8). Guide qi by will to the simulated spot.

(3) Time

Do the exercise once or twice a day, 24 or 48 respiratory cycles each time.

Guidance of Qi in Fixed Form

Guidance of qi in fixed form is carried out on the basis of practice of Double—Nine Yang Exercise, at a time when qi can oscillate in Dantian naturally. With a proper hand posture,the practitioner directs qi oscillating in Dantian to flow to the hands and makes qi vibrate there in a certain form with different frequency under the control of will; at the same time, the internal qi is released along with the vibration. The feature of this kind of guidance of qi is that qi is guided in fixed form when the practitioner assumes a static state and is oscillating when he assumes a dynamic state and qi flows bit by bit.

1. Standing Vibrating with Palms Closed to Guide Qi

(1) Posture

Take a standing—vibrating posture. Keep feet shoulder—width apart. Bend the arms to set the palms closed in front of the chest, fingertips pointing upward and elbows and wrists at the same level. Picture supporting an object on the head. Draw in the chest and straighten the back. Relax the hips and knees. Rest the tongue on the palate. Close the eyes slightly (Fig. 5—5).

(2) Guiding Qi

Breathe naturally and concentrate the mind on Dantian. When

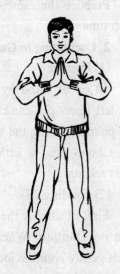

Fig. 5—5 Standing Vibrating with Palms Closed to Guide Qi

the motion of qi in Dantian is felt (a sensation of warmth and qi circulation), guide qi by will to the palms and the fingertips through the Three Yin Channels of Hand during exhaling; when inhaling, have the mind follow qi back to Dantian along the Three Yang Channels of Hand. When the internal qi is circulating freely, keep the attention on the palms and the fingertips with gentle natural breathing. One will feel the palms hot, the fingertips thicker, distending and tingling. Lead the vibrating qi in Dantian to the fingertips and make the fingers vibrating slightly as if something were coming out of them bit by bit.

(3) Time

Practice the exercise once or twice a day, 3 − 10 minutes each time.

2. Oscillating to Guide Qi

(1) Posture

Sit on or stand by a bed. Rest the left hand naturally on the left knee; put the right hand on the bed, the periphery of the palm touching the bed but the centre of it suspended, with the elbows bent a little, shoulders and elbows dropped and wrist relaxed.

(2) Guiding Qi

First of all, get the breath even and concentrate the attention on Dantian. When qi in Dantian is activated, turn the waist gently counterclockwise or clockwise. When inhaling, lift qi to the chest, the intrinsic qi vibrating and ascerding little by little from Dantian and finally reaching the palms along the arms on exhaling. The vibration of the intrinsic qi make the palms tremer rhythmically, and the frequency and force of the tremer will change with mind concentration. Practise repeatedly. When qi gets to the palm, fills the palm and seethes there, one will feel as if there were an inflating ball under the hand. Yet qi is always centred on the Inner Laogong (P 8), gathering together without dispersion.The motion of qi and the movements of the hand are in perfect harmony.

The exercise is usually done in a sitting or a standing posture. The hand poses required for the training of guiding qi in vibrational fixed form include middle–finger–propping (the other fingers bent) or a spreading–palm (the five fingers touching something). After some practice of the exercise when the right hand can vibrate in fixed form, one can practise guiding qi in different frequency, different intensity and different wave peak.

(3) Time

Do the exercise 1 − 2 times a day, 30 − 60 minutes each time. Generally, the skill can be preliminary mastered in three months.

Guiding Qi in Circle and Spiralty

Guiding qi in circle and spiralty is to lead the internal qi to whirl inside the body and guide it to the palms or the fingertips to be emitted in circular or spiral form. It is characterized by the flowing of qi in a circle when the practitioner is in a static state and in spiralty when he is in a dynamic state.

1. Making Three Points Circular to Guide Qi

(1) Posture

Stand vibrating. Light a stick of sanitary incense and put

the burner (or an object) on a table. Stretch the two hands naturally, the three points——the Inner Laogong (P 8) of both hands and the tip of the burning incense forming an equilateral triangle. Draw a circle mentally based on the centre and the three points of the triangle and guide qi to fill the circle (Fig. 5–6).

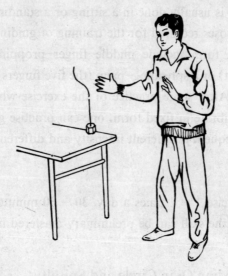

Fig. 5–6　Making Three Points Circular to Guide Qi

(2) Guiding Qi

After you have drawn the circle mentally, get the breath natural and concentrate the attention on Dantian. When qi in Dantian is activated, lead qi to the Inner Laogong (P 8) of both hands. Exhale lightly to emit qi towards the incense tip so as to make the three points attract one another. Picturing holding a ball with the hands, move the hands in response to the sense of qi; while one hand pulls, the other pushes or vice versa alternately.

In this exercise, a tree or a flower can also be taken as an object to make the three points circular.

(3) Time

Do the exercise once or twice a day, 5 – 30 minutes each time.

2. Guiding Qi in Spiralty

(1) Posture

Any of the three postures (standing, sitting and lying) will do. The standing posture is taken hereof as an example.

Stand feet apart, place the right hand in front of the right side of the chest with the elbow bent, palm facing forward and fingertips pointing upward.

(2) Guiding Qi

On guiding qi, get qi in Dantian to turn inside the body counterclockwise in spiralty (qi following mind concentration) through the chest and the upper extremities to the palms. Make qi in Dantian to spiral(taking the navel as the centre) synchronously with that in the palms (taking the Inner Laogong as the centre). Beginners should do it slowly and increase the speed gradually and naturally. The turning is flexible and one should not be too anxious for quick results. The exercise can also be carried out with the index and middle fingers or only the middle finger stretched. Qi is turned to whirl from the smallest to the largest circle, or vice cersa, or in other ways.

(3) Time

The skill of guiding qi described above can not be mastered overnight; it should be practised frequently, making full use of the standing, lying and sitting postures.

Cold and Heat Guidance of Qi

This form of qi—guiding exercise is to give the part where qi is emitted the function of producing coldness or hotness through breathing and mind concentration. It conforms to the treatment principle of TCM in terms of " treatingthe cold—syndrome with hot—natured drugs and heat—syndrome with cold— natured drugs".

1. Heat Guidance of Qi

(1) Posture

Take a standing, lying or sitting posture. Sitting posture is hereof taken as an example.

Sit on a square stool on requirement for qigong practice with the left palm resting naturally on the left thigh, and the right palm stretched on the bed or a table with the centre of the palm suspended. Take natural respiration, close the eyes gently and prop the tongue against the palate.

(2) Guiding Qi

Make the breath even and concentrate the mind on Dantian. Imagine that qi in Dantian is as hot as the burning sun and spreads all over the body. Collect qi back into Dantian and turn it into light and heat. Then shift qi of the light and heat to the chest, the arms and further to the palms and the fingertips, and imagine that it is burning and giving off heat between the palm or fingertips and the object touched and penetrating into the object.

(3) Time

Practise the exercise when there is sun light, facing south or east, 20 — 40 minutes each time.

2. Cold Guidance of Qi

(1) Posture

Refer to the posture in "Heat Guidance of Qi".

(2) Guiding Qi

Cold guidance of qi should also begin with the regulation of even breathing and concentration of mind on Dantian. Gather qi from the heels and the point Yongquan (K 1) and direct it via the chest and arms to the palms, imagining that the palms are as cold as ice. Concentrate the mind on the coldness there and guide it to penetrate into the object the hand touches. The practitioner should not imagine that his whole body is such cold, nor should he direct such cold into his body lest it affect the coordination of qi activities.

(3) Time

Practise the exercise facing west or north at night, 20–40 minutes each time.

Guiding Qi of the Five Elements

Guidance of qi of the Five Elements is one subject of the ancient specialty "Zhuyou", which combines the Five Elements with the five zang–organs (the heart, liver, spleen, lung and kidney), the six–character formulae, time, direction and finger–nail pressing in general exercise and guiding and emitting qi. With this method, qi is divided into five kinds: wood (liver), fire (heart), earth (spleen), metal (lung) and water (kidney), and in clinical practice, methods of guiding qi is determined by the deficiency and excess of the viscera and the philosophy of interrestraint of the Five Elements.

When one is skilled in this exercise, he can continue to practise it in combination with guidance of qi in fixed form, making three points linear to guide qi, making three points circular to guide qi and other qi−guiding methods, to create a qi−emitting complex.

1. Guiding Water−qi

(1) Posture

Take a T−shaped standing posture with the right foot behind the left, and with the chest drawn in, the back straightened, the abdomen contracted, the knees relaxed, the tongue rested against the palate, the eyes slightly closed and the neck straightened picturing supporting an object on the head.

(2) Method

First, press deeply with the left thumb the Shen (the ninth of the Twelve Earthly Branches) or the You (the tenth following Shen) stripe (water stripes) (Fig. 5−7), and put the right hand in front of the chest in a hand gesture of sword−fingers or flat−palm. Then inhale qi in front of the left hand and send it by will to the kidneys and then to Dantian to get it mixed with qi there. When exhaling, lift

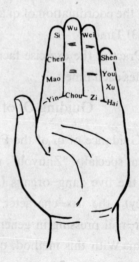

Fig. 5−7   The Sequence of the Earthly Branches on the Palm

the mixed qi in Dantian, with the thumb pressing the Hai or Zi stripe (water stripes) and uttering "chui" in a very low sound, to send it (the water—qi) out of the body by way of the sword—fingers or the palm of the right hand.

(3) Time

The exercise can be done facing west and south during the period of Hai(9—11 pm), Zi (11 pm — 1 am), Shen (3 — 5 pm) or You (5 — 7 pm), or it can be practised in cooperation with other Daoyin (dynamic) exercises, 36 respiratory cycles each time.

2. Guiding Metal—qi

(1) Posture

(Refer to that described in "Guiding Qi of Water".)

(2) Method

Press the mid—stripe of the thumb deeply with the left index finger, imagining that there is a golden building inlaid with jade which is glittering like the rising sun. Guide qi by will to the Lower Dantian and Zhongwan (Ren.12) to get qi there mixed with that inhaled by nose from the universe. Then press the Shen or You stripe (metal stripes) deeply with the left thumb and exhale while uttering "si", to guide qi out of the body by way of the palm of the right hand.

(3) Time

Practise the exercise facing west during the priod of Shen (3 — 5 pm) and You (5 — 7 pm) or Chen (7 — 9 am), Xu (7 — 9 pm), Chou (1 — 3 am) or Wei (1 — 3 pm), for 36 respiratory cycles each time.

3. Guiding Wood—qi

(1) Posture

(Refer to that described in "Guiding Water—qi".)

(2) Method

—243—

With the left thumb pressing deeply the Hai or Zi stripe (water stripes) of the same hand, inhale the liver—qi from the side of the left elbow and the chest and guide it into the chest to get it mixed with that taken in by natural respiration. When exhaling, press the Yin or Mao stripe (wood stripes) deeply with the left thumb while uttering " xu" to get qi out of the body by way of the sword—fingers and the palm of the right hand.

(3) Time

Practise it facing east or northeast during the period of Yin (3 − 5 am), Mao (5 − 7 am), Hai (9 − 11 pm) or Zi (11 pm − 1 am), for 24 or 48 respiratory cycles.

4. Guiding Fire—qi

(1) Posture

(Refer to that described in "Guiding Water—qi".)

(2) Method

Press the Yin or Mao stripe (wood stripes) deeply with the left thumb and inhale the liver—qi from the left elbow and the side of the chest into the lung to get it mixed with that rising from the Lower Dantian. When exhaling, press the Si and Wu fire stripes while uttering "ke" to guide qi out of the body by way of the sword—fingers or the palm of the right hand.

(3) Time

Practise it facing east, southeast or south during the period of Yin (3 − 5 am), Mao (5 − 7 am), Si (− 11 am) or Wu (11 am − 1 pm), for 14 or 28 respiratory cycles.

5. Guiding Earth—qi

(1) Posture

(Refer to that described in "Guiding Water—qi".)

(2) Method

Press the Zi or Wu fire stripe deeply with the left thumb and gather qi all over the body in the region of Zhongwan (Ren 12), and then lift it to the lung to get it mixed with that inhaled from the universe. When exhaling, press the mid—stripe of the left thumb deeply with the left thumb and utter "hu" to guide qi out by way of the sword—fingers or the palm of the right hand.

(3) Time

Practise it facing south, southeast or east during the period of Yin (3 — 5 am), Mao (5 — 7 am), Si (— 11 am) or Wu (11 am — 1 pm), for 10 or 30 respiratory cycles.

Chapter Six   Emission of Qi

Emission of qi is also called "emitting outgoing-qi" (Fafang Waiqi), and in an antient term, "distributing qi" (bu qi). It is a method adopted by those experienced in training qi and guiding qi, who direct their intrinsic qi to the palms and the fingertips or to other parts of the hand to emit it to the channels and points of the patient.

Section One   Hand Gestures in Emission of Qi

Five-Thunder-Fingers (Wuleizhi Shi)

Hand Gesture: The four fingers are bent to the centre of the palm and the thumb is bent and rested on the nails of the four fingers (Fig. 6-1).

Essentials: The four fingers are bent yet propped against the thumb, while the thumb pressing down to close tightly with the four fingers, with the centre of the palm hollow. Qi is gathered in the palm. This kind of qi-guiding-gathering skill should be practised constantly.

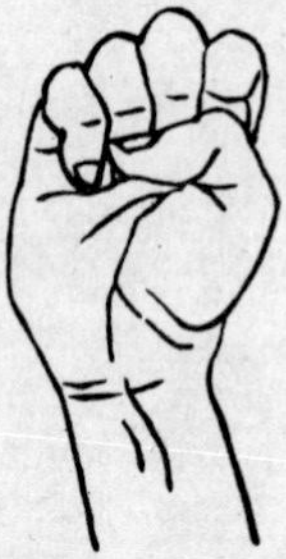

Fig. 6-1   Five-thunder-fingers Hand Gesture

Application: The hand gesture was used to guide and gather qi before emitting it onto the magic figures (left) in ancient times. On emitting qi, the practitioner should exhale and suddenly stretch the five fingers to form a flat—palm, a spreading—claw or a dragon—mouth hand gesture, or he can stretch out the index and middle fingers to make a sword—fingers hand gesture or only the middle finger to make a " middle—finger—propping". When the emission of qi is finished, he should inhale and resume the five—thunder—fingers hand gesture, with qi gathered in the centre of the palm.

Buddha's—Warrior—Attendant—Fingers (Jingang zhi Shi)

Hand Gesture: Make a tight fist, with the thumb put down on the nails of the small and index fingers, the middle finger on the thumb, the ring finger on the first segment of the middle finger, and the index finger on the nail of the ring finger. (Fig 6 — 2).

Essentials: The index, ring and small fingers and the thumb should be bent forcefully and strength is gathered between them. The middle finger is bent naturally without exertion to allow qi to reach its tip.

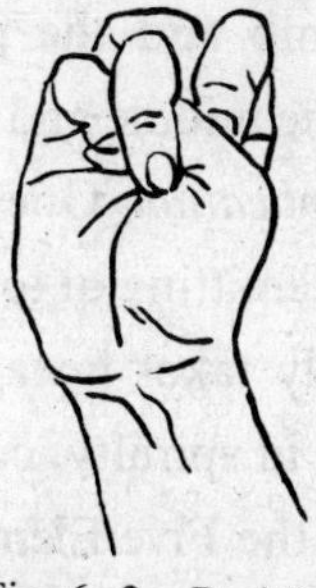

Fig. 6—2 Buddha's—warrior—attendant Hand Gesture

Application: This hand gesture is the main method used in ancient times to guide and emit qi onto the magic figures. The practitioner should take a breath and move the four fingers first before emission of qi to direct qi to the middle finger, then stretch the middle finger or turn the hand gesture into middle–finger–propping to emit qi. When ending the emission of qi, take in a breath and gather qi in the palm, then send it down to Dantian.

One–Finger–Meditation (Yizhichan Shi)

Hand Gesture: The index finger is stretched, the middle, ring and small bent naturally, the thumb bent and put gently on the middle and ring fingers (Fig. 6–3).

Essentials: With the index finger stretched, qi is gathered between the middle and ring fingers. The emission of outgoing–qi from the index finger is regulated by the force produced by the pressure of the thumb and the propping out of the middle and ring fingers.

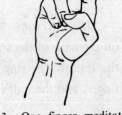

Fig. 6–3　One–finger–meditation
Hand Gesture

Application: One–finger–meditation is the main hand gesture for emitting qi toward the points and the painful localities. It usually takes linear guidance of qi, guidance of qi in fixed form or in spiralty, cold and heat guidance of qi and guidance of qi of the Five Elements as the main qi–guiding methods. Qi is emitted with the index finger of the therapist on or off the body surface of the disordered part of the patient, and with hand manipulations of pushing, pulling, quivering, leading and others.

Flat—Palm (Pingzhang Shi)

Hand Gesture: The five fingers are stretched naturally (Fig. 6—4).

Essentials: The stretching out of the five fingers should be natural without tention. The degree of tightness of the palm should be regulated by the alternation of gentle crooking and stretching of the five fingers and the tension and relaxation of the wrist.

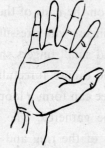

Fig. 6—4   Flat—palm
Hand Gesture

Application: Flat—palm is the main hand gesture for emitting outgoing—qi to the channels,the points and the disordered part of the patient. Qi—guiding methods used include linear, circular or cold and heat guidance of qi, guidance of qi in fixed form and guidance of qi of the Five Elements. Qi is emitted with the hand of the therapist on or off the body surface of the recipient by means of pushing, pulling, rotating, quivering, leading and fixing manipulations. The five—thunder—fingers can also be used to direct qi first and then it should be changed into flat—palm to gather qi in the centre of the palm,with the periphery of the palm as the qi—guiding circle and the Inner Laogong (P 8) as the qi— emitting spot. The emission of qi can be done with one palm or both palms together.

Sword—Fingers (Jianjue Shi)

Hand Gesture: The middle and index fingers are kept close

together, the ring and small fingers bent naturally and the thumb laid gently on their nails (Fig. 6–5).

Essentials: The thumb should be put on the nails of the ring and small fingers with pressure and the ring and small fingers should support the thumb forcefully so that the three can form a loop where qi is to be gathered. The degree of tension of the ring and small fingers may be regulated by the force the practitioner exerts. Qi is guided to the tip of the index and middle fingers.

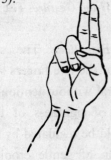

Fig. 6–5 Sword–fingers Hand GestureOthers Nature The Human Body

Application: Sword–fingers was the main qi–guiding and emitting hand gesture used to distribute qi onto the magic figures in ancient times.The index finger is taken as the liver–wood, and the middle finger, the heart–fire. The joining of the two fingers with each other can activate qi of wood and fire, which is of yang nature, simultaneously. So sword–fingers is the main hand gesture for guiding yang–heat.The qi–guiding methods required include linear guidance of qi, guidance of qi in fixed form, heat guidance of qi and guidance of qi of the Five Elements. On emission of qi, qi is firstly gathered in the loop formed by the thumb and the ring and small fingers, and then emitted through the tip of the index and middle fingers, which are placed on or off the body surface of the disordered part of the patient, by way of pushing, pulling, leading, fixing and other manipulations.

Middle—Finger—Propping (Zhongzhi Duli Shi)

Hand Gesture: The middle finger is stretched and the rest are bent naturally (Fig. 6–6).

Essentials: The wrist may either be bent or stretched naturally. The degree of tension of the middle finger is adjusted by the degree of force produced by bending the rest fingers, so is the speed of circulation of qi.

Application: Middle—finger—propping is derived from the Buddha's—warrior— attendant—fingers hand gesture, so on emission of qi, the latter may be assumed first. Qi is guided with linear, fixed or heat method or that of guidance of qi of the Five Elements, and is emitted with pushing, pulling, quivering, leading and fixing manipulations, with the tip of the middle finger on or off the disordered part of the patient.

Spreading—Claw (Tanzhua Shi)

Hand Gesture: The five fingers are half—stretched naturally (as if to touch something) (Fig. 6–7).

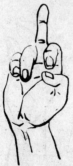 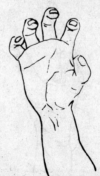

Fig.6—6 Middle—finger—propping   Fig.6—7 Spreading—claw
      Hand Gesture   Hand Gesture

Essentials: The five fingers are firstly stretched to make a flat—palm hand gesture, then the joints of the fingers are bent slightly (the joint connecting the fingers and the palm still stretched). The degree of tension of the palm and fingers is adjusted by the bending and stretching of the wrist and fingers.

Application: The guiding of qi is carried out with the five—thunder—fingers, followed by the flat—palm. Qi is first gathered in the centre of the palm and then emitted from the five fingers in a straight line toward the qi—receiving spot. The methods of qi guidance include linear, fixed, cold and heat and that of the Five Elements, and the emission of qi is performed through the pushing, pulling, quivering and rotating manipulations, with the tip of the fingers of the therapist on or off the part being treated.

Dragon—Mouth (Longxian Shi)

Hand Gesture: The four fingers or only the middle and index fingers are close to each other with the thumb separated and facing them (Fig. 6—8).

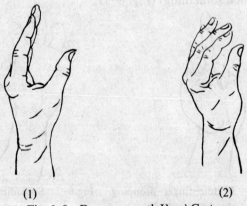

(1)   (2)

Fig. 6—8   Dragon—mouth Hand Gesture

Essentials: The four fingers should be stretched naturally and the thumb should be separated naturally from them and set facing them or only facing the index and middle finger as if a dragon keeping a ball in its mouth. The intensity of qi and force between the thumb and the four fingers is regulated by the gentle movement of the joints of the fingers.

Application: This hand gesture is transformed from the qi—guiding method of the five—thunder—fingers. Qi is emitted from the five fingers and gathered together between the thumb and the four fingers. Linear, fixed, circular and cold and heat guidance of qi as well as guidance of qi of the Five Elements can be adopted, and qi is emitted by hand manipulations such as pushing, pulling, quivering, rotating and fixing with the fingertips of the therapist on or off the qi—receiving part. This hand gesture is often used to emit qi toward the needle inserted in the body of the patient or toward some special parts such as the fingers, ears, shoulders or a tumor or mass.

Bird—beak (Quezui Shi)

Hand Gesture: The thumb is stretched and set opposite to the index, the middle, the ring or the small fingers to form a shape of an open bird beak (Fig. 6—9).

Essentials: The thumb is stretched to face any one of the other four fingers as if a bird holding food in its mouth, with the rest three straight, whose tension and relaxation can regulate the degree of tension between the thumb and the opposite finger.

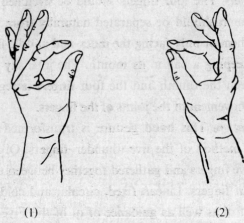

(1)   (2)

Fig. 6-9   Bird-beak Hand Gesture

Application: The five fingers match with the Five Elements and the five viscera, i.e., the thumb stands for earth and matches with the spleen, the index finger for wood and with the liver, the middle finger for fire and with the heart, the ring finger for metal and with the lung, and the small finger for water and with the kidney. And because metal combines with water, which stands for yin, and wood combines with fire, which stands for yang, the combination of the index and middle fingers represents yang and that of the ring and small fingers represents yin. However, the kidney—yang is the yang aspect of yin and the liver—yin is the yin aspect of yang, so they are further divided into two aspects——yin and yang. The thumb stands for earth and matches with the spleen, so if it combines with the four elements of the four fingers, i.e., metal, water, wood and fire, it can accumulate qi of all the five fingers. In a sense, the thumb (earth) can form a hand gesture with any of the other four fingers and the qi emitted with such hand gestures bears the nature of the Five Elements and the yin and yang. For example, qi emitted with the bird—beak gesture formed by the thumb and the middle finger is yang—qi within the heart, which has the function of replenishing yang and regulating the heart.

Bird—beak is derived from the dragon—mouth hand gesture, so the accumulation of qi in the palm should be preceded by the latter and followed by the linear, fixed, circular, cold and heat guidance of qi as well as guidance of qi of the Five Elements. Qi is emitted with the fingertips of the therapeutist touching or off the qi—receiving part with pushing, pulling, rotating, quivering, leading and fixing manipulations. The method is often applied to emission of qi toward the needle inserted in the body of the patient or toward some certain points or parts.

Section Two   The Hand Manipulations in Emission of Qi

Distant Emission of Qi

Distant Emission is the main approach of outgoing—qi therapy, referring to the skill in emitting outgoing—qi through proper guidance of qi and with the hand gesture of the therapist kept 10 − 100 centimetres away from the qi—receiving points or parts (the distance may be adjusted depending on the capability of the therapist for emitting qi).

1. Pushing

Hand Gesture: Flat—palm, one—finger—meditation, sword—fingers, dragon—mouth and bird—beak can be assumed for emission of qi with pushing manipulations.

Procedure: Select a proper hand gesture. Locate the hand about 10 − 100 centimetres off the point or region to be treated. Make two points or three points linear or three points circular to guide qi slowly. When the sensation of qi is attained, push the hand gently with "internal strength" to emit qi to the region being treated or to the related points.

Application: Pushing is the essential manipulation for opening the qi−receiving points or parts of the patient to get his qi activated and replenished. During the treatment, when the therapist has achieved a feeling of attraction or repulsion between the hand of the therapist and the points of the patient, the patient will feel an invisible qi rushing against him as well, or feel local hotness, condensation or stickiness, tingling and distention, or the flow of active qi. Some patients may incline his body or the related part spontaneously in the hand−pushing direction of the therapist. This manipulation is often applied in combination with the pulling, quivering, leading and rotating.

2. Pulling

Hand Gesture: Flat−palm, one−finger−meditation, sword−fingers, dragon−mouth, bird−mouth, etc.

Procedure: Select a proper hand gesture. Position the hand off the region to be treated. Guide qi slowly with the qi−guiding methods of making two points or three points linear or three points circular. When the sensation of qi has been achieved, pull the hand gently with "internal strength" to emit qi to the affected area.

Application: Pulling is essential for opening the qi−receiving points or parts to expel the pathogenic factors out of the body of the patients. During treatment, the therapist may feel the attraction of qi between his hand and the point or the part of the patient, or feel the pathogenic factors being pulled out from the point or part manifested by the sensations of coldness and chilliness, dryness–heat and tingling and heaviness. The manipulation is usually applied together with the pushing, leading and rotating. For instance, the combination of pushing and pulling in guidance of qi can open the points of the patient and make qi inside and outside the body interflow, and the combination of pulling and quivering may facilitate the patient's qi activities, guide his qi to flow and may promote and induce his spontaneous dynamic phenomenon.

3. Rotating

Hand Gesture: Flat–palm, dragon–mouth, bird–beak , one–finger–meditation, sword–fingers, etc.

Procedure: Select a suitable hand gesture and keep the hand off the affected area.Apply spiral qi–guiding method to guide qi slowly. When the sensation of qi is attained,rotate the hand clockwise or counterclockwise to guide qi to flow in spirally way and emit it into the affected area, or into the related points. One can also use the methods of making three points circular to guide qi slowly, and when the sensation of qi is attained, pull one hand and push the other with " internal strength" to make circular motion to emit qi to the affected area.

Application: Rotating is the main manipulation for activating the channel qi and guiding qi to circulate up and down and all around. The emission of qi by flat–palm preceded by guidance of qi by making three points circular to the points such as Jianyu (LI 15), Dazhui (Du 14) and Mingmen (Du 4) may induce the patient's body to turn and sway. This manipulation has the function of activating the channel qi, regulating the fu and zang organs and balancing yin and yang. It is especially effective for allaying pain when combined with the quivering.

4. Quivering

Hand Gesture: Flat—palm, spreading—claw, dragon—mouth, bird—beak, one— finger—meditation, sword—fingers and middle—finger—propping.

Procedure: Select a suitable hand gesture and locate the hand off the region to be treated. Adopt the method of guiding qi in fixed form to guide qi slowly. When the feeling of qi is attained, quiver the hand lightly to emit qi to the region being treated or to the related points.

Application: In clinical application, qi will be most easily activated when the frequency of hand quivering of the therapist is made synchronized with the frequency of qi vibrations of the patient. So this manipulation is mainly used to emit qi to activate the patient's channel qi, and can be combined with the pushing, pulling, rotating, and leading manipulations.

5. Leading

Hand Gesture: Flat—palm, one—finger—meditation, sword—fingers, dragon—mouth, bird—beak , etc.

Procedure: Select a suitable hand gesture. Position the hand off the region to be treated and guide qi slowly. When the sensation of qi is attained, emit qi toward the affected area, and lead the channel qi to flow with or against the course of the channels, leftwards or rightwards and upwards or downwards, decided according to the severity of illness.

Application: When the channel and point qi has been activated with other hand manipulations, the therapist should seize the opportunity to make use of the leading method to guide qi and make its flow smooth and regulated. So leading is the common manipulation for guiding the circulation of channel qi, regulating the excess and deficiency of yin and yang and sending qi back to its origin.

6. Fixing

Hand Gesture: One−finger−meditation, sword−fingers, flat−palm, dragon−mouth and bird−mouth.

Procedure: Select a proper hand gesture. Position the hand off the region to be treated and guide qi slowly. When the sensation of qi is attained, use one or several qi−emitting methods to make fixed emission of qi toward the region being treated.

Application: In this manipulation, the hand of the therapist is fixed toward the point or part to be treated and qi is emitted in a direct line. The method has the function of opening the point, facilitating qi activities and restoring and replenishing qi. For example, fixed emission of qi to Mingmen (Du 4) can tonify the kidney and strengthen yang and, to Dantian, can nourish the genuine qi.

Massage Manipulations in Emission of Qi

Massage manipulation for emitting qi, or qigong−massage is a modern term, referring to the emission of qi with the hands or fingers of the therapist touching the diseased part of the patient. By combining massage with his skill of qi−guidance, the therapist directs his internal qi to the fingers and palms, and emit qi while exerting strength of massage to adjust the "strength" and qi of the patient so that the quality of treatment can be improved. Besides, the function of qi emitted with the hand off the body surface of the patient is different from that emitted with the hand touching it. In the former, qi of the patient tends to be activated and balanced easily and both the therapist and patient can get a strong feeling of qi; while in the latter, the channels are easily dredged and yin and yang are often adjusted more quickly because of the stimulation produced by the strength of the hand on the channels and points, although it is not as efficient as the former in activation and regulation of qi activities. So in clinical practice, neither of the two should be neglected, and only when they are combined with each other properly, can the quality of outgoing-qi therapy be ensured. Introduced hereafter are a dozen common massage manipulations used in emission of qi.

1. Vibrating

Hand Gesture: Flat-palm, one-finger-meditation, middle-finger-propping, dragon-mouth, sword-fingers, bird-mouth, etc.

Procedure: Select a proper hand gesture and lay the hand or fingers on the parts to be treated or on the related points. With the waist as the axis, turn the body slowly clockwise and counterclockwise to guide the vibrating qi in Dantian to go through the chest and arms to the palms or fingers, which also vibrate to emit qi.

Application: Depending on the conditions of qi activities and the severity of illness of the patient, the therapist should make use of will and respiration to adjust the frequency and amplitude of vibration, the shape and nature of qi and the amount of strength and qi. When flat–palm hand gesture is taken, the therapist should gently touch the part to be treated with only the periphery of his palm and emit qi with the Inner Laogong (P 8) as the centre, to make the force produced by the vibrations of the hand and qi emitted from Laogong (P. 8) a single entity. This may bring about desirable results in activating and regulating the qi activities of the patient. For instance, emitting qi with this technique toward Baihui (Du 20) may results in ascending of yang; toward Dazhui (Du 14) and Mingmen (Du 4) may activate qi of the Du Channel; toward Dantian can facilitate and supplement qi in Dantian and can lead qi back to its origin; and toward Zhongwan (Ren 12) may replenish qi and regulate the stomach and induce sleep. Sword–fingers and one–finger–meditation are often adopted to emit qi directly to the points, such as Zhongwan (Ren 12), Qihai (Ren 6), Jingming (UB 1) and Yintang (Extra 1). Dragon–mouth and bird–beak are often used to emit qi toward the needles inserted into the points. In any case , the therapist should have his hand touch the body surface of the patient very gently or try to touch it but not really touch it. Hard pressure should be avoided lest the guiding and emitting of qi be hindered.

2. Kneading

Hand Gesture: One–finger–meditation, sword–fingers, flat–palm or thumb–flat.

Procedure: Select a proper hand gesture and apply it to the parts to be treated. By combining will with respiration, guide qi with heat or spiral qi— guiding method or guidance of qi of the Five Elements to the palms and fingers and then conduct rotatory kneading forcefully and emit qi simultaneously to the patient.

Application: When guiding qi in spiralty is adopted, the whirling frequency of qi should synchronize with that of hand kneading, which can be achieved most easily by combining the frequency of pulse and respiration. The kneading force is determined according to the severity of illness and it is generally believed that more force should be exerted by therapists who stress strength in regulating the patient's qi and less by those who emphasize guidance of qi for that purpose. Kneading manipulation is often used to emit qi to the points of the hand, chest, abdomen and extremities.

3. Rubbing

Hand Gesture: Flat—palm or the flat of the four fingers.

Procedure: Rest the palm or the flat of the four closed fingers gently on the point or the part to be treated. Guide qi to the palm or the flat of the four fingers with vibrating, spiral, cold and heat qi—guiding methods and guidance of qi of the Five Elements. Then rub the body surface of the patient and simultaneously emit qi.

Application: This manipulation is often used in combination with guidance of qi in spiralty. Generally, the hand pressure should not be too hard and the rubbing should be conducted along with the frequency of pulse and respiration. Having the function of dredging the channels and regulating and activating qi, rubbing is often used to alleviate pain in the chest, abdomen and extremities.

4. Scrubbing

Hand Gesture: Flat—palm or the flat of the four fingers.

Procedure: Rest the palm or the flat of the four closed fingers on the part to be treated. Guide qi to the palm or the fingers with heat and cold qi— guiding methods and guidance of qi of the Five Elements. Then push—scrub the affected part in a straight line while emitting qi.

Application: Scrubbing is the manipulation for guiding qi to flow in or against the direction of the channel course or to flow all round the body. With the function of clearing and activating the channels and collaterals, promoting the flow of qi and relaxing the tendons and balancing yin and yang, it is often used to treat disorders of the head and face, chest, abdomen, back and waist and the extremities.

5. Pressing—deeply

Hand Gesture: Flat—palm, one—finger—meditation, sword—fingers, or thumb tip, thumb joint and middle finger joint.

Procedure: Select a proper hand gesture and apply it to the point or the part to be treated. Guide qi to the palm and fingers with spiral, cold and heat and quivering qi—guiding methods. Then press hard while emitting qi. The manipulation can also be performed in cooperation with others such as plucking, kneading and pressing—intervally.

Application: Pressing—deeply has the function of dredging the channels, collaterals and points and relieving spasm and pain. It can be applied to all points of the body.

Auxiliary Hand Manipulations

They refer to other common massage manipulations, which are taken as accessory treatment methods and often applied prior to or after the emission of qi to facilitate the opening and closing of points, relax the muscles, relieve spasms, detach adhesion, lubricate the joints, dredge the channels and collaterals, regulate yin and yang, guide the flow of qi and adjust the body for ending the treatment.

These manipulations, although taken as accessory in outgoing–qi therapy, are very important for regulating the "strength" of the organism. One typical example is the treatment of prolapse of lumbar intervetebral disc, which is manifested by a series of symptoms due to compression of the sciatic nerve by pulpiform nucleus. Because the reposition of the pulpiform nucleus is very difficult with only regulation of qi of the patient, accessory manipulations such as repeated pressing , pulling–obliquely and rocking are necessary in this case. However, the dislocation of the pulpiform nucleus will certainly cause obstruction or disorder of qi flow, so regulation of qi should be not neglected. This is why it is believed that the treatment of the disease should be carried out with adjustment by "strength" as the main approach and the regulation by qi as the assistant.

1. Tapping

Tap with the middle finger or the three closed fingers (thumb, index, middle) or the five fingers lightly along the channels or at the points.

2. Nipping

Nip and press the points and the disordered parts with the thumb nail.

3. Patting

Pat with the palm (fingers stretched) on the disordered region, or along the channels, or on the points.

4. Hitting

Make a hollow fist and beat with its back or other aspects on the disordered region, or along the channels, or on the points.

5. Pressing—intervally

Press on the disordered region or along the channels or on the points with the tip of the thumb or the palm, or the joint of the bent thumb or index finger.

6. Stroking

Push and stroke with one palm or both palms along the channels or on the points or the affected area.

7. Plucking

Pluck the selected points with the fingers or the joint of the bent fingers.

8. Rubbing—to—and—fro

Press a certain part from both sides with the two palms or with the flat of the thumb and the index and middle fingers. Rub the part to and fro gently by exerting force symmetrically.

9. Rocking

Rock or pull to and fro the joints of the extremities with one hand holding the near end of the limb and the other hand holding the far end.

10. Rolling

Roll with the lateral side of the back of the hand on the healing region, with the forearm and the wrist turned, bent and stretched repeatedly, to make the strength produced through manipulations act continuously on the points or the disordered parts.

11. Pulling—obliquely

Hold the two far end of one limb or a certain part of the body respectively with the two hands and pull it in opposite directions.

Section Three   The Forms of Qi
on Emission

Clinical experience in emitting qi indicate that in treatment with outgoing—qi , one of the keys to success is to emit qi in different qi forms according to needs. Qi is emitted in three basic forms ; linear, fixed and spiral. Having grasped the three forms, one can apply them flexibly in clinical treatment in accordance with the conditions of the illness, e.g., one may apply one form, or two forms in combination, or develop some special forms on the basis of the three. The application of the three basic forms can be put into practice in combination with the cold and heat guidance of qi and guidance of qi of the Five Elements so that a combined qi—guiding—emitting process can be developed.

Linear Form: Qi emitted in linear form flows like longitudinal or transverse wave. The methods of making two points or three points linear or other similar qi—guiding methods are taken as the basic skills in training of the linear form emission of qi. Pushing, pulling, fixing, leading and other hand manipulations are generally adopted. Because patients vary in sensitivity to the longitudinal or transverse wave of qi flow, the therapist should try carefully to understand the influence of different waves on the patient during clinical practice. Qi emitted in linear form is relatively mild which often gives the patient a sensation of constriction, tugging, warmth, coldness, tingling and heaviness or cause the patient's spontaneous dynamic phenomenon. It is a basic form for inducing the channel qi, supplementing its deficiency and purging its excess.

This form requires the hand manipulations for emitting qi, i.e., pushing and pulling the hand in a longitudinal or transverse straight line, to be stable and slow, breathing to be deep and long and will to follow the movement of the hand.

Fixed Form: This is the most common qi form in which qi usually flows like spaced or dense waves or like a chain of pearls. It is carried out with vibrating and fixed qi-guiding method as the basic skills, and can be also conducted with various hand manipulations to form a combined qi-emitting complex with which, for example, qi emitted can flow in linear longitudinal successive waves. Emiting qi this way gives marked stimulation to the activities of qi in the channels, points and Dantian. The patient often has a sensation of quivering, hotness, tingling, radiation transmission and qi circulation and develops spontaneous involuntary dynamic phenomenon.

The method usually requires one to take an upright sitting posture or a horse stance and natural and slow respiration. With the waist as the axis and the abdomen as the pump, qi inside the body is made of vibrate and flow to the part of the hand where qi is emitted to the diseased part of the patient. Qi emitted flows like pearls, coming out one after another, or like spaced or dense successive waves. Will should follow the vibration of the qi flow and give guidance to its flowing direction.

It merits special attention that when one carries out fixed emission of qi, one must not hold his breath or make his hand vibrate by vibrating his muscles, otherwise stagnation of qi will occur, resulting in stuffiness in the chest, pain in the hypochondria, sharp pain in the arms as if there is fracture, or laceration of the muscles.

To have a good grasp of this qi—emitting method, one should first master the qi—vibrating method to ensure that qi is emitted naturally. Generally, one should do the exercises in the order of training qi (Double—Nine Yang Exercise), guiding qi (Pile—driving Vibrating Exercise) and hand manipulations. A good grasp of this method is no easy thing for though one can expect to have a basic grasp of it in 3 — 6 months if he perseveres in doing the exercises, he can not expect to apply it skillfully to clinical treatment with only 3 — 6 month's practice.

Spiral Form: It is developed from the method "guiding qi in spiralty". Qi emitted this way goes spirally (clockwise or counterclockwise) toward the affected area and penetrates deep into the body of the patient. Clinical application proves that it has special effective function in regulating qi activities, and most of the patients may get a feeling of qi penetration and that of light, sound and mild electric shock.

The emitting of qi is accompanied by natural respiration and spiral mind concentration. Qi starts whirling from the vortex in Dantian and moves in loops linked one with another to the part of the hand where it is emitted. The therapist should not begin to emit qi until he feels the whirling flow of it.

The learning of this skill needs not only constant practice of qi rotation in Dantian but also the synchronized qi rotation in Dantian and in a certain hand gesture. It is essential to cultivate a fixed conditioned reflex so that when qi in Dantian begins to rotate, it begins to whirl at the hand gesture simultaneously. Only then, can one start to apply the method to clinical treatment.

Chapter Seven   An Outline
of Treatment

Section One   Function and Principles
of Outgoing—qi Therapy

1. The Functions of Outgoing—qi Therapy

Because outgoing—qi (waiqi) therapy has a wide range o
indications which generally involves a variety of diseases of internal medicine, surgery, osteologic injury, pediatrics,obstetrics
and the five sense organs, its function is no doubt diversified.
Based on the features of outgoing—qi, its effect can be summarized as follows.

(1) The Reinforcing and Reducing Function

One of the basic principles in traditional Chinese medicine
is "to treat deficiency syndromes with tonification method and
excess syndromes with purgation and reduction". Tonification
means to supplement the insufficiency and strengthen the body
resistance while purgation and reduction means to reduce the
excess and expel the pathogenic evils. The final aim of the
methods is to balance yin and yang and regulate the physiological functions of the organism. outgoing—qi therapy is practised
in the light of the TCM philosophy in explanation of illnesses
concerning the zang and fu organs, yin and yang and deficiency
and excess. Qi is emitted to a certain part with the methods of
cold and heat guidance of qi and guidance of qi of the Five El-

ements together with manipulations such as pushing, pulling, rotating, leading, quivering and fixing, which, after a certain duration of emission, can produce the function of reinforcing the body resistance, replenishing the zang and fu organs and supplementing the mind and improving intelligence, to mention but a few. For example, for patients with insufficiency of qi in the Middle—jiao manifested by pale complexion and weakness of the extremities, linear guidance of qi and pushing, pulling and fixing manipulations can be taken to emit qi toward the points Zhongwan (Ren 12), Dantian and Pishu (UB 20) to produce the function of replenishing qi and reinforcing the Middle—jiao. Modern animal experiments have proved that outgoing—qi can improve the immunity of the animals markedly. The same result is observed in animal swimming tests, which shows that the animals which have received outgoing—qi have higher immunity level and better adaptive capability to adverse circumstances. All these fully explain the "tonifying" function of outgoing—qi.

Emission of qi with purgation and reduction methods can expel pathogenic evils. This includes two aspects. One is that outgoing—qi functions on the pathogenic factors (viruses, bacteria and other pathogenic agents) directly to expel them. A large amount of clinical and other kind of experiments have been done which have proved that outgoing—qi can kill the gram—positive and gram—negative bacteria and hepatitis B virus or suppress their reproduction. The other aspect is to expel pathogenic evils (the meaning of pathogenic here is different from the westen medical meanigs of viruses, bacteria and other agents), which is termed in TCM as "discharging morbid qi", meaning to dispel the pathogenic evils out of the body by way of channels and points with linear qi—guiding method and manipulations such as pulling and leading. This is a special approach different from the purgation with traditional medicines, acupuncture and massage (Tuina).

(2) The Function of Activating the Channel Qi

Under pathogenical conditions, qi of the viscera and channels may be weak and stagnated manifested by symptoms of listlessness, general asthenia or hypofunction of certain organs and tissues. This may be adjusted by outgoing—qi emitted with corresponding qi—guiding methods and hand manipulations, which can stimulate the qi activities and make qi active and circulatory continuously, so that the function of the viscera and tissues per se can be reinforced.In the case of weak and hypofunctional lung qi, guidance of metal—qi and pushing, quivering and leading manipulations can be adopted to emit qi so as to activate the lung—qi and make the channel qi flow freely over. This may improve the function of the lung. Experiment shows that when qi is emitted toward the heart of a toad, the heart rate of the toad may be slowed down and the ventricular systole time may be prolonged, resulting in decreased heart energy consumption and increased stroke output.

(3) The Function of Dredging the Channels and Allaying Pain

Stagnation of qi and stasis of blood will make the channels obstructed, and "obstruction of the channels may result in pain". Pain may also be caused by outside pathogenic factors, trauma, inflammation, muscular spasms, adhesive degeneration and other factors. In these circumstances, the virtue of outgoing—qi therapy, which usually needs pushing, pulling and leading manipulations, lies in dredging the channels, promoting blood circulation to remove stasis, relieving spasms and allaying pain. Determination of nail fold microcirculation proves that the number of capillary loops of nail fold of those who have received outgoing—qi increases, their blood circulation is speeded up and the circulation mode improved from indistinct to distinct. This explains the theory that outgoing—qi can promote blood circulation, remove blood stasis and dredge the channels. Experiments reveal that when qi is emitted toward the Oddi's sphincter of rabbit, the degree of tension of the sphincter is reduced, which facilitates the discharge of the bile and gallstones and alleviates pain and inflammation.

(4) The Function of Regulating Qi Activities

Every organ of the human body has its specific circulatory principle of qi (message). When the normal function of the organ is affected, the circulation of qi may be disturbed and the disturbance of qi in one organ may influence the functional balance of the whole qi system, even that of the whole body, outgoing— qi therapy in this case may help correct the qi disorder of the organ and further regulate the qi activities of the whole body to balance yin and yang and bring about recovery of the diseased part of the organ.

2. The Principles of Treatment

The principle of treatment in TCM is different from the method of treatment. It refers to the principle with universal instructive significance laid down for clinical cases in line with the basic TCM theory and the philosophy of Yiyi (Application of the Book of Changes to Medicine) and Qigong. Any one of the specific methods of treatment is confined by and pertain to a certain principle of treatment. It is of great significance to have a correct grasp of the principle of outgoing—qi therapy.

(1) Searching for the Primary Cause of Disease in Treatment

"Treatment must aim at the cause of the disease". This is one of the most fundamental principles of TCM in terms of differential diagnosis and treatment. Searching for the primary cause means to understand the nature of the disease and treatment is aimed at the most important etiological and pathological aspects of the diseases.In clinical treatment with outgoing—qi, the phrase means outgoing—qi treatment with certain qi—guiding methods, hand gestures and manipulations aimed at the most important aspect determined by overall and comprehensive analysis of all the data of the disease, which are sorted out from complex clinical symptoms and signs with the " four diagnostic methods". " the eight principal syndromes serving as guidelines in diagnosis" and "disease determination with outgoing—qi" in combination with some clinical examinations of modern medicine.

In clinical application of this principle, the extent of importance of the incidental and fundamental aspects of the disease must be determined so that the relationship between "routine treatment" and " treatment of a disease contrary to the routine" and that between " treatment aimed at etiology" and "treatment aimed at manifestations" can be handled correctly.

(2) Regulating Yin and Yang

The cause of a disease, fundamentally speaking, is the relative imbalance of yin and yang, and this imbalance may be manifested by various pathological changes, i.e., "the excess of yang brings about heat syndromes, the excess of yin brings about cold syndromes, the dificiency of yang causes cold syndromes, and the deficiency of yin results in heat syndromes". It is for this reason that the saying "treatment must aim at the cause of the disease and be based on the theory of yin and yang" has been given priority ever since the ancient times. In clinical outgoing—qi therapy, the prinple of "treating yin for yang disease and treating yang for yin disease" must be adhered to, and satisfactory curative effect can only be achieved when emphasis is put on regulting yin and yang all over the body including the organs and tissues to restore their balance.

(3) Strengthening the Body Resistance to Eliminate Pathogenic Factors

The course of the origination and development of a disease is in essence the process of the struggle between the body resistance and the pathogenic factors. During this process, if the vital energy of the body is sufficient for resisting the pathogenic evils, disease will not occur, otherwise pathogenic evils will get into the body causing illness. The same is explained in Neijing (Canon of Internal Medicine), which states: "Pathogenic evils can not invade into a person whose healthy energy is fully preserved" and "Whenever the body is exposed to the evils, deficiency of vital energy must be present". Therefore the final aim for treatment is to change the balance of force between the healthy and pathogenic factors, and by reinforcing the vital energy and eliminating the evils, to cure the disease . In outgoing—qi therapy, certain qi—guiding methods and qi—emitting manipulations as well as self Qigong exercise are adopted to strengthen the constitution and improve the body resistance so that the pathogenic evils can be expelled and the illness can be cured.

(4) Combining Qi Regulation with Strength Regulation

Diseases are usually caused by congenital and acquired disorders, stagnation and insufficiency of qi or by injuries of the organs and tissues.So in diagnosis and treatment with outgoing—qi, the first important thing is to find out whether the disease is due to qi disorder or due to organic disorder so that the main aspect of regulation, e.g., regulation mainly with outgoing—qi or that mainly with strength or the combination of the two, can be determined. For instance, in the treatment of lumber pain due to disorder of the small joint caused by external injuries, the therapist should first reposition the joint with strength produced through hand manipulations, and then remove qi stagnation resulting from the joint disorder by emission of outgoing qi, and only in this way satisfactory curative effect can be obtained. If the syndrome, for example, palpitation or abdominal distention, is caused by disorder of qi activities, regulation of qi activities through emission of outgoing—qi is enough to relieve the symptoms.

(5) Combining Outgoing—qi Therapy with Self Qigong Exercise

Because the regulation and activation of the patient's internal qi through emitting outgoing—qi are closely related to the patient's qi quality and mental status, the combination of outgoing—qi treatment by the therapist with qigong exercise by the patient himself is advised in order to ensure a better sensitivity to outgoing—qi by the patient and to make this sensitivity easy to synchronize with outgoing qi to achieve resonance in the treatment. In case of replenishing qi, better effect can be gained when the emission of outgoing–qi is carried out with the patient's cooperation in mind concentration and inspiration. While in case of expelling pathogenic evils with outgoing–qi, quick results can be achieved if the patient at the same time expels distractions, exhales and imagines that the pathogenic qi is being expelled from the point selected by the therapist for emission of outgoing–qi. It is more effective if the patient does self Qigong exercise in cooperation.

(6) Applying Treatment in Accordance with Seasonal Conditions, Local Conditions and the Physique of Individuals

Various aspects should be taken into consideration in treatment of a disease, as the origination and progress of the disease may be affected by many factors, such as the climatic variations with the four seasons, the geographical and environmental characteristics, the age, sex, physique, living habits and profession of the patient as well as his degree of sensitivity to outgoing–qi. To achieve the desirable curative effect, a carefull selection of the time, direction, qi–guiding methods, hand manipulations and qi forms is necessary.

Section Two   The Sensation and Effect of Qi

1. The Sensation of Qi

Sensation of qi is actually the response to qi by both Qigong therapist and patient during outgoing–qi therapy. A Qigong therapist can diagnose the disease of the patient and adjust the procedures of treatment according to his feeling as well as the patient's feeling of qi.

(1) The Sensation of Genuine Qi

The message of genuine qi is often manifested as a slightly warm, cold, tingling, constricting or dragging sensation, or that of the flow of qi. In most cases, the direction, density, nature and wave type of the genuine qi can be sensed. When the therapist receives the genuine qi, he may have a sensation of relaxation and comfort in the extremities.

(2) The Sensation of Turbid Qi

Dirtyy qi is also termed evil qi or pathogenic qi. The sensation of turbid qi is otherwise named "pathogenic message" acquired by the therapist during his emission of qi to the patient, which is different from pathogenic factors of infectious disease in modern medicine. According to clinical experience, the pathogenic message can be classified as:

Cold Feeling: The qi felt is especially cold. It may be so cold that when one gets such feeling of qi, his fingertips get cold immediately, and the coldness transmits from the fingertips upwards, causing even shivering and contraction of the sweat pores. This will give one a particular feeling of cold and discomfort. Cold feeling often serves as a message of deficiency and cold syndromes such as rheumatism, rheumatoid disease, deficiency of kidney—yang and cancer.

Feeling of Dryness—heat: The message of qi reacts on the body or the hands of the therapist who gets a feeling of dryness—heat which makes him fidgety as if he were near a fire and being scorched. It may serve as an indicator of syndromes of excessheat and hyperactivity of fire due to yin deficiency.

Feeling of Soreness and Numbness: The therapist may experience an uncomfortable feeling of local soreness or pain, heaviness, numbness and itching. The feeling of soreness and numbness often indicates syndromes of hyperactivity of the liver —yang and exuberance of the wind, cold, dampness or phlegm evil, arthralgia syndrome and cancer.

Feeling of turbidity : Such turbidity can be felt when the therapist is standing opposite the patient or when he is emitting qi towards the patient. It gives one an undescribable offensive feeling. It is often felt when the flat—palm hand gesture is used to detect a disease.

Other Kinds of Feeling: Other factors such as the seven emotions (joy, anger, melancholy, anxiety, grief, fear and terror) and the six climatic conditions (wind, cold, summerheat, dampness, dryness and fire) in excess will also cause illness. During detection and treatment of such illness, the therapist may feel these evils of different nature and response to them correspondingly. For example, he may have a special feeling of joy if the disorder of the patient is due to excessive joy.

After detection and treatment of diseases, the therapist must apply certain manipulations to prevent and expel the pathogenic qi, otherwise he himself may develop the symptoms of the illness of the patient in corresponding locations. For instance, if the patient has headache or pain in the hepatic area, the therapist may have a feeling of discomfort, numbness, itching or pain in his head and hepatic region too. So in clinical practice, a deep understanding and correct judgement of the pathogenic evils is compulsory.

2. The Effect of Qi

When a qigong therapist emits qi to treat patients, most of

the patients may get some effect of qi manifested as follows.

(1) Qi–sensitive Effect

When the therapist emits qi, some patients may gradually get the feeling of qi manifested as cold, hot, depressing, towing, creeping, tingling, heavy, light, floating, sinking, distending and aching. This represents a kind of qi– sensitive effect occurring when qi circulates in the channels and acts on the affected area to reach the focus. The most commom sensation of qi is cold, hotness, depressing, towing and tingling. Our experience in clinical practice shows that 60 – 70% of the patients may get the sensation of qi after one or several times of treatment.

(2) Photoelectric Effect

On receiving outgoing–qi, some patients may get some photoelectric effect manifested by a sensation of electric shock in the extremities. Others may see photopictures of different shapes, most of which are circular, patchy or lightening–like.

(3) Sound Effect

Some patients may hear some kinds of sound when they receive outgoing–qi, such as " la–la" , " long–long" or "zhi–zhi".

(4) Smell Effect

Some patients may smell a special odor on receiving outgoing–qi. The odor usually varies with individuals. It may be the fragrance of sandalwood or that of flowers.

(5) Dynamic Effect

When the therapist emits qi, the patient may immediately or gradually show dynamic phenomenon— — spontaneous movement of a certain part of the extremities or of the whole body, or muscular tremers, contraction and stiffness or movements of the extremities in large amplitude. The phenomenon is known as spontaneous moving Qigong activated and induced by outgoing—qi.

Clinical myoelectric tests on part of our patients shows that the myoelectric potential of those having dynamic effect on the muscles or muscular groups is more than double that of those who contract their muscles voluntarily.

Clinical observations on more than 400 cases have demonstrated that 2—3% of the patients developed the phenomenon of dynamic effect on the muscles and extremities.

The above—mentioned are the common phenomena of qi effect, of which phenomenon of qi—sensitive effect occurs most frequently, dynamic phenomenon occurs in a few patients and other phenomena occur rarely. Some patients may get no qi—sensitive effect at all yet can get the same curative effect.

The phenomenon of effect of qi represents a special dynamic state of the sense or other organs of the patients who have received outgoing—qi. It is rather a factor that decides the sensitivity of a certain organ or the tissues of the patient than the pure therapeutic effect produced by qi working on the diseased site. Some patients may show no apparant effect of qi but recover very quickly after several courses of treatment and gain sensation of qi gradually. Some may have no marked therapeutic effect though they show strong qi effect. This is indeed a rather complicated and mysterious problem which awaits further studies.

Annex: The Phenomenon of Syncope Induced by Qi

A few patients may sweat all over with faster heart rate and dizziness followed by syncope as can be seen in fainting during acupuncture when they are under outgoing–qi treatment or have received qi while waiting for treatment.Some patients may get syncope as well although they may have no apparent sensation of qi and dynamic phenomenon. In this case the therapist should make the patients lie supine, unbutton the collar and carry out digital pressing on Baihui (Du 20), Mingmen (Du 4), Jianjing (G B 21) and Yintang (Extra 1), and grasping manipulation on Jianjing (G B 21), Quchi (L I 11), Hegu (L I 4) Chengshan (U B 57) and Taichong (Liv 3), followed by guiding qi to flow along the Ren and Du Channels and then back to its origin (Dantian). The patients can recover quickly this way.

In some patients, illness may improve markedly after the syncope induced by activation of qi. The therapist should then take advantage of this to carry out regulatory treatment to gain better results. Discontinuation of treatment because of syncope should be avoided lest the good opportunity for regulation and treatment by outgoing–qi be missed. However he should not try to pursue such phenomenon. Close observation is required during treatment to ensure sufficient emission of qi with no induction of syncope.

Section Three　　The Discharge of Turbid Qi

Su Wen – Yi Pian Ci Fa Lun (Plain Questions – The Unpublished Issue on Acupuncture) states: "To enter the room of an infectious case,one should firstly imagine that the green qi comes out from the liver, flows leftwards toward the east and turns wood, then imagine that the white qi comes out from the lung, flows rightwards to the west and becomes metal, then imagine that the red qi comes out from the heart, flows upwards to the south and becomes fire, then imagine that the black qi comes out from the kidney, flows downwards towards the north and becomes water, and lastly imagine that the yellow qi comes out from the spleen, gathers in the centre and becomes earth. When the protection of the body with the Five Elements is done, one can imagine that there is a sparkling light like the Big Dipper above his head. Then one can enter the room of the patient, safe and protected". This is a method adopted in *Nei Jing (Canon of Internal Medicine)* of application of will to guiding qi of the five zang—organs (solid organs), making qi substantial and leading qi back to its origin to prevent invasion by pathogenic qi. During emission of qi, the filthy (pathogenic) qi from the patient is easy to, by chance of qi emission, enter the body of the therapist and interfere with his qi circulation. This pathogenic message may also be transmitted into the body of normal people or other patients. However, those who have not practised Qigong and whose qi circulation is not yet so smooth, the points not open and the exchanges of qi in and outside the body not good, are not prone to the interference of this message because they have a natural "barrier", or they are not sensitive to the message because the degree of sensitivity of their mentality (perceptive ability) is poor; while those who are experienced in Qigong can percieve and differentiate all kinds of qi message because of their strong perceptive ability. So whenever the pathogenic turbid qi enters their body, they may sense it.

When the turbid qi enters the body, it will interfere with

the normal qi circulation, causing disorders in part of or the whole qi circulatory system. In mild cases, qi may stagnate in a certain part (e.g., shoulder, arm, chest, back), causing tingling pain, cold, contraction, heaviness, soreness and distention and stuffiness in the chest; or may interfere with the mental activity causing dizziness, headache, heaviness in the head, vexation and restlessness. In severe cases, the victim may for some time have all the symptoms the patient has yet positive signs can not be detected on physical examination. Vigilance should be aroused in those who develop the symptoms of the patient after they perceive the turbid qi.

It is very important for a doctor who treats patients with outgoing—qi to possess the ability to prevent and expel the turbid qi so that it can rarely or can not at all disturb his qi activities. Damage of qi activities is often seen in those who treat patients with outgoing qi after they have gained some qigong knowledge with no experience, even in those who are veteran in Qigong practice, and the interference of turbid qi is often an important factor of the damage.

When a therapist perceives the interference by turbid qi, he must expel it with proper hand manipulations and readjust his own qi activities. If the dirty qi invades into his fingers, or into a certain channel or certain points, he should guide qi by will to the points, the channel and the fingers and then relax locally and quiver the hands to discharge the turbid qi while exhaling

The therapist should be able to stop the turbid qi before it reaches Dazhui (Du 14) at the back, Tianzhu (Ren 22) and Quepen (St 12) in the front and Fengfu (Du 16) and Fengchi (G B 20) in the superior. The proper way is to expel it when it has just reached the fingers, wrists, elbows and at most the shoulders.

If the therapist is not able enough to expel the turbid qi at the right time because he is not skilled or his internal qi is not substantial, the turbid qi may enter his body by way of finger to wrist and then elbow, or from Baihui (Du 20), Tanzhong (Ren 17), Fengchi (G B 20), Yintang (Extra 1) and Yongquan (K 1) and cause adverse reactions. At this time, the therapist should not persist in emission of qi but should close it with normal procedures and expel the turbid qi by turning the wrist, rubbing the hands and face and moving the shoulders until he feels no discomfort. If the turbid qi can not yet be discharged, he should practise Qigong exercises to regulate his qi activities first and then he may succeed in expelling turbid qi.

Section Four   Outgoing—Qi Diagnosis

In outgoing—qi therapy, the diagnosis is confirmed based on the comprehensive analysis of the data gained with the four TCM diagnostic methods (inspection, auscultation, interrogation and palpation) and the eight principles (yin and yang, exterior and interior, cold and heat and deficiency and excess) and based on the detection of diseases by outgoing—qi which usually reveals the intensity, density and circulating direction of the healthy qi as well as the intensity and nature of the pathogenic qi. Then curative measures can be taken in terms of determination of the channels and points to emit qi toward, the qi—guiding methods, hand gestures and manipulations and treatment procedures.

1. Methods of Disease Detection with Outgoing-qi

There are a variety of methods concerning the diagnosis of diseases by induction of qi between the therapist and the patient and by specific physiological functions, such as perspective, remote sensing, hand detection and physical (body) observation.

(1) Flat-palm Detection (Hand Sensing Method)

There is a qi field around everybody, and when certain organs and tissues are affected, changes will take place in the corrresponding regions of the qi field around the body surface. Detection of the changes with the palm for diagnosis is termed flat-palm detection.

The following is the procedure of flat-palm detection: Ask the patient to take a standing, upright sitting or lying posture and set the whole body relaxed, mind concentrated and breath natural. Position the palm 10 − 100 centimeters from the patient with the Inner Laogong (P 8) or the fingertips facing the patient's body surface. Emit qi faintly and then conduct slow pushing, pulling and leading manipulations to detect qi of the patient from, firstly, the upper and lower, left and right and anterior and posterior aspects , and then from the body surface of the corresponding regions of the internal organs and tissues. Make comparisons between the sensations gained in different places to find out the part where qi is felt abnormal and decide the nature of it. Analyze the sensations on the basis of the relationship between the eight principles (yin and yang, exterior and interior, cold and heat, deficiency and excess) and the Yao image (yin and yang lines) and the parts, internal organs and the healthy and pathogenic factors to deduce the location, nature and severity of the disease.

For example, a great difference in intensity of qi between the two sides of the Stomach Channel of Foot—Yangming in the anterior aspect of the body means the imbalance of qi circulation between the left and right side. The deficiency and cold syndrome of the spleen and stomach may be manifested by a cold and contracted sensation in the epigastric region.

The location and nature such as pathogenic or healthy, cold or heat, deficiency or excess and so forth can be expressed by the six Yao image (yin and yang lines) which constitute the sixty—four diagrams (hexagrams). Specifically, the hexagram Qian ☰ (the 1st of the sixty—four hexagrams; yang lines) symbolizes the qualities of the yang aspects——male, fu—organs (hollow organs),positive and so forth;Kun ☷ symbolizes the opposite qualities——female, zang—organs (solid organs), negative, etc. This principle is used to indicate the status of qi equilibrium. Then the symbol "○" is used to symbolize the qi sensation in or around the body, which, with the symbol "−"(taken as the diaphragm) added to it, indicates the region of the chest and abdomen; with the symbol" | "at its top on the middle, indicates the head; with " = " added to each of its sides,indicating the upper and lower limbs. In this way,the position of the three Yao at the head, three at the chest and abdomen, three at the lower limbs and three at the upper limbs are illustrated clearly. Then words such as male, female, zang—organs or fu—organs are written below the related one of the six hexagrams like Qian and Kun to express the qualities of the diagram in terms of male, female, zang—organs, fu—organs and the parts of the body.

The location and the nature of qi detected with outgoing—qi are expressed with the moving lines of the six hexagrams,of which the position of the lines symbolizes the specific part or organs of the body, and the principle of the lines (yin or yang) symbolizes the attributes as to whether they are pathogenic or healthy, negative or positive. To add "+", "++" and "+++" inside "○" indicates the extent of the healthy qi in terms of weak, moderate, strong; while to add "−", "=" and "≡" in "○" indicates the extent of pathogenic qi in terms of mild, moderate and severe. And when the above symbols are added on the right of the moving lines (the lines corresponding with the parts or organs where qi is sensed), they express the nature of qi (pathogenic or healthy) and its extent.

For instance, moderate extent of densified and cold qi is detected at the surface of the thoracic region of a male patient. As Qian represents male and the 5th Yao line correspondes to the thoracic region, the nine—five line of Qian ䷀ hexagram moves to the position of six—five (yang turns into yin because cold means yin) and the hexagram becomes Dayou ䷍. So ䷍ should be recorded and then "○" should be drawn below it to express that the record is taken with six Yao lines as a whole, and " = " should be drawn to the right of the six—five line to express that the pathogenic qi detected is moderate. If moderately dense and dry—hot pathogenic qi is detected in this patient, the record should be taken with the same method except that the nine—five line remains unmoved as the original Qian hexagram, which means that the pathogenic evil at the nine—five region is of yang nature and is moderate. The method may also be used to record the results of qi detection at the

3rd Yao of the upper limbs and of the head, the 3rd Yao of the abdomen—chest and the head, the 3rd Yao of the lower limbs and the abdomen—chest or the results detected on the right and left and at the anterior and posterior aspects of the body based on the six Yao lines. Again, strong dry—heat, densified, aching and distending qi is detected at the hepatic region or at the related points of a female patient. As Kun represents female and the six—three line matches with the liver, the six—three line of the Kun hexagram ☷ ☷ moves to the position of the nine— three Yao and the hexagram becomes Qian ☰ ☷ (the 15th of the sixty—four hexagrams). After this is taken, the word "female" is written below the hexagram to show the sex and " ☰ " drawn to the right of the nine—three line to indicate the severe extent of pathogenic yang (yang Yao).

(2) Body Detection Based on Biological Correspondence

According to the law of bio—hologram, a bit of qi of the patient may be a message of the whole qi system. When the therapist receives a little amount of qi of the patient and infuses it through out his body, he may get some abnormal feelings in the locations that correspond to that of the patient, the feelings by which he judges the location and nature of diseases.

The following is the procedure of this method: Stand facing the patient. Emit qi by will toward the Baihui (Du 20) point of the patient and infuse it from Baihui (Du 20) to Yongquan (K 1). Then lead qi from the patient's Yongquan (K 1) to yours and guide it to flow upward to your Baihui (Du 20) to form one circulatory cycle of qi between you and the patient. Then infuse qi of this cycle throughout your body and try to feel the reaction of it carefully. The locality where you have abnormal feelings and the feature of the feelings are representative of the locality and nature of the illness that the patient suffers from. The versed therapist may emit qi out of his Laogong (P 8) of one hand toward a certain point of the patient, and accept qi with Laogong (P 8) of another hand and infuse it all over the body to make the diagnosis.

(3) Hand Diagnosis, Foot Diagnosis and Ear Diagnosis

The law of bio-hologram holds that one part of the body contains the message of the whole (including various parts, the viscera, qi and blood), and the local message may reflect the condition of the whole body. Such parts may include the hand, foot, eye, nose, ear, face, etc. The locations on these parts that represent the other different parts and organs are termed as points or zones, or respectively, as hand points (Fig. 7—1), foot points (Fig. 7—2), ear points (Fig. 7—3) and so forth.

The following is their procedure: Take the diagnosis through hand points as an example. The therapist first swings his hands or rubs one of his hands with which he is going to detect diseases gently with another to get its sensitivity even; then he leads qi of the patient by will into the palm, spreads qi over it (concentration on one point should be avoided) and try carefully to sense the reaction of the patient's illness on his palm. He may then get some kinds of special sensation at the points on his palm, which indicates the location of the diseases of the patient. The different sensations such as distention, heaviness, numbness, hotness, itching and throbbing correspond with the feature of the diseases the patient suffers from.

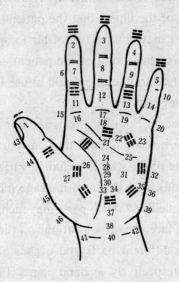

Fig. 7-1   An Illustration of Points for Hand Diagnosis

1.spleen—earth   2.liver—wood   3.heart—fir   4.lung—metal
5.kidney—water   6 / 13 / 26 / 35.large intestine   7.left brain
8.brain   9.right brain   10 / 12 / 31.small intestine
11.gallbladder   14 / 37.urinary bladder   15.left shoulder
16.left cheek   17.nose   18.mouth   19.right cheek
20.right shoulder   21.stomach   22.left lung   23.right lung
24.the whole body   25.heart   27.vitality / mentality   28.navel
29.veneral diseases   30.uterus   32.elbow   33.left kidney
34.right kidney   36.knee   38.reproductive organs   39.hip
40.waist   41.left lower limb   42.right lower limb
43.the back of the head   44.cervical vertebra   45.chest
46.sacrolumbar region

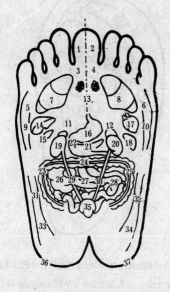

Fig. 7-2　An Illustration of Points for Foot Diagnosis

1 / 2.head　3 / 4.thyroid gland　5 / 6.shoulder　7 / 8.lung

9 / 10.elbow joint　11 / 12.adrenal gland　13.spine　14.liver

15.gallbladder　16.stomach　17.heart　18.spleen　19 / 20.kidney

21.pancreas　22.duodenum　23 / 24 / 25.large intestine

26 / 27 / 28. small intestine　29 / 30.urine duct　31 / 32.knee cap

33 / 34.thigh　35.urinary bladder　36.right foot　37.left foot

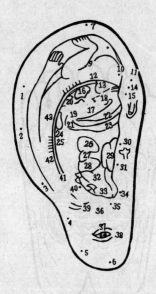

Fig. 7−3   An Illustration of Points for Ear Diagnosis

1−6.helix   7.ear apex   8.uterus   9.Shenmen (H 7)of Hand−
Shaoyin   10.sympathetic nerve   11.external reproductive organ
12.sacrolumbar vertebra   13.urinary bladder   14.urinary tract
15.the lower segment of rectum   16.kidney   17.small intestine
18.large intestine   19.duodenum   20.gallbladder   21.stomach
22.diaphragm   23.esophagus 24.liver   25.spleen   26 / 28.lung
27.heart   29.trachea   30.antilobium apex   31.adrenal gland
32.thyroid gland   33.endocrime system   34 / 35.eye   36.tongue
37.eye   38.cheek   39.teeth   40.Pingchuan (Extra)   41.subcortical
system   42.cervical vertebra   43.thoracic vertebra

Alternatively, the therapist may ask the patient to get breathe evenly, concentrated and turn one of his palms upward while keeping it relaxed. He then moves his index or middle finger (5 − 10 cm off the patient's palm) gently from one hand point of the patient to another. The point where he gets the special feeling represents the location of diseases of the patient, and different feelings represent different features of the disorders.

Another method is to make the diagnosis while the patient is waiting to see the doctor. The therapist leads the patient's qi ·by will to his own hand, foot or ear to feel the reaction on the points to make diagnosis.

(4) Diagnosis by Observing Qi

Ask the patient to take a sitting or standing posture with the whole body relaxed, breath even, distractions expelled and mind concentrated on the location of his disorder. Observe with the naked eyes the space within 30 cm radius around te patient while concentrating the mind on the Upper Dantian. Then transparent or opaque qi flow or mass of different density and colour (red, white, yellow, green, blue, black, etc.) may be observed, which may be taken as the basis for determination of the location and feature of diseases.

(5) Detection by Will

It refers to diagnosis through observation of the image of the patient by will. The therapist firstly observes the image of the patient as a whole, then imagines a sketch picture of the patient in mind and further imagines his interior. If the part or organ that the therapist imagines is darkish or gives him a feeling of turbibness, it will be the location of diseases.

The sense of smell, the sense of taste, straight perspective and remote sensing are also useful diagnostic techniques. The points and zones for diagnosis are also indicated in emission of qi or in stimulation by pressing, kneading and needling.

2. Differentiation of Symptoms and Signs

Generally, hectic fever, flaccidity, perspiration, vexation and so forth are included in the yang and heat syndromes; chills, contracture or rigidity and stagnation are included in the yin and cold syndromes. Deficiency syndrome is manifested by contracted, numb and weak feeling of qi; excess syndrome by distending, turbid, outflowing, tingling and densified qi. Soreness and distention are indicators of swelling due to external injury. Lightness and superficiality reveal exterior syndrome while heaviness and deepness suggest interior syndrome. Turbidity flowing with the course of channel means transmission of pathogenic qi to the interior which should be prevented in time, and that flowing against the course of channel means the initial generation of pathogenic qi. Thinness indicates insufficiency; denseness means accumulation of pathogenic qi or stagnation of qi. Knottiness and sluggishness represent stagnation of qi and stasis of blood. Disorderliness indicates disorder of qi activities. The feeling of joy, anger, anxiety, sorrow or fright means that the pathogenic factors of the patient have influence on others.

Qi of diffe rent viscera have different colours. The heart—qi is red, lungqi white, spleen—qi and stomach—qi yellowish green, liver—qi green, gallbladder— qi blue, and kidney—qi dark purple. Qi of the healthy organ is clear, lucid and clean while that of the diseased organs darkish, grey and turbib. Whether an organ is disordered and the extent of disorder may right be revealed by these colours of qi.

The diagnosis of diseases with outgoing—qi must be combined with the four diagnostic methods of TCM (inspection, auscultation and olfaction,interrogation, and pulse feeling and palpation) as well as modern techniques using instrument Detection of qi may reveal the general conditions of genuine qi, pathogenic qi and other approximation , which can only be taken as one aspect in diagnosis of a disease. Comprehensive analysis of all the data acquired with various techniques should not be neglected. Deliberate mystification of the detection of diseases by the use of outgoing—qi alone may lead to forfeiture of the chance for treatment.

Section Five   The Number of Times Required for Treatment

The number of times required for treatment or for emission of outgoing—qi is often calculated in respiratory cycles. One option is the duration of time.

1. The Number of Yin and Yang

The therapeutic dose required for regulation of yin and yang, expressed as number of respiratory cycles, is calculated on the basis of the number of Yin or yang channels (or the yin and yang aspect of diseases) matching with the number of yin and yang related to the River Chart, the Five Elements, the Luo River Graph and the Acquired Eight Diagrams. For example, the number of yang is used to calculate the respiratory cycles for tonification or purgation of the yang channels; the number of yin for that of the yin channels. Table 7—1 provides a general basis for calculation.

Table 7—1 The Number of Yin and Yang

	Initial	Young	Old
Yang	9	$27(3 \times 9)$ or $49(7 \times 7)$	$81(9 \times 9)$
Yin	6	$18(3 \times 6)$ or $36(6 \times 6)$	$64(8 \times 8)$

2. The Number Related to the River Chart and the Five Elements

The number in the River Chart and the Five Elements is described as: " Heaven—one generates water and results in Earth—six; Earth—two generates fire and results in Heaven—seven; Heaven—three generates wood and results in Earth—eight; Earth—four generates metal and results in Heaven—nine; and Heaven—five generates earth and results in Earth—ten". One, two, three, four and five are the generating numbers of yin and yang of the Five Elements while six, seven, eight, nine and ten are those of resultant numbers of yin and yang. The number of respiratory cycles required for treatment of disorders of the five viscera comes from the multiplication of the resultant numbers (the base numbers) by their multiples. This approach is mainly applied to disorders related to the interpromotion and interconstraint of the Five Elements,or to put it differently, to whether the mother—organ should be tonified or the child—organ should be purged (Table 7—2).

Table 7—2   The Generating and Resultant Numbers Related to the River Chart and the Five Elements

Five Elements	Water	Fire	Wood	Metal	Earth
Generating Number	one	two	three	four	five
Resultant Number	six	seven	eight	nine	ten
Five Viscera	kidney	heart	liver	lung	spleen

3. The Number Related to Acquired Eight Diagrams and the Luo River Graph

It refers to the number of the respiratory cycles required for treatment of the disorders of the five viscera, which comes from the numbers in the Acquired Eight Diagrams and the Luo River Graph in combination with those of the Five Elements and their attributing viscera. This approach is mainly used in the interrestraint between the Five Elements and the viscera (Table 7—3).

Table 7—3   The Number Related to the Acquired Eight Diagrams and the Luo River Graph

Eight Diagrams	Qian	Kan	Gen	Zhen	Xun	Li	Kun	Dui
Orientation	north-west	north	north-east	east	south-east	south	south-west	west
Five Elements	metal	water	earth	wood	wood	fire	earth	metal
Viscera	Large intestine	kidney, urinary bladder	stomach	gall-bladder	liver	heart, small intestine	spleen	lung
Numbers in Luo River graph	6	1	8	3	4	9	2&5	7

4. The Length of the Channels and the Respiratory Cycles

This calculation may be taken as a reference in treatment, mainly concerning with the conduction and activation of the circulation of the channel qi. During one respiratory cycle (one inhalation, one exhalation), the channel qi flows about 6 cun (Table 7—4).

Table 7–4   The Length of the Channels and
the Number of the Respiratory Cycles

Channels	Length (in chi)	Respiratory Cycles Required	Ourflow of Qi over the Length of Channels (in cun)
The Three Yang Channels of Hand	5	9	4
The Three Yang Channels of Foot	8	14	4
The Three Yin Channels of Hand	3.5	6	1
The Three Yin Channels of Food	6.5	11	1
The Du & Ren Channels	4.5(each)	8	3

The above–mentioned number of treatment times is expressed in number of respiratory cycles for emission of outgoing–qi. Clinically, it should be decided based on the location of the diseases and on the nature of them (yin or yang, deficiency or excess, and exterior or interior) to ensure sufficient therapeutic dose. For example, diseases due to deficiency of yin should be treated with tonification method by emitting qi for 6, 18 or 64 respiratory cycles; deficiency of lung–metal should be treated by replenishing the mother–organ spleen–earth, with emission of qi for 10 respiratory cycles; adverse flowing of yang–qi due to excess of liver–wood should be suppressed by emitting qi for 7 respiratory cycles; and stagnation of qi or deranged flow of qi in the Lung Channel of Hand–Taiyin should be corrected by emitting qi for 6 respiratory cycles or the mul-

tiple of 6 defined by the yin channels. However, clinical treatment calls for determination of all this in the light of the facts;
flexibility is advisable. Rigid adherence to the formalities
should be avoided.

Section Six   The Tonification, Purgation, Regulation and Guidance and the Closing Form of Treatment

1. Tonification and Purgation

To reinforce the deficiency and reduce the excess is a radi-
cal curative measure used in every field of TCM. In
outgoing–qi therapy, satisfactory effect can be anticipated only
when the doctor adheres to the principle of " treating
asthenia–syndrome with tonification, sthenia–syndrome with
purgation and non–asthenia–non–sthenia syndrome with regulation along the channels". Introduced here are the major
methods of tonification and purgation adopted in outgoing–qi
therapy.

(1) Tonification and Purgation with Respiration

This is a definition in which tonification and purgation are
classified according to which respiration methods (exhalation
or inhalation) the therapist adopts in emission of qi.
Tonification means that the therapist exhales when he guides
his own qi and emits it into the channels, points and the internal organs and tissues of the patient, purgation meaning that
he inhales when he guides and emits qi to lead qi of the patient
to flow following that of the therapist or pull the pathogenic
evils out of the body of the patient. During treatment, the pa-

tient should cooperate with the therapist by means of respiration. He should first assume a proper posture, expel distractions, relax all over and concentrate the mind on the location which the therapist will emit qi to. When the therapist exhales and emits qi toward him (tonification), he should inhale to take in the therapist's qi naturally from the designated location, and when the therapist does the opposite (purgation), he should exhale to get qi out in the same way.

(2) Tonification and Purgation with Emission of Qi along and against the Course of the Channels

Zhen Jiu Da Cheng(*A Complete Works in Acupuncture and Moxibustion*) states, " The classics say that puncturing along the direction of the channels yields tonifying effect,while going against it induces purgation". This is also a principle of outgoing-qi therapy, i.e., emitting and guiding qi along the course of the Fourteen Channels means tonifying, and against them, reducing. In TCM, the Three Yang Channels of Hand run from the hands to the head, the Three Yin Channels of Hand from the chest to the hands, the Three Yang Channels of Foot from the head to the feet, and the Three Yin Channels of Foot from the feet to the abdomen and chest. So the deficiency and excess of the Twelve Regular Channels can be readjusted according to the course of them, while that of the Two Extra Channels——the Ren Channel and the Du Channel can be done according to the course of the "small circle of qi" described in qigong exercises.

During treatment, the patient should assume a proper posture, relax the whole body, expel distractions, concentrate his mind on the manipulations of the therapist and regulate his breath to cooperate with the treatment by exhaling qi toward the focus of the disease mentally.

(3) Tonification and Purgation with Rotative Hand Manipulations

According to the attributes of yin and yang, the upper part of the body is yang and the lower is yin; the left is yang and the right yin; the back is yang and the abdomen yin. But concerning sex, there is some difference in circulation of qi, blood, yin and yang: in male, the left is yang, the right yin; the back is yang and the abdomen yin; while in female, the right is yang and the left yin; the abdomen yang and the back yin. In short, male and female have three pairs of yin and yang each , which determine the difference in turning clockwise and counterclockwise for tonification and purgation.

As for the direction of rotation, for a male, making cycles with the hand against the trunk from the top to the left and bottom to the right following yang is tonification, and the opposite direction against yang and along with yin is purgation; and for a female, making circles from the top to the right and bottom to left along with yang is tonification and the opposit against yang and along with yin is purgation. And because the body gathers yang—qi from the extremities and yin—qi from the five zang—organs, and the outside is yang and inside is yin, guiding qi from outside into inside means tonification, and vice versa, purgation.

2. Regulation and Guidance

Regulation is a uniform reinforcing—reducing technique which is applicable to asthenia—sthenia syndromes (asthenia accompanied with sthenia or vice versa) to readjust the deficiency and excess of yin and yang. If qi goes adversely upward densely, the therapist should guide it downward. The same principle is applicable to the deficiency or excess of qi in the left or right side of the body. Regulation also includes purgation after tonification and vice versa.

The method of guidance is used when stagnation of qi and stasis of blood or disorders of the channel qi develop, to, by guiding manipulations, regulate the channel qi and dredge the channels and collaterals to facilitate qi circulation or lead qi back to its origin.

3. The Closing Form of Treatment

(1) The Closing Form for the Patient

When the therapist emits qi to the patient, the patient will respond as if he himself were doing the exercises. So when the treatment is over, the therapist should relax the patient by restoring the patient's qi back to its origin by means of hand manipulations such as finger—pressing, tapping, percussing, rubbing and rocking, as the condition of the patient requires.

(2) The Closing Form for the Therapist

To stop emitting qi, the therapist should direct his qi slowly back to Dantian and draw his hands back from the patient (resume the hands from the qi—emitting gesture), and then readjust his mind, breathing and posture properly, relax all over and get the genuine qi to its origin. If he is affected by pathogenic qi, he should first expel it and then carry out the readjustment.

Chapter Eight   Treatment of Diseases

Section One   Internal Syndromes

Common Cold

Etiology

1.Wind—Cold Syndrome Due to Exogenous Evils

The Wind—cold usually enters by way of the body surface, and because the skin and body hair are connected with the lung, it may cause failure of the lung to keep the lung—energy pure and descendant and obstruction of the sweat pores, resulting in wind—cold syndrome.

2. Wind—Heat Syndrome Due to Exogenous Evils

The Wind—heat usually enters the body by way of the mouth and nose, and because the nose is the orifice to the lung, it may also cause failure of the lung to keep the lung—energy pure and descendant and failure of the sweat pores to expel pathogenic evils, resulting in wind—heat syndromes.

Symptoms

1. Wind—Cold Syndrome Due to Exogenous Evils

Severe aversion to cold, slight fever or absence of fever, headache, soreness and pain in the extremities, nasal obstruction with discharge, low—voice speaking, itching of the throat, cough with thin and clear phlegm, pale tongue with thin coating and tense, superficial pulse. Detection with flat—palm hand gesture reveals a sensation of dense, cold and obstructed qi around the head and imbalance of qi between the upper and the lower and the left and right aspects of the body.

2. Wind—heat Syndrome Due to Exogenous Evils

Severe fever, slight aversion to cold, headache, sweating, sore throat, cough with yellowish thick phlegm, thin, white or slightly yellow tongue coating and rapid, superficial pulse. Detection with flat—palm reveals dense, hot and tingling sensation of qi around the head and apparent imbalance of qi between the upper and the lower or the left and the right aspects of the body.

Treatment

1. Emission of Outgoing—Qi (Waiqi)

(1) With the patient sitting, pinch and knead Yintang (Extra 2), Kangong (Extra) and dig—grasp Quchi (LI 11) and Hegu (LI 4) to open up the points and normalize the functional activities of qi. Assume the flat—palm gesture and pushing and pulling manipulations to emit qi toward Yintang (Extra 1) and Taiyang (Extra 2). Then use pulling and leading manipulations to guide qi to flow downward along the Ren Channel and the Stomach Channel of Foot—Yangming to both feet, 3 – 7 times are sufficient for expelling the wind—cold or wind—heat out from the feet.

(2) Press and knead Fengfu (Du 16),Dazhui (Du 14),Fengmen (UB 12) and Feishu (UB 13). Emit qi toward Dazhui (Du 14), Fengmen (UB 12) and Feishu (UB 13) with flat—palm gesture and pushing—pulling manipulation. Then guide qi to flow downward along the Urinary Bladder Channel

of Foot—Taiyang with pulling and guiding manipulations to kake the functional activities of qi balanced.

(3) Lastly, press and knead Fengchi (GB 20), Dazhui(Du 14) and Fengmen(UB 12), dig—grasp Quchi (LI 11) and Hegu (LI 4) and shake the two upper limbs to end the emission of qi.

Modification: In the case of wind—cold syndrome, add heat qi—guiding method to emit qi to Fengmen (UB 12) and Dazhui (Du 14) and guide qi downward along the Urinary Bladder Channel of Foot—Taiyang to facilitate the qi activities of the patient; in case of wind—heat syndrome, add cold qi—guiding method to emit qi to Feishu (UB 13), Dazhui (Du 14), Fengchi (GB 20) and guide qi to flow along the Stomach Channel of Foot—Yangming to facilitate qi activities; for patients with- nasal obstruction, add middle—finger—propping hand gesture and quivering manipulation to emit qi to Yingxiang (LI 20) and Shangen (Radix Nasi) for 9 respiratory cycles; and for those with cough, chest stuffiness and abundant phlegm, add flat—palm or sword—fingers hand gesture and quivering manipulation to emit qi to Shanzhong (Ren 17), Zhongfu (Lu 1) and Yunmen (Lu 2) for 8 respirotary cycles.

2. Qigong—Acupuncture

Insert the filiform needles into Taiyang (Extra 1), Quchi (LI 11) and Hegu (LI 4), then apply the dragon—mouth hand gesture and pushing, pulling and leading manipulations to emit qi to the points and guide qi to Hegu (LI 4).

3. Self Qigong Exercise as Accessory Treatment

(1) Daoyin Exercise for Expelling Pathogenic Wind from the Body Surface (Qufeng Jiebiao Daiyin Gong)

Take the upright sitting posture. Relax all over, close the

eyes slightly, expel distractions and breathe naturally.

Pushing the Forehead: Put the index, middle and ring fingers of both hands close to each other and push the forehead with them from the midpoint of the two eyebrows straight upward to the front hairline 24 − 50 times, then push from the midpoint of the forehead sidewards 24 − 50 times. Push with more force while exhaling and less while inhaling. Try to feel the flowing of qi beneath the hands while pushing.

Kneading−Motioning Taiyang (Extra 2): Put the middle fingers against the point Taiyang (Extra 2) and press and knead−motion them counterclockwise 24 − 50 times.

Sweeping the Gallbladder Channel: Put the four fingers close to each other and curve them slightly. Scrape with the fingertips along the Gallbladder Channel from above the ears backwards via the frontal angle of the forehead towards the back of the head 5 − 10 times.

Bathing the Nose: Rub the dorsal sides of the thumbs against each other till they are hot. Rub with them the sides of the nose gently up and down. Rub 5 times during each inspiration and each expiration for altogether 9 respiratory cycles.

(2) Diaphoretic Exercise by Holding the Head (Pannao Fahan Gong)

Sit cross−legged on bed. Put the hands on the region of Fengfu (Du 16) and Fengchi (GB 20) at the lower part of the occipital bone with the fingers interlocked, and rub for 9 respiratory cycles. Then with hands holding the back of the head, bend forward until the head reaches the bed. Set the body straight and restart the whole procedure till sweat is reduced.

Cough

Etiology

1. Cough Due to Exogenous Evils

It is often caused by invasion of the lung by exogenous pathogenic factors. The wind—cold or wind—heat as pathogenic factors usually invades the body surface externally and injuries the lung internally, causing obstruction of the lung—qi and impairment of the purifying and descending function of the lung, resulting in cough.

2. Cough Due to Internal Injury

Apart from lesions of the lung itself, it is often involved in diseases of other internal organs. For instance, dysfunction of the spleen in transport may result in damp phlegm accumulation and obstruction of the lung—qi; stagnation of the liver—qi may cause the liver—fire to attack the lung; hyperactivity of fire due to yin deficiency of the liver and spleen may also involve the lung. All this may result in failure of the lung to perform its purifying and descending function, and the reversed flow of qi causes cough.

Symptoms

1. Cough Due to Exogenous Evils

Wind—cold type is manifested by abundant white, thin phlegm, stuffy nose with discharge, thin and white tongue coating and superficial pulse; Wind—heat type by cough with thick sticky phlegm, sore throat, thirst, fever, thin yellow coating and rapid superficial pulse. Detection with flat—palm reveales a sensation of dense, cold qi or that of imbalance of qi between the left and right sides.

2. Cough Due to Internal Injury

The phlegm—dampness type is manifested by cough with abundant white and sticky phlegm, stuffiness in the chest, white greasy tongue coating and soft, slippery pulse, while that due to invasion of the lung by the liver—fire manifested by choking cough due to adverse flow of qi, flushed complexion, dry throat, hypochondriac pain due to cough, thin yellow tongue coating with little fluid and rapid, wiry pulse. Flat—palm detection reveals dense, obstructed and tingling and distending sensation of qi at the region of the chest and abdomen.

Treatment

1. Emission of Outgoing—Qi (Waiqi)

(1) Ask the patient to assume a sitting posture. Press—knead Tanzhong (Ren 17), Feishu (U B 23), Zhongfu (Lu 1), Yunmen (Lu 2) and Fengmen (U B 12).

(2) Use the flat—palm gesture and pushing, pulling and quivering manipulations to emit qi towards Shanzhong (Ren 17), Zhongfu (Lu 16), Yunmen (Lu 2) and Feishu (U B 23) for 6. or 12. respiratory cycles respectively, and to guide qi from Zhongfu (Lu 1) and Yunmen (Lu 2) to flow along the Lung Channel to the hand to get qi balanced between the upper and the lower.

With flat—palm hand gesture and vibrating and quivering manipulations, emit qi to Shanzhong (Ren 17) and Zhongwan (Ren 12) for 14 respiratory cycles, and guide qi to flow downward along the Stomach Channel of Foot—Yangming with pulling and leading manipulations to make qi activities balanced between the upper and the lower.

Modification: In case of cough due to exogenous evils, add the manipulations of opening Tianmen (Extra, life pass) pushing Kangong (extra), motioning Taiyang (Extra 2) and pressing—kneading Fengchi (GB 20) 24. times each. For cough due to internal injury with phlegm caused by dampness retention due to dysfunction of the spleen—yang, add flat—palm hand gesture and pulling and leading manipu— lations to emit qi toward Zhongwan (Ren 12) and guide qi down to Fenglong (St 40) along the Stomach Channel of Foot—Yangming. Then emit qi with flat— palm gesture and vibrating and quivering manipulations toward Zhongwan (Ren 12) and Dantian for 24 respiratory cycles.

In case of failure of the lung to main keep its purifying and descending function caused by the liver—fire attacking the lung, add flat—palm gesture and vibrating and quivering manipulations to emit qi toward Ganshu (UB 18), Zhangmen (Liv 13) and Qimen (Liv 14) for 11 respiratory cycles, and then guide qi down to the lower extremities along the Liver Channel of Foot—Jueyin and the Gallbladder Channel of Foot—Shaoyang with pushing and leading manipulations, to get qi balanced.

2. Qigong—Acupuncture

Insert the filiform needles into Shanzhong (Ren 17), Neiguan (P 6), Hegu (LI 4) and Feishu (UB 13). Then apply dragon—mouth or bird—beak hand gesture and pushing, pulling and rotating manipulations to facilitate qi activities of the patient and balance qi between the needles.

3. Self Qigong Exercise as Accessory Treatment

(1) The Exercise of Rubbing the Chest and Uttering "Si" (Moxiong Sizi Gong) Take the standing or upright sitting pos-

ture. Tap the upper and lower teeth against each other 36 times while stiring the saliva with the tongue. Swallow the saliva 3 times during the tapping and sent it mentally down to the lung and to the skin and hair and lastly to Dantian. Then push with the flat— palms on the respective sides of the chest and inhale slowly. Utter "si" during exhaling with the two hands rubbing the chest at the same time, for 7 respiratory cycles.

The exercise is effective for lowering the lung—qi and clearing away the lung—fire. It is indicated for cough due to exogenous evils and should be done 2 — 4 times a day.

(2) The Exercise of Taking White Qi (Fu Baiqi Gong)

Take the same posture and do the same teeth tapping and saliva swallowing as mentioned above. Then imagine white qi. Inhale the white qi through nose and fill the mouth with it. Send it slowly down during inspiration to the lungs and then spread it all over the skin and hair. Repeat the procedure 7 times.

The exercise has the function of tonifying the lung—qi and is indicated for patients with deficiency of the lung—qi. It should be done 2 — 4 times a day.

(3) The Lung Regulation Exercise (Lifei Gong)

Patting—Thumping the Back: Raise the right arm and rest the centre of the palm against Dazhui (Du 14) and pat it 9 times, accompanied by teeth—tapping. Do the same with the left palm, and then thump both the back and the chest with the two hollow fists alternately 9 times, accompanied by tapping the teeth.

Soothing the Chest Oppression to Regulating Qi (Shuxiong Tiaoqi Gong): Push—rub the chest with the left palm first from the upper—left side of the chest obliquely downward to the pit of the stomach 9 times. Do the same with the right palm to the right side of the chest.

Removing Fire in the Lung and Resolving Phlegm: Put the two palms on the infraclavicular fossa of their respective side and push slowly downwards to the lower abdomen of the same side 9 times.

Regulating Qi and Dredging the Channels: Push with the left palm from the right side of the chest to the fingertips via the right shoulder and the medial aspect of the arm, then from the dorsal side of the fingertips back to the chest via the anterior—lateral aspect of the arm and the shoulder,9 times. Do the same with the right hand upon the left side another 9 times. The manipulation is indicated for cough due to either exogenous evils or internal injury and should be performed 2 — 4 times a day.

Asthma

Etiology

Asthma is mostly caused by retention of damp phlegm in the lung. When a person is affected by exogenous evils, disorder of qi in ascending, descending, flowing in and flowing out will develop, and phlegm will ascend with qi and adversely obstruct qi, leading to obstruction of the air passage manifested by symptoms of dyspnea and rales. The disease may also result from obstruction of the lung due to phlegm retention caused by failure of the spleen to transport, or from failure of the kidney to regulate qi because of kidney insufficiency. So the etiology of the disease is ascribed to the dysfunction of the three: the lung, the spleen and the kidney.

Symptoms

1. Wind—Cold Type Due to Exogenous Evils

The main symptoms are shortness of breath, cough and expectoration of abundant thin, clear phlegm with foam accompanied with superficial wind—cold syndrome, white tongue proper with thin coating, and superficial, tense or taut, slippery pulse.

Flat—palm detection may reveal dense and cold qi sensation at the chest and thin, scattered at the lower abdomen and the lower extremities.

2. Accumulation of Phlegm—Dampness in the Lung

This is manifested by shortness of breath, cough, abundant thick and sticky expectoration, stuffiness in the chest and epigastric region, white greasy tongue coating and wiry, slippery pulse.

Flat—palm detection reveals that qi is dense and sluggish at the thoracic and epigastric region and imbalanced in density between the upper and the lower.

3. Insufficiency of the Lung and Spleen Qi

The manifestations include dyspnea, shortness of breath, spontaneous perspiration, aversion to wind, expectoration of clear, thin phlegm, weak—voice speaking, lassitude, loss of appetite, loose stool, pale tongue and feeble pulse.

Flat—palm detection reveals that qi is thin at the chest and dense at the lower limbs.

4. Insufficiency of the Lung and Kidney Yin

The main symptoms are dyspnea, shortness of breath, dry

throat and mouth, dry cough or cough with little expectoration, hectic fever, night sweating, reddish tongue with no coating and rapid, thready pulse. In some patients, there may be hemoptysis and hoarseness.

Flat−palm detection may reveal dense and sluggish qi at the chest and the upper and lower abdomen.

Treatment

1. Emission of Outgoing−Qi (Waiqi)

(1) Conduct digital press−kneading first on Dingchuan (Extra), Tiantu (Ren 22), Shanzhong (Ren 17), Guanyuan (Ren 4) and Feishu (UB 13).

(2) With flat−palm hand gesture and vibrating and quivering manipulations, emit qi to Dingchuan (Extra) and Feishu (UB 13) with the palm touching the body surface of the patient for 14 or 28 respiratory cycles. Then with the palm off the body surface, guide qi along the Du Channel and the Urinary Bladder Channel of Foot−Taiyang down to Mingmen (Du 4) and Shenshu (UB 23) repeatedly 3 − 7 times.

(3) Emit qi toward Tiantu (Ren 22), Shanzhong (Ren 17), Zhongfu (Lu 1) and Yunmen (Lu 2) with middle−finger−propping or sword−fingers hand gesture and vibrating and quivering manipulations. Then with the fingers off the body surface of the patient, guide qi to flow downward from the chest to the abdomen along the Stomach Channel of Foot−Yangming and the Ren Channel to make qi weak in the upper and strong in the lower.

Modification: In case of wind−cold syndrome due to exogenous evils, add opening Tianmen (Extra), pushing Kangong (Extra), motioning Taiyang (Extra 2) and sweeping the Gallbladder Channel at the head. For accumulation of phlegm—dampness in the lung, add emitting qi with flat—palm toward Zhongfu (Lu 1) and Yunmen (Lu 2) and guiding qi with pulling and leading manipulations toward the fingertips along the Lung Channel of Hand—Taiyin to facilitate the channel qi and expel the pathogenic factors. For insuffiency of the lung and spleen qi, add emission of qi with flat—palm and vibrating and quivering manipulations toward Qihai (Ren 6), Zhongwan (Ren12), Feishu (UB 13) and Pishu (UB 20) for 9 or 18 respiratory cycles respectively. And for insufficiency of the lung and kidney yin, add emission of qi with flat—palm and vibrating and quivering manipulations toward Guanyuan (Ren 4), Shenshu (UB 23) and Feishu (UB 13) for 6 or 12 respiratory cycles respectively.

2. Qigong—Acupuncture

Insert the filiform needles into Dingchuan (Extra 17), Tiantu (Ren 22), Shanzhong (Ren 17), Neiguan (P 6) and Lieque (Lu 7), then with dragon—mouth gesture and pushing, pulling and rotating manipulations, emit qi and guide qi downward.

3. Self Qigong Exercise as Accessory Treatment

(1) The Exercise for Relieving Asthma and Guiding Qi Take a sitting or standing posture, expel distractions, close the eyes slightly and relax all over. Firstly, push with the face of the index, middle, ring and small fingers from the sternal notch to the xiphoid process repeatedly 36 times. Then when exhaling, push with the right palm from the thoracic midline to the left 5—10 times and pause when inhaling, for altogether 10 respiratory cycles. Do the same pushing with the left palm to-

ward the right side for another 10 respiratory cycles. Lastly, push—rub with the two palms from the subaxillary regions to the sides of the abdomen 10 − 20 times.

(2) The Exercise for Relaxing the Lung

This should be done when asthma attacks. Sit or stand with all distractions removed. Relax the muscles of the chest and back and then the whole body first, then take in a deep breath and say "relax" silently, and simultaneously imagine that the lungs are relaxed to facilitate qi to descend along the bilateral sides of the body to the soles. Repeat the procedures a certain number of times till the attack of asthma is relieved.

(3) Modification

Patients with insufficiency of the lung—qi should do the above exercises in combination with "taking white qi", and those with domination of pathogenic factors, in combination with "rubbing the chest and uttering 'si'"(Refer to "Cough").

Gastralgia

Etiology

1. Hyperactive Liver—Qi Attacking the Stomach

Emotional factors such as worry, anxiety or anger may cause stagnation of qi which, being functionally impaired, often flows transversely instead of downward to the stomach and cause stagnation of qi there, resulting in stomachache.

2. Cold of Insufficiency Type of the Spleen and Stomach

Cold may originate from the interior of the body if a person has congenital insufficiency of yang in the Middle—jiao (function of the spleen and stomach), and stomachache will occur whenever the diet is improper or cold evil attacks.

Symptoms

1. Hyperactive Liver—Qi Attacking the Stomach

The victim often has distention and fullness in the epigastric region, abdominal pain which involves the hyperchondria, frequent eructation or eructation with vomiting of sour or bilious fluid, thin white tongue coating and wiry, deep pulse.

Flat—palm detection reveals dense and tingling and distending qi at the epigastric and hypochondriac regions.

2. Insufficiency Type Cold of the Spleen and Stomach

It is manifested as dull pain in the stomach which may be relieved by pressure, vomiting of clear fluid, preference for warmth and aversion to cold, lassitude, white tongue coating and feeble, soft pusle.

Flat—palm detection may reveal dense or thin and cold qi at the epigastric region.

Treatment

1. Emission of Outgoing—Qi (Waiqi)

(1) Ask the patient to lie supine and relax all over, dispel distractions, get breath even and guide qi by will to the painful area of the upper abdomen when exhaling.

(2) Knead Lanmen (the ileocecal junction) with the right hand and press Jiuwei (Ren 15) with the middle finger of the left to regulate the patient's qi activities.

(3) Press the stomach lightly with a flat—palm and emit qi with quivering manipulation for 14 respiratory cycles. Then emit qi to Zhongwan (Ren 12) and Qihai (Ren 6) with middle—finger—propping gesture and vibrating manipulation

—316—

for 14 respiratory cycles. Lastly push the abdomen with the palms separately and straightly and then rub and knead it.

(4) Emit qi toward Zhongwan (Ren 12) with the flat—palm off the patient's body surface and with pushing, pulling and quivering manipulations for 14 respirotary cycles, then guide the channel qi to flow to the Lower Dantian along the Ren Channel or the Stomach Channel of Foot—Yangming to make qi balanced between the upper and the lower.

(5) Ask the patient to lie prostrate , then knead with the flat of the thumb the points of Pishu (UB 20), Weishu (UB 21), Ganshu (UB 18) and the Urinary Bladder Channel and the Du Channel. Then emit qi with the flat—palm gesture and vibrating and quivering manipulations toward Pishu (UB 20) and Weishu (UB 21) for 14. respiratory cycles, and guide qi to flow along the course of the channels.

Modification: In case of hyperactive liver—qi attacking the stomach, add emission of qi to Ganshu (UB 18) for 11 respiratory cycles with the flat—palm gesture and pulling and leading manipulations and guide qi with pulling manipulation toward the lower extremities along the Gallbladder Channel of Foot—Shaoyang and the Liver Channel of Foot—Jueyin to dis-perse the stagnated qi and get it balanced between the left and right and the upper and lower. In case of cold of insufficiency type of the spleen and stomach, add emission of qi to Zhongwan (Ren 12), Dantian and Pishu (UB 20) with the flat—palm gesture, pushing and leading manipulations and the methods of heat guidance of qi or guidance of earth—qi.

2. Qigong—Acupuncture

Insert the filiform needles into Zhongwan (Ren 12) and

Zusanli (St 36) and then emit qi to them with pushing, pulling and rotating manipulations to get qi balanced.

3. Self Qigong Exercise as Accessory Treatment

(1) The Psychosomatic Relaxation Exercise

Sit or stand quietly. Relax the body in an orderly way from the head to the chest, the abdomen, the back, the waist and the lower limbs and lastly relax the epigastric region again, imagining "quiescence" when inhaling and murmuring "relaxation" when exhaling, for 5 – 10 minutes.

(2) The Exercise of Taking Yellow Qi

Sit quietly breathing naturally and distractions expelled. Get the upper and lower teeth tapping each other 36 times while stirring the saliva with the tongue. Swallow the saliva 3 times after the tapping and at each time send it down to Zhongwan (Ren 12) mentally. Then imagine yellow qi. Breathe in the yellow qi through nose, fill the mouth with it and, during exhaling , send it slowly down to Zhongwan (Ren 12) and then disperse it through to the extremities and the skin and hair. Repeat the procedures 10 times.

This exercise is indicated for insufficiency of the spleen and stomach.

(3) The Exercise of Rubbing the Abdomen and Exhaling Qi

Take the same posture and conduct the same teeth–tapping and saliva–swallowing as mentioned above. Then put the right palm gently on the epigastric region. Inhale slowly to get the mouth filled with qi, and murmur "hu" when exhaling while rubbing the abdomen with the right palm clockwise for altogether 11 respiratory cycles.

This exercise is indicated for syndrome of excess type, hyperactive liver—qi attacking the stomach as well as stagnation of the cold pathogen in the stomach.

(4) The Daoyin Exercise for Regulating the Spleen and Stomach

Pushing the Abdomen: Rub the palms against each other to get them warm, then overlap them (right above the left in male and vice versa in female) and put them below the right breast.Push from the chest downward to the right side of the lower abdomen when exhaling and reposition the palms when inhaling 10 times. Do the same along the midline and the left side of the chest and abdomen 10 times respectively.

Rubbing the Abdomen: Rub the palms against each other to get them warm and put them overlapped on the abdomen with the Inner Laogong (P. 8) against the navel. Rub clockwise and counterclockwise 36 times respectively while guiding qi to circulate with the movement of the palms.

Case One

Wu, female, aged 48, came for the first visit on April 14, 1979.

Complaints   Pain in the epigastric area for 2 years which was more severe in the second year and radiated to the back and the hypochondria, accompanied by gastric discomfort with accid regurgitation, dizziness and insomnia. Frequent administration of Western and traditional drugs failed to take effect.

Examination   Physical examination revealed soft abdomen, impalpable liver and spleen, tenderness in the right—upper abdomen, reddish tongue proper with thin yellow coating (thick yellow coating at the root of the tongue) and deep, taut pulse. Flat—palm detection revealed densely stagnated, tingling and distending qi at the upper abdomen, and densely stagnated qi between the 8th and 12th thoracic vertebrae of the right side of the back. Barium meal examination showed irritable symptoms of the duodenum with local tenderness and bad filling, and dotted soybean—sized niches beside the greater curvature at the duodenal fundas.

Diagnosis   Gastralgia (Duodenal ulcer).

Treatment   Qi was emitted with flat—palm hand gesture and pushing, pulling, rotating, quivering, leading and fixing manipulations to the points Shangwan (Ren 13), Zhongwan (Ren 12), Liangmen (St 21), Shiguan (K 18), Ganshu (U B 18), Weishu (U B 21) and Pishu (U B 20), once every other day.

Course of Treatment   Emission of qi twice relieved the pain in the stomach and turned the stools normal and sleep even. All the symptoms and signs disappeared after 15 sessions of treatment. Barium meal examination showed normal duodenum. The follow—up visit in 1980 found no relapse and the patient was healthy.

Case Two

Gao, female, 35 years old, came for the first visit on May 18, 1982, who was given an outpatient number of 121651.

Complaints   Distending pain in the abdomen for 8 years which had been aggravated in the last three months, accompanied with preference for warmth and aversion to cold, aggravated pain after taking cold food or even abdominal discomfort at the sight of cold food, dizziness, vertigo, insomnia, cold extremities, lassitude and watery stools.

Examination   Physical examination found fullness of the abdomen, slight tenderness in the upper abdomen, impalpable liver and spleen, reddish tongue proper with thin yellow coating and thready, taut pulse. Flat—palm detection revealed dense, stagnated and tingling qi at the epigastric and hypochondriac regions. Barium meal examination showed prolapse of the stomach and reduced gastric tension; the lowest point of the lesser curvature was 3 cm below the inter—iliac—crest line.

Diagnosis   Gastralgia (Gastroptosis)

Treatment   Emision of qi was performed with flat—palm gesture and pushing, rotating, leading and fixing manipulations toward Zhongwan (Ren 12), Liangmen (St 21), Baihui (Du 20), Pishu (U B 20), Weishu (U B 21) and Zusanli (St 36); then needles were inserted into Zhongwan (Ren 12) and Zusanli (St 36) and qi emitted toward the needles with dragon—mouth gesture and pushing, rotating and leading manipulations. The treatment was carried out once every other day.

Course of Treatment   During emission of qi the patient felt warm in the epigastric region and the warmth went along the Ren Channel and the Stomach Channel. During emission of qi to the needle inserted in Zusanli (St 36), the patient felt that a warm flow of qi ran from the point to Shangwan (Ren 13) along the Stomach Channel.The symptoms were obviously · alleviated after 5 sessions of treatment, and disappeared after 20 times. Barium meal examination showed that the stomach was normally repositioned and the disease was completely cured.

Vomiting

Etiology

1. Invasion of the Stomach by Pathogenic Factors

Invasion of the stomach by wind—cold, summer dampness and turbid qi may all cause failure of descending of the stomach—qi, which in turn leads to vomiting.

2. Improper Diet

Overeating or taking raw, cold or contaminated food may cause stagnation of food in the stomach and make the impaired stomach—qi to rise adversely resulting in vomiting.

3. Insufficiency of the Spleen and Stomach

Vomiting may also be caused by abnormal ascending of qi due to phlegm—dampness and obstruction of the stomach—qi resulting from dysfunction of the stomach in digestion and transport.

In short, vomiting is most commonly related to the stomach. Any factors that impair the stomach and affect the descent of the stomach—qi may be the cause of vomiting.

Symptoms

1. Vomiting Due to Invasion of the Stomach by Pathogenic Factors

Sudden vomiting which is often accompanied by aversion to cold and fever, white thin tongue coating and superficial pulse. Flat—palm detection often reveals cold or hot or turbid and dense qi sensation at the gastric region.

2. Vomiting Due to Improper Diet

Vomiting of sour and foul food, belching, anorexia,

fullness of the abdomen that may be aggravated by intake of food, vomiting that can relieve the discomfort of the stomach, thick greasy tongue coating and slippery pulse. Flat— palm detection may reveal dense, stagnated and heavy qi sensation at the gastric region.

3. Insufficiency of the Spleen and Stomach

It is manifested by vomiting after intake of more food than usual, pallor, lassitude, watery stools, pale tongue and feeble pulse. Flat—palm detection often reveals thin and slightly tingling sensation of qi at the gastric region and all the other parts of the body.

Treatment

1. Emission of Outgoing—Qi (Waiqi)

(1) Conduct digital kneading on Pishu (UB 20), Weishu (UB 21), Shanzhong (Ren 17), Zhongwan (Ren 12), Neiguan (P 6) and Zusanli (St 36) first.

(2) Emit qi with the flat—palm gesture and pulling and leading manipulations to Pishu (UB 20) and Weishu (UB 21) and guide qi to circulate downward to the lower limbs along the Urinary Bladder Channel to get it balanced between the upper and the lower. Then emit qi to Shanzhong (Ren 17), Zhongwan (Ren 12) and Liangmen (St 21) and guide qi to flow toward Zusanli (St 36) along the Ren Channel and the Stomach Channel of Foot—Yangming to make the stomach—qi descend.

(3) Emit qi to Shenque (Ren 8) with flat—palm gesture and pushing, rotating and leading manipulations, and then with Shenque (Ren 8) as the centre, push—rotate counterclockwise to lead the stomach—qi to descend.

Modification :

In case of invasion of the stomach by pathogenic factors and improper diet, add flat—palm hand gesture and pulling and leading manipulations to lead qi out of the stomach or lead it to Zusanli (St 36) and discharge it there. In case of insufficiency of the spleen and stomach, add flat—palm and vibrating and quivering manipulations to emit qi to Zhongwan (Ren 12), Pishu (UB 20) and Guanyuan (Ren 4) for 14 reapiratory cycles respectively.

2. Qigong—Acupuncture

Insert the filiform needles into Neiguan (P 6), Zusanli (St 36) and Zhongwan (Ren 12) and emit qi and guide the pathogenic qi to Neiguan (Ren 4) and Zusanli (St 36) with dragon—mouth hand gesture and pulling, leading and rotating manipulations.

3. Self Qigong Exercise as Accessory Treatment

(1) The Exercise for Regulating the Stomach and Checking the Adverse Flow of Qi Push with the face of the index, middle and ring fingers from the sternal notch to the xiphoid process 36 times, followed by kneading Shanzhong (Ren 17) 36 times. Then when exhaling, push with the four fingers or the palm from the xiphoid process to the pubic symphysis along the abdominal midline 36 times. Lastly push with the face of the four fingers of both hands from Zhongwan (Ren 12) obliquely to either side of the abdomen 36 times.

(2) The Exercise for Regulating the Chest, Abdomen and Stomach to Send Down the Abnormally Ascending Qi

Take a lying or sitting posture, breathe naturally, close the eyes slightly, expel distractions and relax all over. Take in a breath while thinking "quiescence", then exhale while thinking "relaxation" to relax the chest and then the abdomen, for 14 respiratory cycles. Apply the same to relaxation of the lungs and the stomach for 14 respiratory cycles to guide the stomach—qi to descend.

Case One

Du, female, aged 6, came for the first visit on August 22, 1979.

Complaints   The patient complainted of vomiting of watery yellowish undigested food in frequent spells (more than 10 in a day) for five days, chest stuffiness, bitter mouth, dry throat, vomiting after drinking water, listlessness and fidgets. Gentamicin, and antiemetic drugs failed to take any effect.

Examination   The abdomen was soft, liver impalpable, the centre of the palms and soles hot, throat congested and neck feeble. The tongue coating looked thin and white (thick and yellow at the root), the pusle was slippery and the body temperature 36.9℃. Flat—palm detection revealed densed, tingling and distending sensation of qi at the epigastric region.

Diagnosis   Vomiting (Acute gastritis).

Treatment   Pushing and kneading massage was carried out on Tianzhugu (UB 10), Zusanli (St 36), Shanzhong (Ren 17), Zhongwan (Ren 12), Tianheshui (Extra, the medial aspect of the forearm), Zusanli (St 36) and Neiguan (P 6), then emission of qi was conducted with flat—palm gesture and pushing, rotating and leading manipulations toward these points and qi was guided to flow along the Yangming Channels to the lower and upper extremities.

Course of Treatment   The patient took in 200 ml of water immediately after the first treatment and was told to take fluid diet. All the symptoms disappeared and the patient recovered after 3 sessions of treatment.

Case Two

Wang, male, a worker of 35 years old, came for the first visit on October 27, 1980.

Complaints   Continous vomiting for more than half a month; stomachache and vomiting due to consumption of alcohol, distention, discomfort and gravistatic pain in the epigastric region after every meal accompanied by frequent vomiting, borborygmus and intestinal flatus from anus; no history of other diseases.

Examination   Physical examination found abdominal distention, tenderness below the xiphoid process, impalpable liver and spleen, thick, greasy tongue coating and taut, slippery pulse. Flat—palm detection revealed a sensation of stagnated, densified qi at the epigastric region. X—ray film showed cross conformation of the esophageal and gastric mucosa, double magenblases and fluid levels with the greater gastric curvature above the lesser. The position of the pyloric antrum was vertically higher than the duodenal bulb, inverting the duodenal bulb.

Diagnosis   Vomiting (Volvulus of stomach).

Treatment   Pushing, kneading rubbing and grasping manipulations were carried out on Lanmen (ileocecal junction), the right Shiguan (K 18), Liangmen (St 21), Qihai (Ren 6), Zusanli (St 36), Pishu (U B 20), Weishu (U B 21) and Jianjing (GB 21); qi is emitted toward these points with the flat—palm hand gesture and the pushing, pulling and leading manipulations, once a day.

Course of Treatment Vomiting and abdominal distention were relieved after the first treatment. All the symptoms disappeared and the patient could take meals normally after the fifth treatment. Reexamination by barium meal on November 17, 1980 revealed a normal stomach, and the patient recovered completely.

Hiccup

Etiology

Hiccup is usually caused by spasm of the diaphragm due to excessive intake of raw, cold or pungent food, emotional depression, and adverse rising of the stomach—qi resulting from liver—qi attacking the stomach.

Symptoms

Hiccup is continuous, usually lasting several minutes or hours and then ceasing without treatment in the mild cases; while in the severe cases, it may lasts days and nights, which seriously interferes with eating and sleep, cousing a state of utter exhaustion in the patient . If hiccup occurs at a time when the patient has been sick for a long time or in a state of severe illness, it serves there as a sign of crisis which deserves special attention.

Detection with the flat—palm hand gesture may gain a sensation of densified and stagnated qi at the chest.

Treatment

1. Emission of Outgoing—Qi (Waiqi)

(1) Ask the patient to sit or stand, face south, relax and

take normal breathing. Pinch Zhongge (Extra, at the end of the line between the first two segments of the middle finger of the thumb side), press and knead Pishu (UB 20), Geshu (UB 17), Shanzhong (Ren 17), Zhongfu (Lu 1) and Yunmen (Lu 2).

(2) Flat—palm hand gesture and pushing—pulling—leading manipulation should be applied to emit qi towards Shanzhong (Ren 17) and Rugen (St 18) and then, guide qi to flow down to the lower limbs along the Stomach Channel of Foot—Yangming, which helps regulate the functional activities of qi. Still then, emit qi toward Pishu (UB 20), Weishu (UB 21) and Ganshu(UB 17) on the back, and guide qi to flow down to the lower extremities along the Urinary Bladder Channel of Foot—Taiyang.

(3) If the patient shows no improvement, emit qi again towards the point Baihui (Du 20) and guide qi to flow to Dantian along the Ren Channel with the flat— palm gesture and pushing, pulling and leading manipulations.

2. Self Qigong Exercise As Accessory Treatment

Sit or stand facing south, keep the feet apart at shoulder—width and relax the whole body. Then with antidromic abdominal respiration, take a deep breath and during exhaling guide qi to flow downward to Dantian and further down to the point Dadun (Liv 1), for a period of 3 or 9 respiratory cycles.

Case

Liu, male, aged 36, came for the first visit on May 23, 1983.

Complaints Hiccup with frequent spells (more than 10 in a day) for two days caused by cold, each spell lasting for 30 —

60 minutes, accompanied by insomnia, hypochondriac pain and discomfort, chest stuffiness, pain in the upper abdomen, lassitude and listlessness.

Examination The tongue coating was thin and white and the pulse deep and slow. Flat—palm detection revealed densified and stagnated qi sensation at the chest.

Diagnosis Hiccup (Phrenospasm).

Treatment Pressing and kneading were conducted on the points Geshu (UB 17), Weishu (UB 21), Ganshu (UB 18), Shanzhong (Ren 17), Huagai (Ren 20), Yunmen (Lu 2), Zhongfu (Lu 1) and Zusanli (St 36) first, and then emission of qi was carried out toward these points with the flat—palm hand gesture and pushing, pulling and leading manipulations.

Course of Treatment Recovery took place after the second treatment.

Diarrhoea

Etiology

Improper diet and exopathogenic factors may cause gastrointestinal dysfunction which results in diarrhoea. The disease is most prevalent in summer and autumn when dampness and heat, the two exopathogenic factors, are rampant. On the other hend, deficiency of the spleen—yang and the kidney—yang, the internal pathogenic factor, may also cause chronic diarrhoea. An old saying holds that deficiency of the kidney leads to frequent defecation, and deficiency of the spleen impairs its normal function in transportation.

Symptoms

1. Diarrhoea Due to Cold

Patients with diarrhoea due to cold generally suffer from intestinal gurgling and abdominal pain, loose stool with undigested food, watery stool, frequent clear urination, and deep and slow pulse. Flat–palm detection often reveals densified and cold qi sensation around the navel.

2. Diarrhoea Due to Heat

As for diarrhoea due to heat, the symptoms include foul smelling, yellow and loose stool, burning sensation in the anal area, thirst, restlessness, dark urine, frequent urination, yellowish tongue coating and wiry and rapid pulse. Flat–palm detection reveals densified, tingling, distending and hot qi sensation around the navel.

3. Diarrhoea at Dawn

Diarrhoea at dawn is due to weakness of kidney–yang which results in indigestion of food. The patient usually defecates (loose stool) 2 – 3 times every day before dawn. Flat–palm detection may reveal cold and thin sensation of qi at the navel and the lower abdomen.

Treatment

1. Emission of Outgoing Qi (Waiqi)

(1) Carry out digital pressing on Pishu (U B 20), Weishu (UB 21) and Dachangshu (UB 25) to open through the Shu points (stream points). Then press and knead, with the tip of the middle finger of the right hand, the point Lanmen (ileocecal junction) while pressing the point Jiuwei (Ren 15) with the tip of the middle finger of the left hand to help normalize the functional activities of qi there.

(2) Apply flat–palm gesture and vibrating and quivering manipalations to emit qi toward Zhongwan (Ren 12), Shenque

(Ren 8) and Guanyuan(Ren 14) for 14 respiratory cycles respectively. Then massage the abdomen 36 times (It has the effect of tonification in a deficiency syndrome and of purgation in an excess one).

(3) Apply flat–palm gesture and pushing, pulling and rotating manipulations to emit qi towards the abdomen and, at the same time, guide qi to rotate clockwise or counterclockwise, and then guide qi to flow downward along the Stomach Channel.

(4) Push from the coccyx up to the seventh thoracic vertebra with the face of the four fingers 300 times, then press and knead the Urinary Bladder Channel (both sides) and the point Zusanli (St 36).

Modification: For patients with diarrhoea at dawn, flat–palm gesture and pushing and leading manipulations should be added to emit qi towards Mingmen (Du 4), Dantian and Shenshu (UB 23) for 9 – 10 respiratoty cycles.For patients with diarrhoea due to cold, add emission of qi to Pishu (UB 20), Shenque (Ren 8) and Guanyuan (Ren 4) with flat–palm hand gesture and pushing and leading manipulations and heat guidance of qi. For diarrhoea due to heat, add emission of qi to Zhongwan (Ren 12) and Tianshu (St 25) with flat–palm gesture, pulling and leading manipulations and the method of cold guidance of qi, to guide the pathogenic qi along the Stomach Channel of Foot–Yangming down to Zusanli (St 36), where it is discharged.

2. Qigong–Acupuncture

Insert the filiform needles into Zhongwan (Ren 12), Tianshu (St 25), Zusanli (St 36) and Neiguan (P 6). Then emit qi to the points and guide qi to flow to Zusanli (St 36) and Neiguan (P 6) with the dragon–mouth hand gesture and the rotating, pulling and leading manipulations to get qi balanced between the needles.

3. Self Qigong Exercise as Accessory Treatment

(1) Patients with diarrhoea due to heat may practise the exercise of rubbing the abdomen and "hu" (exhaling) qi;those with diarrhoea due to cold may practise the exercise of taking yellow qi (Refer to "Gastralgia").

(2) The Exercise of Automatic Circulation of Qi for Relieving Diarrhoea

Lie latericumbent, relaxed and quiet, with the breath even and tongue rested against the palate. Lead qi to circulate with the navel as the centre. The moving starts during inhaling from the point left of and beneath the navel clockwise to the point right of and above the navel, and during exhaling, from this point to the starting point to complete a counterclockwise circle. Guide the circulation of qi round the navel from the smallest circle to the largest for 81 rounds. Continue the guidance of qi from the largest circle to the smallest from the sides of the abdomen to the navel for another 81 rounds. This procedure requires the patient to contract the anus and abdomen during inhalation and relax them during exhalation. Beginners of this exercise may at first try to direct qi to rotate with the help of respiration and the movement of the abdominal muscles. As soon as they are skilled they will be able to direct the intrinsic qi to rotate round the navel by will alone.

Case

Wang, female, aged 38, came for the first visit on June 20,

1982.

Complaints　Repeated diarrhoea (2 − 4 episodes a day) for successive 8 years. Defecation was urgent with indigested food. Other complaints included discomfort in the abdomen, preference to warmth and aversion to cold, abdominal gurgling and diarrhoea that would occur after intake of even a small amount of cold food or drinks or even at the sight of them, dribbling clear urine, insomnia and lassitude.

Examination　Physical examination revealed emaciation, cold extremities, pale complexion, soft abdomen with the liver and spleen impalpable, pale tongue proper with thin, white coating and deep, thready pulse. Flat−palm detection revealed densified and cold sensation of qi at the abdomen.

Diagnosis　Diarrhoea (Irritable / allergic colitis).

Treatment　Emission of qi was carried out with flat−palm gesture and pushing, rotating, leading and quivering manipulations toward the points of Pishu (UB 20), Dachangshu (UB 25), Shenque (Ren 8), Guanyuan (Ren 4), Tianshu (St 25) and Zusanli (St 36).

Course of Treatment　On emitting qi to Shenque (Ren 8) and Tianshu (St 25), the patient felt warmth on the abdomen and a flow of warm qi descending to the lower extremities along the Stomach Channel. Diarrhoea was relieved after the first treatment and cured completely after 17 sessions of treatment.

Constipation

Etiology

1. Constipation of Excess Type

It is usually due to accumulation of heat in the stomach and intestines caused by exuberance of yang in the body and consumption of pungent or hot food, or due to impairment of the body fluid and obstruction of fu—qi (qi of the hollow organs) resulting from intense heat inside the body, or due to stagnation of qi and failure of fluid transportation caused by emotional depression.

2. Costipation of Deficiency Type

It is mostly seen in those who have just recovered from an illness or have just given birth when they are still deficient with qi and blood, or in those suffering from insufficiency of yang—qi of the Lower—jiao and accumulation of yin—cold, which makes it difficult for the intestine to perform normal transporting function.

Symptoms

1. Constipation of Excess Type

Difficult defecation or reduced frequency of defecation (once every 3 — 5 or 6 — 7 days) of dry and hard stools, feverish body, thirst, poor appetite, taut or slippery, replete pulse and thin, greasy or yellow dry tongue coating. Flat— palm detection may reveal stagnated, hot and distending sensation of qi.

2. Constipation of Deficiency type

Dry and hard stools hard to pass, pale and dim complexion, mental fatigue and palpitation due to deficiency of qi, cold pain in the abdomen, preference to warmth and aversion to cold, feeble, thready or deep, slow pulse and pale tongue with thin coating. Flat—palm detection may reveal sparse, cold, tingling and distending and stagnated sensation of qi.

Treatment

1. Emission of Outgoing Qi (Waiqi)

(1) Press and knead Dachangshu (UB 25), Shenshu (UB 23) and the eight liao points of Shangliao (UB 31), Ciliao (UB 34), Zhongliao (UB 33) and Xialiao (UB 34) to break through the Shu points (stream points). Then, push from the 4th lumbar vertebva down to the end of coccyx 50 times.

(2) Break through the point Lanmen (Extra, ileocecal junction) and Jiuwei (Ren 15) by pressing and kneading them with the thumbs and the middle fingers of both hands. Then, emit qi with flat—palm gesture and vibrating and quivering manipulations towards the points Zhongwan (Ren 12) and Liangmen (St 21) for 14 respiratory cycles, and emit qi with the dragon—mouth hand gesture and vibrating and quivering manipulations towards the point Tianshu (St 25) for 14 respiratory cycles, followed by guiding qi to rotate counterclockwise with the flat—palm gesture and rubbing manipulation.

(3) Emit qi with flam—palm gesture and pushing, pulling and rotating manipula— tions to Zhongwan (Ren 12), Shenque (Ren 8), Tianshu (St 25) and Guanyuan (Ren 4). Then guide qi to rotate counterclockwise with rotating, quivering and leading manipulations to facilitate the functional activities of qi and to lead qi to flow to the lower extremities along the Stomach Channel of Foot— Yangming.

Modification: For treatment of constipation of excess type, add emission of qi with flat—palm hand gesture, cold qi—guiding method and counterclockwise rotating, quivering and leading manipulations for 14 respiratory cycles; for treatment of constipation of deficiency type , add emission of qi with flat—palm hand gesture, the method of guiding water—qi and vib rating and quivering manipulations to Dantian and Shenshu (UB 23) for 8 or 16 respiratory cycles each.

2. Qigong—Acupuncture

Insert the filiform needles into Tianshu (St 25), Zhigou (SJ 6), Shangjuxu (St 37) and Dachangshu (UB 25) and emit qi with dragon—mouth or bird—beak hand gesture and pushing, pulling and rotating manipulations to regulate qi activities and balance it between the needles.

3. Self Qigong Exercise as Accessory Treatment

(1) The Automatic Qi Circulation Exercise for Bowel Movement

Lie supine, relaxed and quiet. breathe evenly and put the tongue against the palate. Taking the navel as the centre of a circle, move the abdominal muscles with qi following will. The moving of qi starts during inhalation from the point right to and beneath the navel clockwise to the point left to and above the navel, and continues to flow forward during exhalation back to the original point to complete the circle. Conduct the moving of qi for 81 circles from the smallest circle at the navel to the largest at the sides of the abdomen. Beginners of the exercise may at first try to direct qi to rotate with the help of respiration and the movement of the abdominal muscles. When skilled, one will be able to guide qi to turn only by will.

(2) Patients with constipation of excess type may practise the exercise of rubbing the abdomen and "hu" (exhaling) qi; and patients with constipation of deficiency type may practise the exercise of taking yellow qi (Refer to "Gastralgia").

Case

Zhang, female, 59, came for the first visit on October 23, 1981.

Complaints   The patient complained of constipation for successive 10 years, which was manifested as dry and hard stools and difficulty in defecation (once every 3 − 4 days), accompanied by dizziness, dryness in the mouth and hypertension for many years.

Examination   Physical examination revealed flushed complexion, fat physique, reddish tongue proper with thin yellow coating and taut pulse, and blood pressure of 140 / 100 mmHg. Flat−palm detection revealed densified, distending and tingling sensation of qi.

Diagnosis   Constipation (Senile constipation).

Treatment   Emission of qi was conducted with the flat−palm hand gesture and counterclockwise pulling, leading and quivering manipulations toward Dachangshu (UB 25), Mingmen (Du 4), Tianshu (St 25), Shenque (Ren 8), Daheng (Sp. 15) and Zusanli (St 36).

Course of Treatment   Stools became soft and bowel movement smooth after the first treatment. The disease was completely cured after the second treatment. Follow−up visit in 1982 found no relapse.

Dysentery

Etiology

1. Dysentery of Damp−heat Type

It is due to impairment of qi and blood of the intestines caused by retention of dampness and heat in the stomach and intestines resulting from invasion of the body by summer—damp—heat (an exgenous factor) or from intake of raw and cold food (an endogneous factor).

2. Dysentery of Cold—damp Type

It is due to retention of cold—dampness in the intestines caused by cold invasion in summer or by careless intake of raw, cold and contaminated food.

3. Chronic Dysentery (Persistent Dysentery)

It often results from prolonged duration of dysentery when the pathogenic factors linger, causing insuffiency of qi of the Middle—jiao and failure of the stomach and spleen to transport, or causing damage of the primordial energy, insufficiency of the kidney—qi and weakened body resistance to prevailing pathogenic factors.

Symptoms

1. Dysentery of Damp—heat Type

It is characterized by abdominal pain, bloody mucous stools, tenesmus, burning sensation of the anus, scanty dark urine, yellowish greasy tongue coating and slippery, rapid pulse. Flat—palm detection may reveal deeply stagnated, dry and hot and strongly distending sensation of qi at the abdomen.

2. Dysentery of Cold—damp Type

It is characterized by passage of whitish purulent stools, preference to warmth and aversion to cold, distending stress of the epigastrium, flat taste in the mouth, absence of thirst, whitish greasy tongue coating and soft, rapid or soft, slow pulse. Flat—palm detection often reveals densified, cold, tingling and distending and stagnated sensation of qi at the abdomen.

3. Chronic Dysentery (Persistent Dysentery)

This is the type of dysentery with a chronic course and a tendency of relapse characterized by lassitude and preference to lying in bed, tenesmus, pale tongue peoper with greasy coating and soft, thready or feeble, large pulse. Flat—palm detectionoften reveals thin, tingling of tensified, cold sensation of qi at the abdomen.

Treatment

1. Emission of Outgoing Qi (Waiqi)

(1) Conduct digital kneading first on the points Pishu (UB 20), Weishu (UB 21) and Dachangshu (UB 25) to open the Shu points at the back; then press— knead Lanmen (Extra,ileocecal junction) with the middle finger of the right hand while press—knead Jiuwei (Ren 15) with that of the left to facilitate the qi activities there; then press—knead Zhongwan (Ren 12), Tianshu (St 25) and Guanyuan (Ren 14).

(2) Emit qi with middle—finger—propping hand gesture and vibrating and quivering manipulations to Zhongwan (Ren 12), Tianshu (St 25) and Guanyuan (Ren 14) for 14 respiratory cycles each. Then rub the abdomen 36 times (this has the effect of tonification in deficiency syndrome and of purgation in excess syndrome).

(3) Guide qi to flow clockwise and counterclockwise for 81 respiratory cycles respectively with flat—palm hand gesture and pushing, pulling, rotating and leading manipulations.

(4) Emit qi with the flat—palm gesture and pushing and leading manipulations to Pishu (UB 20), Weishu (UB 21) and Dachangshu (UB 25), then guide qi downwards to the lower

extremities along the Urinary Bladder Channel of Foot—Taiyang.

Modification: Add the method of heat—guidance of qi to treatment of dysentery of cold— damp type and cold—guidance of qi to treatment of damp—heat type. For chronic type, add flat—palm gesture and pushing and leading manipulations to emit qi to Dantian, Mingmen (Du 4), Weishu (UB 21) and Pishu (UB 20) and guide the channel qi toward the lower extremities to balance qi.

2. Qigong—Acupuncture

Insert the filiform needles into Hegu (LI 4), Tianshu (St 25) and Shangjuxu (St 37). Then guide the pathogenic qi of the patient to go out from these points with dragon—mouth or bird—mouth hand gesture and pushing, rotating and leading manipulations.

3. Self Qigong Exercise As Accessory Treatment

(1) The Exercise for Guiding Qi to Rotate Automatically

Lie supine, relaxed and quiet. Get the breath even and the tongue against the palate. Taking the navel as the centre of a circle, move the abdominal muscles with qi following will. The moving of qi starts during inhalation from the point right to and beneath the navel clockwise to the point left to and above the navel, and continues to flow clockwise during exhalation to the original point to complete the circle. Conduct the moving of qi for 81 circles from the smallest circle at the navel to the largest at the sides of the abdomen, then guide qi to rotate counterclockwise for another 81 circles in the same way. Beginners of the exercise may at first try to direct qi to rotate with the help of respiration and the movement of the abdominal muscles. When skilled, one will be able to guide qi to turn only by will. The above method is suitable for chronic dysentery. Patients with dysentery of cold–damp type should guide qi to rotate only clockwise for 81 circles and those with dysentery of damp–heat type, only counterclockwise for 81 circles.

(2) The Turbidity Elimination Exercise (Dihui Gong)

Take a sitting or lying posture. Relax all over with the tongue against the palate, the eyes slightly closed, and the breath even.

Imagine that qi whirls in by mouth via stomach and circulates in void to make the genuine qi fill the large intestine and drive the virulent heat–evil to wind from left to right clockwise and revolve through the intestines, and then come out of the anus. Then inhale and contrat the anus gently to close it. Guide the genuine qi to wind from right to left counterclockwise in the opposite direction through the intestines and finally come out from the upper orifice of the stomach. Repeat the procedures 5 – 10 times.

After the exercise, concentrate the mind on Dantian for a moment to get the genuine qi back to its origin, then rub the abdomen gentally with the hands to end the exercise.

Disorders of the Biliary Tract

Etiology

Disorders of the biliary tract mainly include cholecystitis, cholelithiasis and ascariasis of the biliary tract. Traditional Chinese medicine holds that the first two diseases belong to the category of "hypochondriac pain" or "jaundice", while the last is called "biliary ascariasis". These disorders are mainly caused by mental depression, excessive intake of fatty food, exopathogenic invasion, stagnation of gallbladder—qi and failure of biliary dredge resulting from stagnation of dampness and heat and obstruction by ascarid. Though causes and symptoms of these disorders are different, qigong exercise for them and treatment with outgoing—qi are almost the same. That is why they are jointly introduced hereof as one.

Symptoms

The onset of these disorders are usually acute, and pain is felt on the right upper abdomen and on the right hypochondrium. Other symptoms are nausea, vomiting,rigor, high fever, yellow stained skin and sclera, or whitish—grey stool when the biliary tract is completely blocked, and tenderness of the gallbladder when breathing deeply. Patients with biliary ascariasis may feel severe colic or a tearing pain below the xiphoid process. The pain is so severe that the patient is wet with sweat, accompanied by nausea and vomiting. If the ascarid has withdrawn from the biliary tract, the pain is relieved immediately but can recur intercurrently. If the ascarid has moved completely into the gallbladder, the pain becomes continuous and distending; jaundice, rigor and high fever may appear; tenderness on the right part of the xiphoid process may be felt upon deep pressing.

Flat—palm detection may reveal stagnated, hot, cold, densified and strong tingling sensation of qi at the gallbladder area.

Treatment

1.Emission of Outgoing—qi(Waiqi)

(1) With the patient in a sitting posture, press and knead the points Pishu (UB 20), Weishu (UB 21), Ganshu (UB 18), Danshu (UB 19), and Dannang (Extra, a point of tenderness 2. cun below the point Yanglingquan, GB 34). Stress is laid on the points of the right side.

(2) Emit qi towards the gallbladder area of the front side for 24 respiratory cycles with the flat–palm hand gesture and pushing, pulling, quivering and leading manipulations. Then pulling and leading manipulations should be used to guide qi to flow downward to the lower extremities along the Gallbladder Channel of Foot–Shaoyang and the Stomach Channel of Foot–Yangming to promote the circulation of gallbladder–qi and regulate qi by relieving epigastric distention and regulating the stomach.

(3) Emit qi towards the points Pishu (UB 20), Weishu (UB 21), Ganshu (UB 18), Danshu (UB 19) and Dannang (Extra) on the right side of the body for 28 respiratory cycles, then emit qi towards the pain location at the front side of the body for 28 respiratory cycles with the flam–palm hand gesture and vibrating and quivering manipulations.

(4) Press the point Danshu (UB 19) on the right side for 12 respiratory cycles. Press and knead downward along the Urinary Bladder Channel of Foot– Taiyang on the two sides of the back and waist 3 times.

Modification: For treatment of ascariasis of the biliary tract, rubbing the abdomen counterclockwise 81 times should be included. Cholelithiasis and cholecystitis are often treated by guiding qi downward to the lower extremities along the Liver Channel and the Gallbladder Channel and by balancing the qi activities between the upper and lower and the left and the right.

2. Qigong–Acupuncture

Insert the filiform needles into Neiguan (P 6), Danshu (UB 19), Dannang (Extra), Yanglingchuan (GB 34) and Zusanli (St 36) and emit qi toward the needles with the dragon–mouth or bird–beak hand gesture and pushing, pulling, quivering and rotating manipulations to get qi balanced between them.

3. Self Qigong Exercise as Accessory Treatment

(1) Rubbing the Chest and "Xu" Qi

Taking a standing or sitting posture. Put the palms against the hypochondria and guide qi slowly to the hypochondria during inhaling, and during exhaling, utter "xu" while rubbing the hypochondria gently with the palms. Do the exercise 10 or 20 respiratory cycles.

(2) Relaxation of the Liver and Gallbladder

Pratise relaxation exercise with a lying or sitting posture. Inhaling, think the word "quiescence" and exhaling, the word "relaxation" to relax in sequence from the head, chest and abdomen, back and waist, the upper limbs and the lower limbs, and then the liver and gallbladder, for 14 or 28 respiratory cycles respectively.

Case

Zhao, male, 43 years old, came for the first visit on April 6, 1983.

Complaints   The patient complained of pain in the gallbladder region for two months, characterized by abdominal distention, persistent dull pain in the right hypochondrium, burning sensation in the stomach, nausea, belching, indigestion which may be aggravated by intake of fatty food, and discomfort in the right—upper limb. Administration of traditional drugs yielded no apparent effect.

Examination   There were tenderness and percussing pain in the right—upper abdomen and reddish tongue proper with thin, yellow coating. Flat—palm detection revealed hot, tingling and densified qi sensation at the right—upper abdomen. Ultrasonogram showed inflated gallbladder with dysfunction of contraction.

Diagnosis   Cholecystitis (the hyperactive liver—qi attacking the stomach).

Treatment   Emission of outgoing—qi was performed with flat—palm hand gesture and pushing, pulling, quivering, rotating and leading manipulations toward Ganshu (UB 18), Danshu (UB 19), Zhangmen (Liv 13), Qimen (Liv 14), Yanglingquan (G B 34), Liangmen (St 21) and Zusanli (St 36).

Course of Treatment   Nausea and vomiting occurred immediately after guiding qi to turn clockwise was performed with the qi—guiding method of making three points circular. So guiding qi to turn counterclockwise was taken instead in combination with guiding qi to go downwards to the lower extremities along the Liver Channel and the Stomach Channel, which resulted in a comfortable sensation in the abdomen. All the symptoms disappeared after 6 times of treatment, and with 3 more times of treatment for consolidation of the effect, the patient recovered completely.

Abdominal Pain

Etiology

1. Abdominal Pain Due to Internal Accumulation of Cold

The pain is induced by cold which may either accumulates internally due to excessive intake of raw or cold food or due to invasion of the navel by pathogenic cold during careless sleeping in the open.

2. Abdominal Pain Due to Dysfunction of the Spleen—Yang

In those who are usually deficient in yang—qi and weak in digestive functions, pain often occurs following invasion, no matter how mild it may be, by cold, or following starvation, overeating and over—exertion.

3. Abdominal Pain Due to Stagnation of Food

The pain is induced by stagnation of qi resulting from mutual interference between the clear and turbid qi caused by failure of the stomach and intestines to digest and transport.

Symptoms

1. Abdominal Pain Due to Internal Accumulation of Cold

The pain occurs abruptly manifested as pain which may be relieved by defecation warm, the stools are and loose and there is, white tongue coating and deep, tense pulse. Flat—palm detection may reveal densified, cold and stagnated sensation of qi at the painful region.

2. Abdominal Pain Due to Dysfunction of the Spleen—Yang

It is characterized by continuous recurrent pain which may be relieved by pressure, loose stools, mental fatigue, aversion to cold, thin white tongue coating and deep, thready pulse. Flat—palm detection may reveal thin, cold and tingling sensation of qi at the painful region.

3. Abdominal Pain Due to Stagnation of Food

It is characterized by gastric and abdominal distention, severe tenderness, aversion to food, acid regurgitation, greasy tongue coating and slippery pulse. Flat—palm detection may reveal intensified, stagnated, heavy and distending sensation of qi at the painful region.

Treatment

1. Emission of Outgoing—qi (Waiqi)

(1) Knead Lanmen (Extra, ileocecal junction) first to open the point,then press— knead Pishu (UB 20), Weishu (UB 21) Zhongwan (Ren 12), Tianshu (St 25) and Zusanli (St 36). Press—knead along the Urinary Bladder Channel of Foot—Taiyang on the back and waist from the upper to the lower 3 — 5 times to open the Shu points.

(2) Emit qi with flat—palm hand gesture and vibrating and quivering manipulations toward Zhongwan (Ren 12), Tianshu (St 25), Pishu (UB 20) and Weishu (UB 21), then guide qi with pushing, pulling and leading manipulations to go from the abdomen and back toward the lower extremities along the Stomach Channel of Foot—Yangming and the Urinary Bladder Channel of Foot—Taiyang to make qi of the two channels balanced between the upper and the lower.

(3) Emit qi with flat—palm hand gesture and pushing, pulling and fixing manipu— lations toward Zhongwan (Ren 12) and Tianshu (St 25) for 14 respiratory cycles, then with pulling and leading manipulations, guide qi of the patient to flow to the lower extremities along the Stomach Channel of Foot—Yangming to get qi balanced between the upper and the lower.

(4) Taking the navel as the centre, rub the abdomen with a flat—palm for 81 respiratory cycles.

Modification: In case of abdominal pain due to internal accumulation of cold, add the method of heat—guidance of qi and guidance of fire—qi; in case of pain due to dysfunction of the spleen—yang, add heat—guidance of qi to emit qi to Pishu (UB 20), Weishu (UB 21) and Mingmen (Du 4); in case of pain due to stagnation of food, add emission of qi with flat—palm hand gesture and rotating and leading manipulations to Zhongwan (Ren 12), Tianshu (St 25) and Guanyuan (Ren 4), to facilitate qi activities of the patient in the upper and the lower.

2. Qigong—Acupuncture

Insert the filiform needles into Zhongwan (Ren 12), Guanyuan (Ren 4), Tianshu (St 25) and Zusanli (St 36), then emit qi toward the needles with dragon—mouth or bird—beak hand gesture and pulling and rotating manipulations, to get qi balanced between the needles.

3. Self Qigong Exercise as Accessory Treatment

(1) The Abdominal Exercise for Regulating Qi

Rest the right palm on Zhongwan (Ren 12) and knead clockwise and counter— clockwise 36 times respectively, then knead around the navel clockwise and counterclockwise respectively 36 times each way. Push with the four fingers of both hands from the xiphoid process to the pubic symphysis along the abdominal midline during exhaling 36 times. Lastly, overlap the hands (the right over the left in male and vice versa in female), apply them to the midpoint of the lower abdomen and knead clockwise and counterclockwise 36 times respectively.

(2) The Exercise of Guiding Qi to Rotate Automatically

(Refer to "Dysentery")

(3) The Exercise of Taking Essence from the Sun (Cai Rijinghua Gong)

The exercise should be done when the sun rises from the horizon.

Stand facing the sun, quiet and relaxed, with the breath even, distractions expelled and eyes slightly closed (not too tightly closed so that the soft, reddish sunlight can be seen). Inhale the sun essence naturally and fill the mouth with it mentally. Stop inhaling and tranquilize the mind, and swallow the essence slowly during exhaling down to Dantian. Do the inhaling and swallowing 9 or 18 times.

This exercise is suitable for patients suffering from dysfunction of the spleen—yang with aversion to cold.

Palpitation

Etiology

Several factors contribute to palpitation. In patients suffering from deficiency of qi and blood and insufficiency of heart—energy, palpitation may occur following sudden mental irritation. It may also be caused by deficiency of the heart—blood that fails to nourish the heart. Internal disturbance by phlegm— fire and disorder of heart—energy may also give rise to palpitation. Another causing factor is the dysfunction of heart—yang that leads to fluid retention.

Symptoms

The patient may note unduly rapid heart beat accompanied, in case of deficiency of heart—energy, with pallor, restless sleep at night, dizziness and vertigo, light red tongue proper and thready, feeble pulse; in case of internal disturbance of phlegm—fire, with fidgets, dreaminess, yellow tongue coating and slippery, rapid pulse; and in case of fluid retention, with epigastric stuffiness, dizziness, salivation, mental fatigue; white tongue coating and taut, slippery pulse. Flat—palm detection may reveal densified, stagnated, tingling or sparse sensation of qi at the precordial region.

Treatment

1. Emission of Outgoing—qi (Waiqi)

(1) First, press—knead Xinshu (UB 15), Ganshu (UB 18), Shanzhong (Ren 17), Jiuwei (Ren 15) and Lanmen (Extra 33) to get these points open.

(2) Emit qi with middle—finger—propping or sword—fingers hand gesture and vibrating and quivering manipulations to Xinshu (UB 15), Ganshu (UB 18), Shanzhong (Ren 17) and Jiuwei (Ren 15) for 6 or 12 respiratory cycles each. Then guide qi back to Dantian.

(3) Emit qi to the precordial region with flat—palm hand gesture and pushing, pulling and leading manipulations. Then guide the channel qi to circulate to the fingertips along the Heart Channel of Hand—Shaoyin and the Pericardium Channel of Hand—Jueyin, to balance qi between the upper and the lower.

Modification: In case of insufficiency of the heart—blood, emission of qi to Geshu (UB 17) and Pishu (UB 20) with flat—palm gesture and pushing and fixing manipulations may be added for 6 or 12 respiratory cycles. In case of internal disturbance of phlegm—fire, add emission of qi to Zhongwan (Ren

12) and Fenglong (St 40) with middle−finger−propping hand gesture and vibrating and quivering manipulations, and guidance of qi from Zhongwan (Ren 12) to Fenglong (St 40) with pulling and leading manipulations. In case of fluid retention, add emission of qi to Weishu (UB 21) and Sanjiaoshu (UB 22) for 14 or 24 respiratory cycles with flat−palm hand gesture and pulling and leading manipulations.Then guide qi to flow to the point of Weizhong (UB 40) along the Gallbladder Channel of Foot−Taiyang to balance qi.

2. Qigong−Acupuncture

Insert the filiform needles into Xinshu (UB 15), Juque (Ren 4), Shenmen (H 7) and Neiguan (P 6) and emit qi toward the needles with dragon−mouth or bird−beak hand gesture and pushing, pulling and rotating manipulations to get qi balanced between the points.

3. Self Qigong Exercise as Accessory Treatment

(1) The Exercise of Taking Red Qi

Take a sitting or lying posture. Relax all over, breathe naturally, expel distractions.

First, tap the upper and lower teeth together 36 times while stiring the saliva in the mouth with the tongue. Swallow the saliva 3 times after the tapping and send it mentally down to Dantian. Then imagine red qi.Inhale the red qi nasally and fill the mouth with it. Send the red qi slowly down to the heart and then to Dantian during exhaling to get the heart and kidney coordinated and then all the channels of the body communicated with each other. Do this 7 or 14 times.

This exercise is suitable for treatment of palpitation due to insufficiency of the heart−blood.

(2) The Exercise of Rubbing the Chest and "Ke" Qi

Tap the teeth and stir the saliva with the tongue as prescribed above. After the saliva is swallowed, put the left palm against the precardium and inhale slowly followed by slow exhale while pronuncing "ke". This is suitable for treatment of retention of phlegm—fire and fluid.

(3) The Exercise of Invigorating the Heart and Guiding Qi

Take the standing or the sitting posture, relax all over,breathe naturally, stick the tongue against the palate. Put the two palms together gently and set them in front of the chest. Keep in "quiescence" for a moment. Then abduct the palms, the two arms stretching to the back along the sides of the body. Keep still for a moment. Turn the palms upwards and lift them beside the chest. Stretch the hands slowly forwards with force focused on the tips of the middle fingers. Clench the fists as if dragging some heavy things. Pull the fists backward along the sides of the body. Turn the palms and arms inward and set the palms closed in front of the chest to end the exercise. It is indicated for palpitation of various causes.

Case

Yan, aged 29, came for the first visit on July 15, 1983.

Complaints Palpitation for a year manifested as self—noted irregular heart rate and paulocardia, cardiac distress, lassitude, restless sleep at night, dizziness, vertigo and listlessness.

Examination Clinical findings showed pale tongue proper with thin, white coating and knotted pulse. Flat—palm detection revealed densified and slight tingling sensation of qi at the precordial region. Auscultation found accentuation of the first heart sound and weakening of the second. Electrocardiographic examinaton showed ventricular extrasystole.

Diagnosis Palpitation (Ventricular extrasystole).

Treatment Emission of outgoing—qi was performed with flat—palm hand gesture and pushing, pulling, quivering and leading manipulations toward the points of Shanzhong (Ren 17), Huagai (Ren 20), Dazhui (Du 14), Xinshu (U B 15), Geshu (U B 17) and Neiguan (P 6).

Course of Treatment The palpitation was alleviated and sleep improved after being treated for twice. All the symptoms disappeared after 15 times of treatment. Electrocardiographic examination revealed normal heart function.

Dysuria

Etiology

Dysuria is termed "Longbi" in traditional medicine and uroschesis in modern medicine. It is often caused by blockage of the urinary tract due to the downward flow of damp—heat,or by disorder of the activities of qi (vital energy) due to insufficiency of kidney—yang and decline of fire from Mingmen (Du 4, the gate of life).

Symptoms

The disease is manifested by distention and pain in the lower abdomen, difficult urination though the patient may have strong desire for urination, accompanied with timidness, weakness of the extremities and deep, thready and weak pulse in case of insufficiency of kidney—qi, and with thirst but no desire for drinking, yellow tongue coating and rapid pulse in case of downward flow of damp—heat. Flat—palm detection may reveal densified, stagnated, tingling and heavy qi sensation at the lower abdomen.

Treatment

1. Emission of Outgoing—qi (Waiqi)

(1) Push the medial aspect of the thigh from the knee to the groin 300 times. Press—knead Baliao (the Eight Liao Points), Guanyuan (Ren 4) and Zhongji (Ren 3).

(2) Emit qi to the prominence of the lower abdomen with flat—palm hand gesture and vibrating and quivering manipulations for 14 or 28 respiratory cycles, then emit qi to the lower abdomen while guiding qi to flow along the Spleen Channel of Foot—Taiyin to Sanyinjiao (P 6) with pushing and leading manipulations for 6 or 12 times.

Modification: In case of insufficiency of kidney—qi, add emission of qi to Shenshu (U B 23) and Mingmen (Du 4) with flat—palm gesture and pushing and fixing manipulations for 11 or 22 respiratory cycles. In case of downward flow of damp—heat, add flat—palm gesture and pulling and leading manipulations to emit qi to Zhongji (Ren 3) while guiding qi to flow along the Spleen Channel of Foot—Taiyin to Yanglingquan (GB 34) in the lower limb for 11 or 22 respiratory cycles.

2. Qigong—Acupuncture

Insert the filiform needles into Zhongji (Ren 3) and Sanyinjiao (Sp 6). Emit qi toward the needles with dragon—mouth hand gesture and pushing and pulling manipulations. Then pull and lead qi in Sanyinjiao (Sp 6) to flow downward.

3. Self Qigong Exercise as Accessory Treatment

Push-rub with the two palms the lumbosacral portion from the upper to the lower 300 times. Then apply the palms (overlapped) against the lower abdomen, and rub clockwise while relaxing the anus and abdomen during exhaling, and stop rubbing and contract the abdomen slightly during inhaling, for 14 or 28 respiratory cycles.

Enuresis

Etiology

It is mostly due to dysfunction of the urinary bladder caused by failure of the kidney and Sanjiao (the three warmers) to control fluid metabolism.

Symptoms

The disease is characterized by involuntary discharge of urine during sleep at night, even several times a night in severe cases. It occurs most commonly in children over the age of three. Enuresis or incontinence of urine in adults is accompanied with listlessness and emaciation. Flat-palm detection often reveals densified,cold and tingling sensation of qi at Shenshu(UB 23), Mingmen (Du 4) and the lower abdomen.

Treatment

1. Emission of Outgoing-qi (Waiqi)

(1) Press-knead Pishu (UB 20), Shenshu (UB 23), Sanjiaoshu (UB 22), Mingmen (Du 4) and Sanyinjiao (Sp 6) first.

(2) Emit qi with flat-palm hand gesture and vibrating and

quivering manipula– tions to Mingmen (Du 4), Shenshu (U B 23) and Dantian for 11 or 22 respiratory cycles and guide qi with pushing and leading manipulations to the lower extremities along the Spleen Channel of Foot–Taiyin and the Kidney Channel of Foot–Shaoyin to get qi regulated between the upper and lower.

(3) Emit qi to Dantian with flat–palm hand gesture and pushing and leading manipulations. Push clockwise to lead the circulation of qi.

2. Qigong–Acupuncture

Insert the filiform needles into Guanyuan (Ren 4), Zhongji (Ren 3), Baihui (Du 14) and Sanyinjiao (P 6). Emit qi and guide qi to circulate clockwise with dragon–mouth hand gesture and pushing and leading manipulations to get qi activities balanced between the needles.

3. Self Qigong Exercise as Accessory Treatment

Practise "the Exercise for Strengthening the Kidney and Arresting Urine".

Stand erect, make fists and apply them against the soft parts at the sides of the waist and turn the waist clockwise and counterclockwise 6 times each. Then take the sitting posture. Put the two hands on the sides of the waist and rub from above to below 36 times. Hold the scrotum with the right hand, apply the left palm to the pubes inferior to the pubic symphysis. Move the two hands up and down simultaneously 81 times. Change hands and do the same for another 81 times.

Insomnia

Etiology

The disease is caused by insufficient generation of blood due to impairment of the spleen—qi and malnourishment of the heart—energy due to deficiency of heart—blood resulting from anxiety and over—fatigue; or by irritability due to incoordination between the heart and the kidney resulting from impairment of the kidney by excessive sexual life; or by irritability due to emotional depression; or by incoordination between the spleen and the stomach resulting from improper diet.

Symptoms

The main symptom is inability to sleep, which, based on different conditions of illness, may be further classified as inability to get into sleep at the beginning, abnormal waking and inability to fall asleep after waking. The accompanying symptoms vary with the causes of the disease. Insomnia due to deficiency of the heart and the spleen is manifested by palpitation, dizziness, vertigo, perspiration and thready and feeble pulse;that due to kidney deficiency is manifested by dizziness, involuntary seminal emission, soreness of loins, reddish tongue proper and thready and rapid pulse; and that due to emotional depression, by discomfort in the epigastrium, belching and acid regurgitation, thick, greasy tongue coating and slippery pulse. Flat—palm detection may reveal thin, tingling and cold sensation of qi around the body in case of deficiency of the heart and the spleen, and densified, scattered, tingling and distending sensation of qi at the head, hypochondria and epigastrium in case of other types.

Treatment

1. Emission of Outgoing—qi (Waiqi)

(1) Knead Lanmen (Extra), Zhongwan (Ren 12) and Guanyuan (Ren 4); Push Tianmen (St 25) and Kangong (Extra); knead Taiyang (Extra 2); knead digitally Pishu (UB 20), Weishu (UB 21), Ganshu (UB 18), Danshu (UB 19) and Zusanli (St 36); and press–knead the Urinary Bladder Channel of both sides.

(2) Emit qi with flat–palm gesture and vibrating manipulation to Baihui (Du 20), Dazhui (Du 14), Mingmen (Du 4), Zhongwan (Ren 12) and Guanyuan (Ren 4) for 9 or 18 respiratory cycles each; emit qi with the middle–finger–propping gesture and vibrating and quivering manipulations to Zhongwan (Ren 12) for 9 respiratory cycles; and emit qi to Baihui (Du 20) and Dantian with the hand off patient's body surface with flat–palm gesture and pushing and leading manipulations, and guide qi to circulate along the Ren Channel.

(3) Emit qi to Touwei (St 8) with flat–palm gesture and pushing, pulling and leading manipulations, and guide qi toward Zusanli (Sp 36) along the Stomach Channel of Foot–Yangming to balance qi.

Modification: For treatment of insomnia due to deficiency of the heart and the spleen, add flat–palm gesture and pushing and leading manipulations to emit qi to Xinshu (UB 15) and Pishu (UB 20) and to guide qi downward along the Urinary Bladder Channel of Foot–Taiyang. For insomnia due to kidney deficiency, add flat–palm gesture and pushing and quivering manipulations to emit qi to Shenshu (UB 23) and Mingmen (Du 4). For insomnia due to emotional depression, add flat–palm gesture and pulling and leading manipualtions to emit qi toward Qimen (Liv 4) and Zhangmen (Liv 3) and to guide the channel qi downward to the lower extremities along the Liver Channel of Foot—Jueyin and the Gallbladder Channel of Foot—Shaoyang. And for insomnia due to incoordination of the spleen and the stomach, add middle—finger—propping hand gesture and vibrating and quivering manipulations toward Zhongwan (Ren 12), Liangmen (St 21) and Zusanli (St 36).

2. Qigong—Acupuncture

Insert the filiform needles into Zhongwan (Ren 12), Shenmen (H 7),Sanyinjiao (Sp 6) and Zusanli (St 36) and emit qi toward the needles with dragon—mouth hand gesture and pushing and leading manipulations to balance qi between the points.

3. Self Qigong Exercise as Accessory Treatment

(1) The Psychosomatic Relaxation Exercise

Take a sitting or lying posture. Relax the whole body step by step by means of concentrating the mind on one part after another, while saying "relax" silently, in the order of the head, shoulders, upper limbs, back, waist, hips, chest, abdomen and the lower limbs. Carry out the relaxation 3 — 5 times with natural respiration.

(2) The Qi Circulation Exercise

Take a sitting or lying posture with breath even, mind concentrated on Dantian and distractions expelled. When a flow of hot qi is felt accumulating in Dantian and rushing toward the coccyx, take antidromic respiration and lead qi to go upwards from the coccyx to Baihui (Du 20) along the Du Channel and then to go downwards via the chest and abdomen and finally back to Dantian along the Ren Channel, to complete a "small circle of qi", which is followed by concentration of the mind on Dantian for a while before ending the exercise.

Case

Meng, female, a 22 year old typist, came for the first visit on April 9, 1983.

Complaints The patient complained of suffering from insomnia for more than a year, which was manifested as inability to sleep, dreaminess, palpitation, irritability, aching–pain and discomfort all over the body, dizziness, heavy sensation in the head, bitterness in the mouth, dryness of the eyes, perspiration, shortness of breath and lassitude of the extremities.

Examination Physical examination found thin, white tongue coating and deep, thready and feeble pulse. Flat–palm detection revealed thin and slightly cold sensation of qi at the chest and head. Electrocardiographic and electro–encephalographic examinations showed no abnormalities.

Diagnosis Insomnia (Functional disturbanc of vegetative nerves).

Treatment Emission of qi was conducted to Tianmen (Extra), Yintang (Extra 1), Taiyang (Extra 2), Pishu (UB 20) and Xinshu (UB 15) with flat–palm and middle–finger–propping hand gestures and pushing, pulling, leading and quivering manipulations.

Course of Treatment On receiving outgoing–qi, the patient presented involuntary forward and backward bending and turning of the body. Recovery took place after 5 times of treatment.

Seminal Emission

Etiology

Seminal emission falls into two kinds, nocturnal emission and spermatorrhoea. Nocturnal emission is usually caused by excess of ministerial fire, exuberance of the heart−yang, deficiency of kidney−yin, overstain and breakdown of the normal physiological coordination between the heart and the kidney, while spermatorrhoea is caused by failure of the kidney in storing reproductive essence and incompetence of orifice for keeping seminal fluid, which is a more knotted syndrome than the former.

Symptoms

1. Nocturnal Emission

It refers to ejaculation when dreaming. It occurs once every 5 − 6 nights or every 3 − 4 nights and is accompanied with the symptoms of dizziness, vertigo, fatigue and abdominal pain. Flat−palm detection often reveals densified, tingling and cold sensation of qi at the head, the waist and the lower abdomen.

2. Spermatorrhoea

Spermatorrhoea refers to ejaculation not related to dream; it may occur at any time or upon thinking of sexual activities. Patients with spermatorrhoea often have lassitude of the extremities and hypomnesis. In severe cases, the disease can last for years. Flat−palm detection usually reveals tingling, thin and stagnated sensation of qi which is of imbalance between the left and right and the upper and lower.

Treatment

1. Emission of Outgoing-qi (Waiqi)

(1) Press and knead Shenshu (UB 23), Xinshu (UB 15) and Mingmen (Du 4),and press Guanyuan (Ren 4), Zhongji (Ren 3) and Sanyinjiao (Sp 6) digitally.

(2) Emit qi, with flat-palm gesture and vibrating and quivering manipulations toward the points Zhongwan (Ren 12), Guanyuan (Ren 4) and Mingmen (Du 4) for a period of 12 respiratory cycles each. Again, emit qi, with flat-palm gesture and pushing, pulling and vibrating manipulations, toward Mingmen (Du 4), and guide qi to flow upwards along the Du Channel to Baihui (Du 20) and then downward along the Ren Channel back to Dantian.

(3) Emit qi, with flat-palm hand gesture and pushing-leading manipulation, towards Baihui (Du 20) for a period of 7 respiratory cycles, and then guide qi to flow along the Ren Channel back to Dantian.

Modification: In case of nocturnal emission, add flat-palm hand gesture and pushing, rotating and leading manipulations to emit qi to Xinshu (UB 15), Pishu (UB 20), Zhongwan (Ren 12) and Jiuwei (Ren 15), and to guide the channel qi down to Shenmen (H 7) and Daling (P 7) along the Heart Channel of Hand-Shaoyin and the Pericardium Channel of Hand-Jueyin; in case of spermatorrhoea, add flat-palm hand gesture and pushing, rotating and leading manipulations to emit qi to Shenshu (UB 23), Mingmen (Du 4), Zhongwan (Ren 12) and Zusanli (St 36) and to guide qi to flow down to Zusanli (St 36) along the Stomach Channel of Foot-Yangming to balance qi between the upper and the lower.

2. Qigong-Acupuncture

Insert the filiform needles into Guanyuan (Ren 4), Dahe (K 12), Jinggong (Extra), Shenmen (H 7), Neiguan (P 6) and Zusanli (St 36). Emit qi with dragon—mouth hand gesture and pushing, pulling and rotating manipulations toward the needles. balance qi round the needles.

3. Self Qigong Exercise as Accessory Treatment

(1) Yang—Recuperation Exercise (Daoyang Gong)

At midnight when the penis is erecting, lie supine with the eyes and mouth closed and the tongue rested against the palate. Bow the waist up and prop the coccyx with the middle finger of the left hand. Make the right hand a fist with the thumb—tip pressing ziwen (the stripe joining the palm and the ring finger). Then stretch the legs, with the toes bending toward the soles forcefully. Take a breath and get the qi inhaled mentally to the back of the body, the back of the head and then the top of the head. During exhaling, get qi down along with exhaling to the Lower Dantian while relaxing the waist, legs, hands and feet with ease. Do the exercise till the penis prostrates. If the penis does not erect at midnight, the practitioner may try to get it erected and then do the exercise.

(2) The Vital Essence Recovering Exercise (Huijing Huanye Gong)

This exercise is indicated for seminal emission and mucous urination.

When urinating, make fists with the thumbs nipping ziwen (the stripe joining the palm and the ring finger), flex the toes toward the soles and clench the teeth. After some water has been passed, draw a sudden breath and simultaneously stop urinating. Contract the glans and penis to hold urine while directing qi up to Mingmen (Du 4), then back to Dantian, with the hands, feet and the whole body relaxed. Restart urination and stop again in the same way. Repeat the procedures 2 or 4 times during one urination period.

(3) The Yang—Recovering Exercise (Huanyang Gong)

This exercise should be done at 7 – 9 pm or 9 – 11 pm. Lie on one side with the body bent. Hold the scrotum with one hand and press the lower abdomen with the other. Carry out up—and—down movement 81. times. Change hands and do the same for another 81 times or do it at other time of the same day. Then rub the hands against each other to get them warm and scrub Shenshu (UB 23) and Yongquan (K 1) with them 81 times respectively.

Impotence

Etiology

Impotence is usually caused by masturbation in adolescence or intemperance in sexual life. Anxiety which impairs the reproductive essence, and constraint, depression and kidney impairment by fright may also give rise to it.

Symptoms

The main symptoms are failure of normal penis erection, or quick ejaculation at sexual impulse. These symptoms may be accompanied by lassitude in the loins and legs, dizziness, vertigo and listlessness and hypomnesis. In severe cases, the disease may last for years. Flat—palm detection often reveals densified, tingling and cold sensation of qi at the lower abdomen and the sacral part.

Treatment

1. Emission of Outgoing-qi (Waiqi)

(1) Press-knead Shenshu (UB 23),Mingmen (Du 4),Guanyuan (Ren 4) and Sanyinjiao (Sp 6) first.

(2) Emit qi with flat-palm hand gesture and vibrating and quivering manipula- tions to Guanyuan (Ren 4) for 12 respiratory cycles, then with middle-finger- propping gesture and the same manipulations to Zhongji (Ren 3) for 12 respiratory cycles, followed by emitting qi with flat-palm ges- ture and pushing and pulling manipulations to Mingmen (Du 4) for 24 respiratory cycles.

(3) Emit qi with flat-palm hand gesture and pushing, pul- ling, rotating and leading manipulations to Mingmen (Du 4) and Dantian for 24 respiratory cycles and guide qi to flow clockwise.

2. Qigong-Acupuncture

Insert the filiform needles into Zhongji (Ren 3), Guanyuan (Ren 4), Sanyinjiao (Sp 6) and Zusanli (St 36), then emit qi to- ward the needles to get qi activities between these points bal- anced.

3. Self Qigong Exercise as Accessory Treatment

(1) Iron Crotch Exercise (Tiedang Gong)

Pushing the Abdomen: Lie supine, overlap the hands with the right above the left, and push with them from the xiphoid process to the pubic symphysis 36 times.

Pushing the Abdomen Obliquely: Lie supine, and push with the palms from the xiphoid process separately and obliquely to the sides of the abdomen 36 times.

Kneading the Navel: Lie supine, overlap the hands and

knead with pressure the navel clockwise and counterclockwise 36 times respectively.

Twisting the Spermatic Cords: Take a sitting posture, pinch—knead the spermatic cords with the thumb and the index and middle fingers 50 times each.

Kneading the Testicles: Sit and grasp both the testicles and penis at the root with the right hand. Put the left palm on the left testicle and knead it 50 times. Change hands and knead the right testicle 50 times.

Rubbing the Testicles: Sit. Hold the testles between the thumbs and the index and middle fingers of both hands and rub—twist 50 times.

Proping the Testicles: Sit, with the tips of the thumbs supporting the testicles of the respective sides. Prop the testicles up toward the groins and then lower them. Do this 3 times.

Swaying the Sand Bag: Stand erect. Make a slipknot at one end of a piece of gauze (33 cm wide, 85 cm long) and tie a sand bag (1.25 kg) to the other end. Get the slipknot looping at the root of the penis and testles with an optimal degree of tightness. Sway the sand bag forward and backward 50 times.

Pounding the Testicles: Stand erect. Make hollow fists of both hands, and pound with the back of the fists on both testicles alternately 50 times each.

Pounding the Renal Regions: Stand erect and pound alternately with the back of the fists on their respective renal regions 50 times each.

Activating the Back: Stand erect. Make hollow fists, relax the joints of the shoulders, elbows and wrists. Sway the waist to lead one fist to pound the chest (palm facing the chest) and the other (the back of the fist) to pound the region inferior to the scapula simultaneously and alternately 25 times for each side.

Turning the Knees: Stand with feet close together. Rest palms on the knees. Turn the knees clockwise and counterclockwise 25 times each.

Rolling the Stick: Sit straight. Put on flat—sole shoes. Step on a round stick and roll it with both feet to and fro 50 times.

Ending of the Iron Crotch Exercise: Sit quietly with palms on the thighs for a while, then stand up and move the body freely to end the exercise.

(2) The Yang—Strengthening Exercise (Qiang Yang Gong)

Hold the penis in one hand with the balanus exposed. Exert to make qi and blood to flow to the balanus several times, with the strength of gripping increased gradually. Slipping of the hand up and down should be avoided. The exercise should be done 2 − 4 times a day.

Case

Bao, male, 29 years old, came for the first visit on May 19, 1983.

Complaints   The patient complained of impotence for 7 years accompanied by dizziness, vertigo, insomnia, hypomnesis, soreness and weakness of the loins and knees and listlessness. He had a history of masturbation and seminal emission. His first marriage failed because of his sexual inability. He was in great agony when he failed to get his wife pregnant three years after his second marriage. After acupuncture and administration of traditional drugs in hospitals in Shanghai, Hangzhou and Beijing failed to take effect, he came to try qigong.

Examination Physical examination found pale tongue with thin, white coating and deep, thready and feeble pulse. The testicles and the penis were normal, with no tenderness. Flat—palm detection with outgoing—qi revealed thin and cold sensation of qi at the points of Mingmen (Du 4) and Shenshu (UB 23).

Diagnosis Impotence (Decline of fire from the gate of life).

Treatment Flat—palm and middle—finger—propping hand gestures and pushing, quivering and fixing manipulations were adopted to emit qi to Dantian, Zhongji (Ren 3), Mingmen (Du 4), Shenshu (UB 23), Zusanli (St 36) and Sanyinjiao (Sp 6). The patient was told to practise the Iron Crotch Exercise.

Course of Treatment The penis could erect voluntarily after 12 times of treatment but the erection was not desirable. Complete recovery took place after 30 times of treatment. He had a daughter in August, 1984.

Premature Ejaculation

Etiology

The disease is often caused by masturbation in adolescence, deficiency of the kidney—qi due to intemperance in sexual life or dampness and heat of the Liver Channel.

Symptoms

Failure of the normal sexual life characterized by ejaculation of semen at the beginning of the sexual act and prostration of the penis immediately after the ejeculation is the main manifestation of the disease.

Premature ejaculation due to deficiency of the kidney—qi have the symptoms of soreness and pain in the waist, weakness of the knees and feeble cubit pulse. Densified, cold and tingling qi may be detected at the lambosacral region and the lower abdomen with the flat—palm hand gesture.

Premature ejaculation due to dampness and heat of the Liver Channel may be accompanied with vexation, bitterness in the mouth, dark urine, urodynia or itching and swelling of the pudendum, and yellow tongue coating and taut, forceful pulse. On flat—palm detection, densified and stagnated qi may be felt at the lower abdomen and around Shenshu (UB 23).

Treatment

1. Emission of Outgoing—qi (Waiqi)

(1) Press—knead Shenshu (UB 23), Guanyuan (Ren 4) and Sanyinjiao (Sp 6) first.

(2) Emit qi with flat—palm hand gesture and vibrating and quivering manipulations to Shenshu (U B 23), Guanyuan (Ren 4), Qichong (St 30) and Guilai (St 29) for 11 or 22 respiratory cycles respectively.

(3) Emit qi to Dantian and guide qi to rotate clockwise with flat—palm gesture and pushing, leading, and rotating manipulations.

Modification: In case of deficiency of kidney—qi, add emission of qi to Dantian with middle—finger—propping hand gesture and vibrating and quivering manipulations for 42 respiratory cycles; in case of dampness and heat of the Liver Channel, add flat—palm gesture and pushing, pulling and leading manipulations to emit qi to Qimen (Liv 4), Zhangmen (Liv 13) and Riyue (GB 24) and guide qi to flow toward

Yanglingquan GB 34) and Taichong (Liv 3) along the Liver Channel of Foot—Jueyin and the Gallbladder Channel of Foot—Shaoyang.

2. Qigong—Acupuncture

Insert the filiform needles into Guanyuan (Ren 4), Sanyinjiao (Sp 6), Taixi (K 3) and Taichong (Liv 3). Emit qi toward these points with bird—beak hand gesture and pushing, pulling and rotating manipulations to balance qi between the points. In case of dampness and heat of the Liver Channel, guide qi toward Yinglingquan (Sp 9) and Taichong (Liv 3) to expel the evils there.

3. Self Qigong Exercise as Accessory Treatment

(1) Practise the Iron Crotch Exercise (Refer to "Impotence").

(2) The Exercise for Strengthening the Kidney—Yang

Hitting the Lumbosacral Region: Hit the sides of the waist and the sacral region with hollow fists when there is a tendency to ejaculate.

Rubbing the Penis and Testicles: Hold the testicles and the penis between the two palms and rub—knead them 36 times each. Practise "hitting the lumbosacral region" when there is a tendency to ejaculate.

Tossing the Penis: Lie supine. Grip the penis by the root with the index and middle fingers of the left hand and toss it onto the interior aspect of the left thigh 36 times. Do the same with the right hand and onto the right thigh for another 36 times. Then grip the penis by the root with the thumb and the index and middle fingers of both hands and toss the penis onto the lower abdomen 36 times.

Kneading the Penis and Pulling the Testicles: Put the index and middle fingers of one hand on the frenulum of prepuce of the penis and the thumb on the coronary edge and pinch—knead the penis with symmatric force; hold the scrotum and the testicles in another hand and pull them downward and backward. The pincing—kneading and pulling should be carried out simultaneously and the movements of the two hands should be coordinative. Release both hands suddenly after 3 — 4 respiratory cycles of practice, and repeat the procedure again several times.

Kneading the Testicles: Lie supine, rest the root of the left palm against the root of the testicles and knead with pressure 81 times. Repeat the procedure with the right palm 81 times.

Vertigo

Etiology

Several factors contribute to the syndrome: hyperactivity of the liver—yang aused by failure of water (kidney) to nourish wood (liver) due to insufficiency of the kidney—yin; insufficiency of qi and blood in the heart and spleen leading to deficiency of the marrow reservior; and stagnation of phlegm—dampness caused by deficiency of the spleen and the stomach which fail to transport.

Symptoms

The syndrome is characterized by severe dizziness and vertigo, blurred vision and nausea, accompanied with soreness of the waist, mental fatigue, flushed complexion, tinnitus, reddish tongue and taut, rapid pulse in case of hyper—activity of the liver—yang; with listlessness, disinclination to talk, anorexia, palpitation, insomnia, pale tongue and thready pulse in case of insufficiency of qi and blood; and with nausea, heaviness in the head, greasy tongue coating and slippery pulse in case of stagnation of phlegm—dampness. Flat—palm detection may reveal densified, cold, tingling, distending and stagnated sensation of qi at the top of the head and the forehead or all over the head.

Treatment

1. Emission of Outgoing—qi (Waiqi)

(1) Press—knead Dazhui (Du 14), Baihui (Du 20) and Taiyang (Extra 2), push— knead Hanyan (GB 4) and Shuaigu (GB 8) and knead with the fingertip Ganshu (UB 18), Shenshu (UB 23), Guanyuan (Ren 4) and Qihai (Ren 6) to open the points and dredge the channels.

(2) Emit qi with flat—palm gesture and vibrating manipulation toward Baihui (Du 20), Dazhui (Du 14), Zhongwan (Ren 12) and Guanyuan (Ren 4) for 12 or 24 respiratory cycles respectively.

(3) With flat—palm gesture and pulling and leading manipulations. emit qi to Touwei (St 8), Liangmen (St 21) and Zusanli (St 36). Then guide the channel qi to flow from Baihui (Du 20) via Zhongwan (Ren 12) to Guanyuan (Ren 4) along the Du Channel; from Touwei (St 8) to Zusanli (St 36) along the Stomach Channel of Foot—Yangming to make qi strong in the lower and weak in the upper, and guide qi with the same method toward the ends of the upper limbs along the Large Intestine Channel of Hand—Yangming to balance qi .

(4) Then knead with the fingertip Baihui (Du 20) and

Taiyang (Extra 2), push Hanyan (GB 4) and Shuaigu (GB 8). Finally pat Baihui (Du 20) and Dazhui (Du 14) and rock the upper limbs to end the exercise.

Modification: In case of hyperactivity of the liver—yang, add flat—palm hand gesture and pushing, pulling and rotating manipulations to emit qi to Ganshu (UB 18), Shenshu (UB 23) and Dantian, and guide qi to flow along the channel or counterclockwise so as to nourish yin and suppress the hyperactive yang; in case of insufficiency of qi and blood, add flat—palm gesture and pushing and fixing manipulations to emit qi to Pishu (UB 20), Geshu (UB 17), Ganshu (UB 18) and Dantian so as to nourish qi and replenish blood; and in case of stagnation of phlegm—dampness, add flat—palm gesture and pushing, pulling and leading manipulations to emit qi to Zhongwan (Ren 12) and Liangmen (St 21), and guide qi to flow toward Zusanli (St 36) along the Stomach Channel so as to dredge the channels and expel the evils.

2. Qigong—Acupuncture

Insert the filiform needles into Yintang (Extra 1), Taiyang (Extra 2), Baihui (Du 20), Touwei (St 8), Neiguan (P 6), Zusanli (St 36) and Taichong (Liv 3). With dragon—mouth or bird—beak hand gesture and pushing, pulling and leading manipulations, emit qi toward the needles and guide qi to Neiguan (P 6) and Taichong (Liv 3).

3. Self Qigong Exercise as Accessory Treatment

(1) The Three—Line Relaxation Exercise

The first line refers to the one from the lateral sides of the head, neck, shoulder and the upper limbs; the second to anterior side of the head, neck, chest, abdomen and the lower limbs; and the third, to the posterior side of the head, neck, back, waist and the lower limbs.

Any of the three postures, standing, sitting or lying, can be taken. To start the exercise, the practitioner should concentrate the mind on the first part of the first line and say " relax" silently, and then on the next part and so on and so forth. Then proceed to the second and third lines. Complete the relaxation of the three lines in sequence. It is indicated for any type of vertigo.

(2) The Exercise of Taking Black Qi

Take a standing or sitting posture, breathe naturally and expel distractions. Conduct teeth—tapping 36 times while stirring the saliva with the tongue. Swallow the saliva 3 times after the tapping and each time send it mentally down to the kidneys and then to Dantian.

Imagine black qi. Inhale it nasally and fill the mouth with it. Send it slowly to the kidneys and then to Dantian during exhaling. Do this 7 times.

The exercise has the function of nourishing the liver and kidney and strengthening yang. It is indicated in patients suffering from deficiency of kidney—yin and hyperactivity of liver—yang.

Hypertension

Etiology

The cause of the disease remains obscure. It may be related to mental stress, mental irritation and heredity. Traditional Chinese medicine has it in the categories of " vertigo" and "headache".

Symptoms

1. Hypertension Due to Hyperactivity of Yang Caused by Deficiency of Yin

This type is manifested by high blood pressure, dizziness, headache, vertigo, tinnitus, insomnia, dreaminess, hot sensation in the heart , the palms and the soles, reddish tongue proper and wiry, thready and rapid pulse. Flat—palm detection may reveal densified and tingling sensation of qi at the top of the head, the anterior and posterior aspects of the body and at the hypochondria, and cold and densified qi sensation at the waist and the lower abdomen.

2. Hypertension Due to Hyperactivity of the Liver—Fire

It is manifested as high blood pressure, vertigo, headache, flushed complexion, bitterness in the mouth, restlessness, constipation, reddened tongue with yellow coating and rapid pulse. Flat—palm detection may reveal hot, tingling and densified sensation of qi at the top and the two sides of the head.

3. Hypertension Due to Deficiency of Both Yin and Yang

The main manifestations are high blood pressure, dizziness, tinnitus, palpitation, short breath, soreness of the loins, weakness of the legs, insomnia, dreaminess, pale or reddish tongue proper with white coating, and wiry, thready pulse. Flat—palm detection may reveal no obvious sensation of qi all over the body.

Treatment

1. Emission of Outgoing—qi (Waiqi)

(1) Push—wipe Yintang (Extra 1) and Kangong (Extra), sweep—wipe Shuaigu (GB 8) and Hanyan (GB 4) and

press—knead Baihui (Du 20), Fengchi (GB 20) and Dazhui (Du 14).

(2) Emit qi with flat—palm hand gesture and vibrating and quivering manipulations toward Baihui (Du 20), Dazhui (Du 14), Mingmen (Du 4) and Zhongwan (Ren 12) for a period of 6 or 12 respiratory cycles respectively; emit qi with middle— finger—propping hand gesture and vibrating and quivering manipulations towards Zhongwan (Ren 12) and Guanyuan (Ren 4) for 6 or 12 respiratory cycles.

(3) With flat—palm gesture and pulling and leading manipulations,emit qi toward Baihui (Du 20) and Touwei (St 8) and guide the channel qi to flow toward Mingmen (Du 4) along the Du Channel and to flow to Neiting (St 44) along the Stomach Channel of Foot—Yangming to make it strong in the lower and weak in the upper.

Modification : In case of hyperactivity of yang caused by deficiency of yin, add flat—palm hand gesture and pushing and rotating manipulations to emit qi to Ganshu (UB 18), Shenshu (UB 23) and Dantian, and at the same time guide qi to go along the channel or to go counterclockwise. In case of hyperactivity of the liver— fire, add flat—palm gesture and pulling and leading manipulations to emit qi to Zhangmen (Liv 13), Qimen (Liv 14) and Riyue (GB 24), and to guide the channel qi to flow toward the lower extremities along the Liver Channel of Foot— Jueyin and the Gallbladder Channel of Foot—Shaoyang to make it strong in the lower and weak in the upper. In case of deficiency due to both yin and yang, add emission of qi to Pishu (UB 20), Shenshu (UB 23), Mingmen (Du 4) and Dantian with flat—palm gesture and pushing and rotating manipulations.

2. Qigong—Acupuncture

Insert the filiform needles into Quchi (LI 11), Waiguan (SJ 5), Zusanli (St 36), Sanyinjiao (Sp 6), Taixi (K 3), Taichong (Liv 3) and Zhongwan (Ren 12). Emit qi toward them with dragon—mouth or bird—beak hand gesture and pushing and rotating manipulations, and guide the channel qi to Taichong (Liv 3) and Waiguan (SJ 5).

3. Self Qigong Exercise as Accessory Treatment

(1) The Bath—Relaxation Exercise

Stand or sit quiet and relaxed all over, with the eyes closed,tongue sticking to the lower gum and distractions expelled. Imagine the feeling of a warm shower: the warm water pouring down onto the head, torso, extremities and the soles. Do the exercise 36 times.

Or, practise the Three—Line Relaxation Exercise (Refer to "Vertigo").

(2) The Exercise of Rubbing the Hypochondrium and "Xu" Qi

Take the standing or sitting posture. Put the palms against the ribs and inhale slowly. Say "xu" during exhalation with the palms rubbing the ribs. Do the exercise for 10 − 20 respiratory cycles.

It is suitable for hypertension due to hyperactivity of the liver—fire.

Hypochondriac Pain

Etiology

Though hypochondriac pain may be caused by different factors such as trauma, stagnation, accumulation and blockage of qi , stasis of phlegm and deficiency or excess of constitution, it is always related to the liver and is commonly seen in patients with hyperactivity of liver—fire or stagnation of the liver—qi.

Symptoms

Hypochondriac pain, which occurs in one side more often than that in both sides.

1. Excess Syndrome

Severe pain with difficulty in cough and breathing is seen in patients with excess syndrome; hypochondriac pain in both sides, wiry pulse, bitter mouth are found in patients with excess syndrome of the liver or excessive fire. Flat— palm detection often reveals heavy, stagnated, tingling and distending sensation of qi at the hypochondria.

2. Deficiency Syndrome

Feeble pulse, dry throat, poor appetite, dull pain or stinging pain are found in patients with deficiency syndrome, including insufficiency of the liver—yin and the kidney—yin, which is often caused by mental depression or hemorrhage.

Treatment

1. Emission of Outgoing—qi (Waiqi)

(1) Conduct digital pressing—kneading on the points Shanzhong (Ren 17), Qimen (Liv 14), Zhangmen (Liv 13), Ganshu (UB 18), Geshu (UB 17) Zhigou (SJ 6) and Yanglingquan (GB 34) to break through them and to promote the circulation of qi and blood in the Liver Channel.

(2) Emit qi with flat—palm gesture and pushing and pulling manipulations toward Qimen (Liv 14), Zhangmen (Liv 13)

and the painful region, then guide qi with leading manipulation to flow from the chest and hypochondrium to the lower extremities along the Liver Channel of Foot—Jueyin and the Gallbladder Channel of Foot—Shaoyang.

Modification: For deficiency syndrome (insufficiency of the liver—yin and kidney—yin), add digital pressing on the point Guanyuan (Ren 4), kneading the point Shenshu (UB 23), and emitting qi with flat—palm gesture and vibrating and quivering manipulations toward the lower abdomen with the point Guanyuan (Ren 4) as the centre for 12 or 24 respiratory cycles. For excess syndrome, add pushing the chest on both sides, digging—grasping Xuelang (the muscles at the anterior sides of the axillary fossa), digitally kneading Ganshu (UB 18), and rocking and rubbing the upper limbs. For pain caused by trauma, add pushing—rubbing the affected side with flat—palm hand gesture and rocking the shoulder joint.

2. Qigong—Acupuncture

Insert the filiform needles into Zhigou (SJ 6) and Yanglingquan(GB 34). Emit qi with dragon—mouth hand gesture and pulling and rotating manipulations, and rotate the hand counterclockwise to guide qi to go downward.

3. Self Qigong Exercise as Accessory Treatment

(1) Pushing the Hypochondrium and "Xu" Qi

Take a standing or sitting posture, relax all over, breathe naturally and expel the distractions.

Get the upper and lower teeth tapping each other 36 times while stirring the saliva with the tongue. Swallow the saliva 3 times after the tapping and each time send it down to the hypochondrium and further to Dantian. Then put the palm on both sides of the ribs. Inhale slowly to make the mouth filled with qi. When exahaling, utter "xu", with the palms rubbing the ribs gently from the upper to the lower 7 times. Do this for 8 respiratory cycles.

(2) Pushing the Chest to Guide Qi

If the pain is in the left side, conduct pushing massage with the right palm starting from the thoracic midline downward to the left 7 times, then from the upper to the lower straightly another 7 times, followed by kneading Shanzhong (Ren 17) and Qimen (Liv 14).

(3) Soothing the Liver and Guiding Qi

Stand relaxed and quiet, the two arms falling naturally on sides, the five fingers raised slightly upwards and the palms pressing downwards with a little force, thinking that qi has been directed to the centre of the palms and further to the fingertips.

Lift the two hands up to the chest with palms facing the front. Push the palms forward until the shoulders, the elbows and the wrists are at the same level. Concentrate the mind on the palms.

Stretch the arms sideways like a bird stretching its wings. With the fingers turned upward, push the arms toward the right and left respectively. Guide qi to the centre of the palms.

Withdraw the hand and set them in front of the chest, with palms upward and the fingertips of the two hands pointing to each other. Adduct the palms and push them down to the pubic symphysis to guide qi back to Dantian. Then drop the hands at the sides of the body to end the exercise.

Headache

Etiology

1. Invasion of the Channels by Pathogenic Wind

The wind—cold pathogen invades the channels in the head and lingers there, resulting in incoordination between qi and blood and obstruction of the channels, which in turn gives rise to headache.

2. Insufficiency of Both Qi and Blood

This type of headache is caused by insufficiency of the channel qi in the marrow reservoir (the brain) due to general debility and insufficiency of both qi and blood.

Symptoms

1. Invasion of the Channels by Pathogenic Wind

(1) Shaoyang Headache (Migraine)

As the Shaoyang Channels run along the sides of the head, pain in one side is the main symptom, which is often accompanied by a sensation of excessive heat in the head and splitting pain, conjunctival congestion, hypochondriac pain, bitterness in the mouth, dry throat, yellow and dry tongue coating, and wiry and rapid pusle. Flat—palm detection often reveals densified, distending, tingling and stagnated sensation of qi at the painful side of the head.

(2) Taiyang Headache (Occiput Pain)

Pain in the occipito—posterior position is the main symptom as the back of the head, the nape and the back of the torso are the areas where the Taiyang Channels spread, which is accompanied by fever, aversion to cold, stiffness and pain in the nape and back, thin and white tongue coating, and superficial and tense pulse. Flat—palm detection often reveals cold, densified and stagnated qi sensation at the occipital area.

(3) Jueyin Headache (Vertex Pain)

Because the Jueyin Channels converge at the vertex, pain in the vertex is the main symptom which is accompanied by vertigo, vexation, quick temper, flushed face, bitterness in the mouth, insomnia, reddened tongue with yellow coating, and wiry pulse. Flat—palm detection often reveal densified, cold, tingling and stagnated sensation of qi at the top of the head.

(4) Yangming Headache (Sinciput Pain)

Pain in the forehead is most obvious because the Yangming Channels go to the forehead along the hairline, accompanied by thirst, dysphoria with smothery sensation, foul breath, constipation, yellow tongue coating and forceful or slippery and rapid pulse. Flat—palm detection may reveal densified, stagnated, tingling and distending sensation of qi at the forehead.

2. Insufficiency of Both Qi and Blood

This type is characterized by general continuous headache, vertigo, heaviness of the head, lassitude, dim complexion, thready and feeble pulse, and thin and white tongue coating.

Treatment

1. Emission of Outgoing—qi (Waiqi)

(1) Push—open Tianmen (life pass, the superficial venules of the palmar side), push Kangong (Extra), knead Taiyang (Extra 2), sweep the Gallbladder Channel (with the fingers), dig—grasp Fengchi (GB 20) and Fengfu (Du 16), and press—knead Baihui (Du 20).

(2) Emit qi with flat—palm gesture and pulling and rotating (clockwise or counterclockwise) manipulations to Baihui

(Du 20) first, then with vibrating and quivering manipulations toward Baihui (Du 20), Dazhui (Du 14) and Mingmen (Du 4) for 6 or 12 respiratory cycles.

Modification: To treat Shaoyang headache (migraine), add flat—palm gesture and pulling and rotating manipulations to emit qi to Shuaigu (GB 8) and Hanyan (GB 4) and guide the channel qi to flow along the Channels of Foot—Shaoyang and Hand— Shaoyang to the ends of the extremities, where the pathogenic wind—cold can be expelled.

To treat Taiyang headache (occiput pain), add flat—palm gesture and pushing and leading manipulations to emit qi toward Fengchi (GB 20) and Tianzhu (UB 10), and guide the channel qi to flow to the upper and lower extremities along the Channels of Hand—Taiyang and Foot—Taiyang.

To treat Jueyin headache (Vertex pain), add flat—palm gesture and pulling and rotating (counterclockwise) manipulations to guide qi to flow clockwise and then downward to the lower extremities along the Gallbladder Channel of Foot—Shaoyang.

To treat Yangming headache (sinciput pain), add flat—palm gesture and pulling and leading manipulations to emit qi toward Taiyang (Extra 2), Touwei (St 8) and Yintang (Extra 1), and guide qi to flow to the lower extremities along the Channels of Hand—Yangming and Foot—Yangming and along the Ren Channel, or guide qi to the Ren Channel.

To treat headache due to insufficiency of both qi and blood, add flat—palm gesture and pushing and leading manipulations to emit qi to Pishu (UB 20), Geshu (UB 17), Shanzhong (Ren 17), Zhongwan (Ren 12) and Guanyuan (Ren 4).

2. Qigong—Acupuncture

According to the location of pain, insert the filiform needles into: Shang— xing (Du 23), Touwei (St 8), Hegu (LI 4) and Ashi points (pressure pain points) in the case of Yangming headache; into Baihui (Du 20), Tongtian (UB 7), Xingjian (Liv 2) and Ashi points in the case of Jueyin headache; into Shuaigu (GB 8), Hanyan (GB 4) Taiyang (Extra 2), Xiaxi (GB 43) and Ashi points in the case of Shaoyang headache; into Fengchi (GB 20), Dazhui (Du 14), Kunlun (UB 60)and Ashi points in the case of Taiyang headache; and into Baihui (Du 20), Qihai (Ren 6), Pishu (UB 20), Ganshu (UB 18), Hegu (LI 4) and Zusanli (St 36) in case of headache due to insufficiency of blood and qi. Then emit qi toward the needles with dragon—mouth hand gesture and pushing, pulling, rotating and leading manipulations to balance qi between the needles.

3. Self Qigong Exercise as Accessory Treatment

(1) The Relaxation Exercise by Body Partitions

Stand or sit with the whole body relaxed, distractions expelled and breath natural. By concentrating the mind on one part after another and saying "relax" silently, relax the whole body in the order of the head, shoulders, back, waist, hips, the upper limbs and the lower limbs. Do the exercise 3 — 5 times.

(2) The Head—Face Exercise

Pushing the Forehead: Push—rub the forehead with the four fingers (close to each other) of the two hands from the midpoint of of the line joining the eye—brows upward to the front hairline 24 — 48 times.

Kneading Taiyang (Extra 2): Knead Taiyang (Extra 2) counterclockwise 24 — 48 times with the middle fingers.

Bathing the Face: Rub the face with the two palms, starting from the midpoint at the forehead sidewards, then downwards, and then upwards along the sides of the nose back to the forehead 24 − 48 times.

Combing the Hair: Seperate the five fingers separated and curve them slightly. Comb the hair with them 24 − 48 times starting from the front hairline backwards.

Sweeping the Gallbladder Channel: Get the four fingers close to each other and slightly curved. Scrape−sweep with the fingertips along the Gallbladder Channel from above the ears backwards via the frontal angle towards the back of the head 10 or 20 times.

Rubbing the Back of the Head: Interlock the fingers of the two hands. Clasp the occipital bone with the roots of the palms and rub the back of the head from the upper to the lower 24 − 48 times.

Diabetes

Etiology

Two main factors contribute to the origination of the disease. The first factor is improper diet including over intake of alcohol and acrid and greasy food, which may cause stagnation at the Middle−jiao (the portion housing the stomach and the spleen), failure of the stomach and spleen to transport and accumulation of heat inside the body which, in turn, may give rise to failure of the yin fluid to nourish the lung and kidney, resulting in diabetes. The second factor is emotional; emotional upsets may lead to stagnation of qi which in turn impairs the body fluid, resulting in yin—deficiency with hyperactivity of the fire—evil, and eventually, diabetes.

Symptoms

1. Diabetes Involving the Upper—Jiao

It is characterized by thirst and polydipsia, dry throat and tongue, frequent micturition, polyuria, reddened tip and margin of tongue, thin and yellow tongue coating and rapid pulse. Flat—palm detection often reveals densified, hot, tingling and sensation of turbid qi at the Upper—jiao (the body cavity above the diaphragm where the heart and lung are located).

2. Diabetes Involving the Middle—Jiao

It is characterized by polyphagia, emaciation or constipation, dry yellow tongue coating and rapid, slippery pulse. Flat—palm detection often reveals hot, tingling, densified, filthy and stagnated sensation of qi at the Middle— jiao (the part holding the stomach and the spleen).

3. Diabetes Involving the Lower—Jiao

This type is characterized by frequent micturition, polyuria, chyluria or urine with sweet smell, weakness and softness in the waist and knees, reddish tongue proper without coating, and deep, thready and rapid pulse. Flat—palm detection often reveals densified, cold, stagnated and tingling sensation of qi at the Lower—jiao (the body cavity below the level of the umbilicus).

Treatment

1. Emission of Outgoing—Qi (Waiqi)

(1) Knead Feishu (UB 13), Pishu (UB 20), Shenshu (UB 23), Zusanli (St 36) and Sanyinjiao (Sp 6); dredge Lanmen (Extra), Liangmen (St 21), Zhongwan (Ren 12) and Guanyuan

(Ren 4).

(2) With flat—palm gesture and vibrating and quivering manipulations, emit qi to Feishu (UB 13), Pishu (UB 20), Shenshu (UB 23), Zhongwan (Ren12) and Guanyuan (Ren 4) for 6 or 12 respiratory cycles.

(3) With flat—palm hand gesture and pushing, pulling and leading manipulations, emit qi to Feishu (UB 13), Pishu (UB 20), Shenshu (UB 23), Tanzhong (Ren 17), Zhongwan (Ren 12) and Guanyuan (Ren 4); and with leading manipulation, regulate the qi activities in the chest and abdomen as well as the back and waist to get qi balanced between the Upper, Middle and Lower jiao.

2 (4) Dig—grasp Jiquan (H 1), Quchi (LI 11) and Hegu (LI 4) and rub and rock the upper limbs to end the treatment with outgoing—qi.

2. Qigong—Acupuncture

Insert the filiform needles into Tanzhong (Ren17), Zhongwan (Ren 12), Guan— yuan (Ren 4), Zusanli (St 36), Sanyinjiao (Sp 6), Taixi (K 3), Taichong (Liv 3) and Zhigou (SJ 6). Emit qi with dragon—mouth hand gesture and pushing, pulling and rotating manipulations to get qi balanced between the points.

Modification: Add emission of qi with flat—palm hand gesture and vibrating and quivering manipulations to Tanzhong (Ren 17), Zhongfu (Lu 1) and Yunmen (Lu 2) for diabetes involving the Upper—jiao; to Weishu (UB 21) and Sanjiaoshu (UB 22) for diabetes involving the Middle—jiao and to Pangguangshu (UB 28) and Zhongji (Ren 3) for diabetes involving the Lower—jiao.

3. Self Qigong Exercise as Accessory Treatment

(1) The Inner Health Cultivation Exercise (Neiyang Gong)

Take a sitting posture and either orthodromic or antidromic abdominal respiration, with the eyes closed and the whole body relaxed. Say silently some sentences such as "I keep quiet", "I am sitting and keeping quiet" and "I keep quiet and I'll be healthy". Inhaling, stick the tongue against the palate and say the first word of a sentence. Hold breath after inhaling and say the words in the middle. Exhaling, release the tongue and say the last word of the sentence. Start the exercise with a shortest sentence. Increase the number of words in a sentence gradually but the sentence should not be as long as to exceed nine words. Example : I (inhale) —— keep quiet and I'll be (hold breath)——healthy (exhale).

(2) The Nine-Turn Exercise for Longevity

First, stand or sit in quiescence with distractions expelled, breath even and the part to be manipulated exposed. Put the fingers below the xiphoid process and knead it clockwise 21 times.

Second, put the hands below the xiphoid process in the same way. Rotate and push the hands clockwise until they get to the pubic symphysis.

Third, separate the hands and rub the abdomen sidewards and then upwards till they are back to the xiphoid process where they meet each other.

Forth, overlap the index, middle and ring fingers of the two hands and push from the xiphoid process down to the pubic symphysis along the Ren Channel 21 times.

Fifth, overlapp the palms and put them on the abdomen

with the Inner Laogong (P 8) touching the umbilicus, and rub clockwise and counterclockwise 21 times respectively.

Sixth, put the left hand below the left ribs with the thumb stretched and pointing forward, and rub with the fingers from the ribs down to the groin 21 times. Do the same with the right hand on the right side another 21 times. Seventh, sit cross–legged after the pushing. Make fists with the two thumbs nipping ziwen (the crease joining the palm and the ring finger). Put the fists on the knees. Turn the chest and abdomen clockwise and counterclockwise 21 times respectively. The turning should be gentle, the breath in natural and the mind concentrated on the knees under the hands.

Hemiplegia

Etiology

Hemiplegia is the sequela of apoplexy caused by up–stirring of liver–wind or by invasion of the channels and collaterals by exopathic wind.

Symptoms

The marked symptoms are wry mouth with distorted eyes, hemiparalysis, retraction of tongue and flaccidity of hand and foot.

Flat–palm detection may reveal tingling, distending, densified and stagnated sensation of qi at the affected side.

Treatment

1. Emission of Outgoing–Qi (Waiqi)

(1) Press–knead Hegu (LI 4), Jiache (St 6), Neiguan (P 6), Quchi(LI 11), Yanglingquan (GB 34) and Weizhong (UB 40);

pinch the fingertips and the sides of the nails of the affected limb.

(2) Press-knead the Urinary Bladder Channel from the upper to the lower part 6 − 7 times.

(3) Emit qi, with flat-palm or sword-fingers hand gesture and pushing, pulling and leading manipulations, towards Yintang (Extra 1) and Baihui (Du 20), and guide the channel qi to flow downward along the Ren Channel. Then with the same manipulations, guide the channel qi from the upper to the lower along the Urinary Bladder Channel of Foot-Taiyang and the Stomach Channel of Foot- Yangming to balance qi.

Modification: If the patient suffers from right side hemiplegia, the following curative method should be added: knead with the fingertips Hanyan (GB 4), Shuaigu (GB 8) and Jiaosun (SJ 20) of the left side; sweep-scrape the affected side of the head along the Gallbladder Channel; then with flat-palm gesture and pulling and leading manipulations, emit qi toward the left side of the head and guide qi to flow from the head to the neck and then cross the neck and continue to flow along the Stomach Channel of Foot-Yangming and the Urinary Bladder Channel of Foot-Taiyang of the right side of the body, to the right foot. This may facilitate the qi activities and balance qi. For treatment of left side hemiplegia, guide the channel qi from the right side of the head to the left side of the body in the same way.

2. Qigong-Acupuncture

When the needles are inserted into the selected points, dragon-mouth or flat- palm hand gesture and pushing, pulling, leading and quivering manipulations should be applied to emit qi toward the points and guide the channel qi to flow downward.

The points should be selected in consideration of the conditions of the patient, e.g., Jianyu (LI 15), Quchi (LI 11), Waiguan (SJ 5) and Hegu (LI 4) in case of upper limb hemiplegia; Huantiao (GB 30), Yanglingquan (GB 34), Fenglong (St 40) and Juegu (GB 39) in case of the lower limb hemiplegia; Tiantu (Ren 22), Yamen (Du 15) and Tongli (H 5) in case of dysphasis; and Dicang (St 34), Jiache (St 6) and Hegu (LI 4) in case of wry mouth with distorted eyes.

3. Self Qigong Exercise as Accessory Treatment

(1) Try to promote movements of the affected limbs.

(2) Gently pat the affected limb from the upper to the lower with the fist of the healthy side, 7 − 9 times as one session, 3 − 5 sessions per day.

(3) Pull the affected limb with the hand of the healthy side. Pull upward, inward and outward when inhaling and release it when exhaling. Imagine that qi is flowing to the affected limb at the same time. Do it 4 − 6 times per day.

Facial Paralysis (Bells Palsy)

Etiology

Also named deviation of the eye and mouth in traditional Chinese medicine, it is usually caused by invasion of the head by pathogenic wind and cold.

Symptoms

The disease is characterized by hemiparalysis of the face manifested as numbness of the affected side, distorted mouth with the corners tilted to the healthy side, half–closed eye with dacryorrhea, and shallowed nasolabial groove. Flat–palm detection often reveals scattered, densified, cold and stagnated sensation of qi at the affected side.

Treatment

1. Emission of Outgoing–Qi (Waiqi)

(1) Press–knead gently Yangbai (UB 14), Chengqi (St 1), Sizhukong (SJ 23), Tongziliao (GB 1), Tinggong (SI 19), Quanliao (SI 18), Yingxiang (LI 20), Jiache (St 6), Yifeng (SJ 17), Fengchi (GB 20) and Hegu (LI 4).

(2) With flat–palm gesture and pushing–pulling–leading or pulling–quivering manipulation, emit qi to the affected side and guide the channel qi to circulate from the anterior to the posterior, or circulate to Hegu (LI 4) along the Large Intestine Channel of Hand–Yangming.

Modificaton: For treatment of the first–stage paralysis, it is advisable to apply gentle pressing–kneading and select flat–palm hand gesture and pushing, pulling and leading manipulations. As for paralysis with a long course, deep pressing–kneading and vibrating and quivering manipulations are desirable.

2. Qigong–Acupuncture

Insert the filiform needles into Dicang (St 4), Jiache (St 6), Qianzheng (Extra), Yangbai (GB 14), Yingxiang (LI 20), Yifeng (SJ 17), Fengchi (GB 20) and Hegu (LI 4). Emit qi with dragon–mouth hand gesture and pushing, pulling and quivering manipulations to the needles to get qi balanced between the points. Guide the channel qi to Hegu (LI 4).

3. Self Qigong Exercise as Accessory Treatment

(1) Push—knead the affected side of the face with the flat of the four fingers, from the corner of the mouth to the ear, from the zygomatic bone to the ear, and from the midpoint of the forehead sidewards to the back of the head 81 times respectively.

(2) Knead Jiache (St 6), Yifeng (SJ 17), Yangbai (GB 14), Sibai (St 2) and Yingxiang (LI 20) with the tip of the thumb 24 times each.

(3) Bathing the Face: Rub the face with the two palms starting from the midpoint of the forehead sidewards, then downwards, and then upwards along the sides of the nose back to the forehead, 24 − 48 times. Rub face in the opposite direction 24 − 48 times.

Arthralgia Syndrome

Etiology

It is caused by attack of the channels by pathogenic evils of wind, cold and dampness due to irregular daily life, weakened wei—qi (superficial qi or body resistence), or due to staying in a draught after sweating, wading in water, exposing to cold weather and long—time lying on damp ground.

Symptoms

1. Migratory Arthralgia

This type is characterized by migratory pain in the limbs which is sometimes ccompanied by fever and chills, yellow and greasy tongue coating and superficial pulse. Flat—palm detection often reveals tingling, distending and densified sensation of qi at the aching region.

2. Cold—type Arthralgia

Symptoms of this type include general or localized pain which may be relieved by warmth and aggravated by cold, white tongue coating and taut, tense pulse. Flat—palm detection often reveals cold, densified and stagnated sensation of qi at the aching region.

3. Damp—type Arthralgia

It is manifested as heaviness and numbness of the limbs and localized arthralgia (e.g., joints of the limbs) which tends to attack in wet days, and soft, slow pulse and white, greasy coating. Flat—palm detection may reveal cold, stagnated, densified, distending and tingling sensation of qi at the aching limb joints.

Treatment

1. Emission of Outgoing—Qi (Waiqi)

(1) Knead Dazhui (Du 14), Feishu (UB 13), Mingmen (Du 4) and Dantian.

(2) With the patient standing, emit qi with flat—palm gesture and pushing, pulling, quivering and leading manipulations to his Dazhui (Du 14), Mingmen (Du 4) and Dantian to facilitate his qi circulation and arouse his spontaneous movements. If the patient presents no spontaneous movements, the therapist should guide and regulate his qi of the Urinary Bladder Channel of Hand—Taiyang, starting from Fengmen (UB 12) and Tianzong (SI 11).

(3) Select the points along the channels, at the far end of the channels and those at the affected area. Emit qi toward the affected part with flat—palm gesture and pulling and leading manipulations, then guide the pathogenic qi to the far end of the extremities to expel it there. The patient should imagine at

the same time that his pathogenic qi is being expelled along with his exhaling. For example, for treatment of knee joint arthralgia, the doctor should firstly conduct pressing, kneading, pushing and rolling massage on Waixiyan (Dubi, St 36), Liangqiu (St 34), Xiyangguan (GB 33) and Yinglingquan (Sp 9), then with flat—palm hand gesture and pulling and leading manipulations, guide the patient's channel qi to flow along the Stomach Channel of Foot—Yangming and the Spleen Channel of Foot—Taiyin to the far end of the lower limbs and expel the wind, cold and dampness evils from Yinbai (Sp 1) and Dadun (Liv 1).

2. Qigong—Acupuncture

Select points at the affected area, at the far end of the channel or near the affected area. Insert the filiform needles into the selected points and emit qi with dragon—mouth hand gesture and pulling, rotating and leading manipulations toward them. Guide qi to flow from the aching point or along the channels to the far end to expel the evils there. For example, to treat arthralgia in the ankle, the points Shenmai (UB 62), Zhaohai (K 6), Ashi point (pressure pain point), Kunlun (UB 60) and Qiuxu (GB 40) should be selected.

3. Self Qigong Exercise as Accessory Treatment

(1) The Exercise for Expelling Wind, Cold and Dampness Stand quiet and relaxed, with the two palms pressing downward, knees slightly bent, eyes slightly closed and tongue stuck against the palate. Inhale first and send qi down to Dantian, and exhale and imagine that the genuine qi is coming out from Dantian and going along the channels directly to the painful area to drive the evil qi out of the body from the points at the

painful area or at the far end of the channel. Do the exercise 81 times.

(2) Six—Form Brocade Exercise (Liuduan Gong)

Form One   Stretching Out Hands to Shut the Cave Door: Set feet apart at shoulders width, the toes pointing inwards to form inverted splayfeet, the waist and legs straight, eyes looking straight ahead, mind concentrated on Dantian and breath natural. Lift the two hands with palms downwards to the two sides of the chest, and push forwards slowly as if shutting a door. Then strain the wrists and the ten fingers to exert traction to the tendons of the arms, 10 times.

Form Two   Stretching Arms and Shrugging Shoulders: Proceed from the last stance. Turn the arms sidewise in opposite directions and keep them at shoulder level, palms facing upward as if carrying a shoulder pole. Stretch the arms backwards and simultaneously shrug the shoulders, 10 times.

Form Three   Pressing Gourd Gently: Draw the hands back to the chest and then drop them to the sides of the legs with palms facing downwards and the fingers of them pointing at the opposite directions and bending dorsally a little. Press downwards forcefully 10 times.

Form Four   Bending Over to Touch Dan (Genuine Qi): Keep the legs straight and bend the waist. With palms facing downwards, cross the arms alternately while pressing the hands down to stroke, 10 times.

Form Five   Holding Mount Taihang by Hands: From the last stance, turn the palms upward as if to fish for something and lift them slowly to Tanzhong (Ren 17) with the back straightened. Adduct the palms and stretch the arms slowly upwards to the top of the head, palms apart at shoulders width. Then stretch the arms and palms forcefully upwards as if to hold up a mountain, 10 times.

Form Six   Snatching the Belt with Hands Alternately: Proceed from the last stance. Cup the hands slightly. Lower the left arm towards the front, and snatch as if to get something. Withdraw the left hand to the chest and snatch with the right hand. Repeat this 10 times.

Flaccidity Syndrome

Etiology

The disease is due to failure to nourish the muscles resulting from over consumption of the lung—fluid caused by invasion of the lung by exopathic wind— heat, or due to the overwhelming of dampness—heat which impairs the Yangming Channels, or due to insufficiency of liver—yin and kidney—yin (essence and energy of the liver and kidney) resulting from lingering illness or intemperance in sexual life.

Symptoms

The syndrome is marked by weakness and limited movement of the lower limbs, accompanied by fever, cough, vexation, thirst, scanty dark urine, reddened tongue proper with yellow coating and thready and rapid pulse in the type of retention of pathogenic heat in the lung; by heavy sensation of the body, turbid urine, hot sensation in the feet which may be relieved by coldness, yellow greasy tongue coating and soft and rapid pulse in the type of overwhelming dampness—heat; and by soreness and weakness of the waist and back, seminal emission and prospermia, dizziness and vertigo, thready, rapid pulse and reddened tongue proper in the type of insufficiency of the liver—yin and kidney—yin.

Flat—palm detection of the three types may reveal densified, distending and stagnated or scattered, tingling and cold sensation of qi at the affected limb.

Treatment

1. Emission of Outgoing—Qi (Waiqi)

(1) For treatment of flaccidity of the upper limbs, select Dazhui (Du 14), Jiquan (H 1), Xiaohai (SI 8), Shaohai (H 3), Quchi (LI 11), Hegu (LI 4) as the main points; for that of the lower limbs, select mainly Mingmen (Du 4), Huantiao (GB 30), Weizhong (UB 40), Yanglingquan (GB 34), Zusanli (St 36) and Chengshan (UB 57). Knead the points with the fingertips first, then roll with the back of the hand upon the affected lower limb.

(2) Then with flat—palm gesture and pushing and leading manipulations, emit qi toward the above points, and guide the channel qi to flow from Dazhui (Du 14) and Mingmen (Du 4) along the Three Yang Channels of Hand or the Three Yang Channels of Foot to the upper or the lower limb to direct the channel qi to the affected part.

Modification: In case of retention of pathogenic heat in the lung, add flat—palm and vibrating and quivering manipulations to emit qi toward Fishu (UB 13) and Dachangshu (UB 25) for 14 respiratory cycles, and guide the channel qi to flow along the Channels of Hand—Taiyang and Foot—Taiyang;in case of overwhelming of dampness—heat, add the same gesture and manipulations to emit qi toward Pishu (UB 20), Weishu (UB

21), Liangmen (St 21) and Tianshu (St 25) for 14 respiratory cycles, and guide the channel qi to flow toward the ends of the extremities along the Channels of Hand—Yangming and Foot—Yangming; and in case of insufficiency of the liver—yin and kidney—yin, add the same gesture and manipulations to emit qi toward Ganshu (UB 18), Shenshu (UB 20) and Dantian for 14 respiratory cycles, and guide the channel qi to flow along the Liver Channel of Foot—Jueyin and the Kidney Channel of Foot— Shaoyin to the toes.

2. Qigong—Acupuncture

Insert the filiform needles into, for the upper limb flaccidity, Jianyu (LI 15), Quchi (LI 11), Hegu (LI 4) and Yangxi (LI 5), and for the lower limb flaccidity, Biguan (St 31), Liangqiu (St 34), Zusanli (St 36), Yinlingquan (Sp 9), Yanglingquan (GB 34) and Jiexi (St 41). Then emit qi toward them with dragon—mouth, bird—beak or flat—palm hand gesture and pushing, rotating and leading manipulations to get qi balanced.

3. Self Qigong Exercise as Accessory Treatment

(1) The Health Promotion Exercise (Qiangzhuang Gong)

Take a sitting or lying posture with the whole body relaxed, distractions expelled, and tongue stuck against the palate.

Take antidromic abdominal respiration and concentration of mind on Dantian. Pull in the abdomen and contract the anus during inhalation to instil qi into Dantian; buldge the abdomen and relax the anus during exhalation to send qi down to Dantian.

(2) The Exercise of the Upper Limbs for Dredging the

Channels

Pounding the Shoulders and Arms: Make the hand of the healthy side a hollow fist and pound with it the external, internal and anterior sides of the affected arm from the shoulder to the wrist 3 − 5 times.

Dredging the Three Yin and Three Yang Channels of Hand: Push−rub with the palm of the healthy side the internal side of the affected arm from the chest along the Three Yin Channels of Hand down to the fingertips, then from the fingertips upwards via the back of the hand along the Three Yang Channels of Hand back to the shoulder, 5 − 10 times.

(3) The Exercise of the Lower Limbs for Dredging the Channels

Patting the Lower Limbs: Pat the affected lower limb with the roots of both palms from the uppermost of the thigh down to the shank 5 − 10 times.

Dredging the Three Yin and Three Yang Channels of Foot: Push−rub the lower limbs with both palms. Exhaling, push−rub downwards along the Three Yang Channels of Foot and inhaling, upwards along the Three Yin Channels of Foot 5 − 10 times.

Lumbago

Etiology

1. Lumbago Due to Cold−Dampness

It is caused by retention of the cold and dampness pathogens in the channels and collaterals leading to impeded or stagnated circulation of qi and blood.

2. Lumbago Due to Kidney Deficiency

It is caused by failure of the kidney to nourish Sanjiao (the three warmers) due to its deficiency resulting from over consumption of the kidney essence by sexual life.

3. Lumbago Due to Trauma

It is due to injury of the muscles and tissues, stagnation of qi and stasis of blood and obstruction of the channels and collaterals resulting from sprain or sudden sprain, contusion and collision injury.

Symptoms

1. Lumbago Due to Cold−Dampness

It is marked by heaviness and pain in the waist which may radiate to the hips and legs or may be accompanied by muscular stiffness and, in chronic cases, the pain is on and off with different degrees and severity. The patient often feels cold at the waist and lumbago, especially in wet and cold days. The tongue coating is white and greasy and the pulse soft Flat−palm detection often reveals cold, densified, tingling and sluggish sensation of qi at the waist.

2. Lumbago Due to Kidney Deficiency

The pain is dull and continuous, accompanied by soreness and weakness of the waist and knees, cold limbs and nocturnal emission. Flat−palm detection often reveals stagnated, cold and tingling sensation of qi at the waist.

3. Lumbago Due to Trauma

The patient has a history of trauma. The pain is splitting and localized, with tenderness and movement limitation. The tongue is often purple and the pulse is deep and uneven. Flat−palm detection usually reveals stagnated, densified, sluggish and distending sensation of qi at the waist.

Treatment

1. Emission of Outgoing—Qi (Waiqi)

(1) Press—roll and press—knead Shenshu (UB 23), Mingmen (Du 4), Yaoyangguan (Du 3), Weizhong (UB 40) and Ashi points (pressure pain points).

(2) With flat—palm gesture and pushing, pulling and leading manipulations, emit qi toward Ashi points, Shenshu (UB 23) and Dachangshu (UB 25), and guide qi to flow along the Urinary Bladder Channel of Foot—Taiyang to the lower extremities to get qi of the patient balanced.

(3) Conduct massage of the waist with oblique—pulling, patting and rubbing manipulations.

Modification: For lumbago due to cold—dampness, add flat—palm gesture, pulling and leading manipulations and the method of heat—guidance of qi to emit outgoing qi and guide the pathogenic qi out of the body. For lumbago due to kidney deficiency, add flat— palm gesture and vibrating and quivering manipulations to emit qi toward Shenshu (UB 23), Zhishi (UB 52), Mingmen (Du 4) and Dantian for 14 respiratory cycles each, and for lumbago due to trauma, add the same gesture and manipulations to emit qi to Ashi points for 28 respiratory cycles.

2. Qigong—Acupuncture

Insert the filiform needles into Shenshu (UB 23), Ashi point, Dachangshu (UB 25) and Weizhong (UB 40). Emit qi with dragon—mouth gesture and pushing, pulling and rotating manipulations to facilitate the channel qi of the patient to balance it.

3. Self Qigong Exercise as Accessory Treatment

(1) Moving the Waist to Reinforce the Muscles

Make hands akimbo and turn the waist clockwise and counterclockwise 36 times respectively.

(2) Thumping the Lumbosacral Region

Thump the sides of the waist, the renal regions and the sacral regions with the two hollow fists alternately 36 times each.

(3) Rub the hands to get them hot and rub the renal region with them from the upper to the lower till the regions feel warm.

Section Two   Surgical and Gynecological Syndromes

Mammary Abscess (Cyst)

Etiology

Mammary abscess is also called mastitis which, as traditional Chinese medicine holds, is caused by stagnation of qi and stasis of blood resulting from tagnation of the liver—qi or the gallbladder—qi and excessiveness and stagnation of toxic heat in the Stomach Channel. Milk stagnation in the mammary glands, which is caused by trauma or extrusion, may give rise to acute mastitis. Acute mastitis infected via baby's mouth is called "chuiru". The disease is commonly seen in women in their lactation.

Symptoms

Local swelling, fever, pain or mass accompanied with general fever or chills, nausea and polydipsia appearing at the first stage. Flat—palm detection often reveals hot, tingling, stagnated and densified sensation of qi at the affected area.

Treatment

Treatment with outgoing—qi is efficacious only at the first stage of the disease. Incision and drainage are needed if abscess develops.

1. Emission of Outgoing—Qi (Waiqi)

(1) Press—knead Shanzhong (Ren 17), Rugen (St 18), Zhongfu (Lu 1), Ganshu (UB 18) and Weishu (UB 21) to open through the points along the Liver Channel, Stomach Channel and the Lung Channel.

(2) Flat—palm gesture and vibrating and quivering manipulations are applied to emit qi, with the point Inner Laogong facing the swollen mass, for 48 respiratory cycles. Then, apply dragon—mouth hand gesture and the same manipulations to emit qi toward the mass for 24 respiratory cycles. Still then, flat—palm gesture and pushing, pulling and leading manipulations should be taken to emit qi toward Ruzhong (St 17) and guide the channel qi to flow downward along the Stomach Channel of Foot—Yangming to dredge the channels and expel the pathogenic factors out of the body.

(3) Gently pinch the affected breast with the thumb, index finger and middle finger to extrude the stagnated milk. This should be done once a day.

2. Qigong—Acupuncture

Insert the filiform needles into Jianjing (GB 21), Fengmen (GB 20), Chize (Lu 5) and Zusanli (St 36). Then emit qi with dragon—mouth gesture and pushing, pulling and leading manipulations toward them and guide the channel qi to Zusanli

(St 36) and Chize (Lu 5).

3. Self Qigong Exercise as Accessory Treatment

(1) Patients at the first stage of the disease may knead by themselves the surrounding area of the swelling gently with the tips of the index, middle, ring and little fingers (close together) and practise the Chest—Hypochondrium Exercise.

(2) "Chui" Qi to Expel the Pathogenic Evils

Sit quietly, get the upper and lower teeth tapping each other, swallow the saliva and regulate the breath even. Inhale to gather qi in the chest and exhale to guide qi to rotate from Rugen (St 18) to the nip while uttering "chui" to dispel the evil qi out by way of the nip. Do this for 12 respiratory cycles.

Case

Wang, female, aged 28, came for the first visit on July 8, 1983.

Complaints   The patient complained of swelling—pain in the left breast for three days with localized redness, swelling, hotness and difficulty in milk discharge.

Examinatioin   A mass 3 × 4 cm in size could be palpated in the internal side of the left breast. The local skin looks red and swelling with tenderness. Flat— palm detection with outgoing—qi found hot, tingling and densified qi at the affected part of the left breast.

Diagnosis   Mammary abscess (Mastitis).

Treatment   Flat—palm and dragon—mouth hand gestures and vibrating, quivering, pulling and leading manipulations were used to emit qi to Shanzhong (Ren 17), Rugen (St 18), Zhongfu (Lu 1), Ganshu (GB 18), Weishu (UB 21) and Zusanli (St 36).

Course of Treatment   On emission of outgoing–qi, the patient felt her breast distending and tingling and a flow of qi rushing from the breast to Zusanli (St 36) along the Stomach Channel of Foot–Yangming. The mass almost disappeared after the first treatment and there remained only mild tenderness. The disease was cured after the second treatment .

Angiitis

Etiology

Angiitis is termed "Tuoju" (gangrene of toe) in traditional Chinese medicine. It is often caused by accumulation of virulent fire–evil and stagnation of qi and blood in the channels and blood vessels, which may result from invasion of cold dampness preventing the vital energy from going downward, over–intake of fatty and pungent food leading to internal generation of purulent fire, or from deficiency of the kidney–yin that fails to suppress the evil fire.

Symptoms

In mild cases, there may be cold and numb sensation at the end of the extremity with changes of the skin colour and intermittent claudication, while in severe cases, there may be muscular atrophy, acronecrosis and chronic ulcer which often lead to severe pain and make the patient sleepless at night and keep sitting with the knees in arms. The arteriopalmus of the affected limb usually weakens or disappears. Flat–palm detection may reveal densified, cold and stagnated qi at the affected limb.

Treatment

1. Emission of Outgoing—Qi (Waiqi)

(1) Roll, knead and rub the affected limb with progressively increased force, then press—knead Jiquan (H 1), Xiaohai (SI 8), Shaohai (H 3), Qichong (St 30), Yanglingquan (GB 34) and Weizhong (UB 40).

(2) For treatment when the upper limb is affected affection, flat—palm hand gesture and pushing, pulling, quivering and leading manipulations should be used to emit qi toward Jiquan (H 1) and guide qi to flow to the fingertips along the Three Yin Channels of Hand; for treatment of the lower limb affection, the same gesture and manipulations are used to emit qi to Dantian, Huantiao (GB 30) and Qichong (St 30) and guide qi to flow to the toes along the Stomach Channel of Foot—Yangming.

2. Qigong—Acupuncture

Insert the filiform needles into Quchi (LI 11), Hegu (LI 4), Biguan (St 31), Yanglingquan (GB 34), Huantiao (GB 30), Weizhong (UB 40), Chengshan (UB 57) and Kunlun (UB 60). Emit qi toward these points and then guide qi to the fingertips or toes with dragon—beak or bird—mouth hand gesture and pulling and leading manipulations.

3. Self Qigong Exercise as Accessory Treatment

(1) Practise the Exercise for Guiding Qi to Rotate Automatically (Refer to "Dysentery"). When qi can rotate following will, guide qi by will to rotate from Dantian downward to dredge the channels and collaterals and facilitate the circulation of qi.

(2) Practise selectively the Exercise of the Upper Limbs for Dredging the Channels and the Exercise of the Lower Limbs

for Dredging the Channels (Refer to "Flaccidity Syndrome").

Dysmenorrhea

Etiology

As one of the common gynecological diseases, dysmenorrhea is mainly due to stagnation of qi and stasis of blood caused either by mental stress such as anxiety and anger or by cold evil affection. It may be classified into two types——deficiency type and excess type.

Symptoms

1. Dysmenorrhea of Execess Type

Patients with dysmenorrhea of excess type have the symptoms of pain in the lower abdomen prior to menstruation or constant pain in the lower abdomin, interior heat, dry mouth, dark violet menstrual blood, advanced menstrual period and taut and rapid pulse. Flat–palm detection often reveals densified, stagnated, distending and tingling sensation of qi at the lower abdomen.

2. Dysmenorrhea of Deficiency Type

Patients with dysmenorrhea of deficiency type have the symptoms of pain in the lower abdomen after menstruation which can be alleviated by warming and hand– pressing, scanty and thin mentrual blood, delayed menstruation period, aversion to cold and fine and slippery pulse. Flat–palm detection often reveals cold, densified and tingling sensation of qi at the lower abdomen.

Treatment

1. Emission of Outgoing–Qi (Waiqi)

(1) Press and knead with the fingertips Qihai (Ren 6), Guanyuan (Ren 4), Zhongwan (Ren 12) and Shenshu (UB 23) to open through these points.

(2) Emit qi, with flat—palm or middle—finger—propping gesture and vibrating manipulation, towards Zhongwan (Ren 12), Qihai (Ren 6) and Guanyuan (Ren 4) for 8 — 16 respiratory cycles. Then conduct rotating massage on the lower abdomen, followed by pressing and kneading Sanyinjiao (Sp 6).

(3) Emit qi towards the Lower Dantian with flat—palm gesture and pushing— pulling—rotating manipulation, and guide qi to whirl around the umbilicus.Rotate clockwise for cases with deficiency syndrome and counterclockwise for those with excess syndrome.

Modification: To treat the execess type, add flat—palm hand gesture and pulling and leading manipulations to guide the channel qi to flow from Dantian (Extra) downward to the lower limbs along the Liver Channel of Foot—Jueyin and the Stomach Channel of Foot—Yangming. To treat the deficiency type, add flat—palm hand gesture and pushing and leading manipulations to emit qi to Guanyuan (Ren 4) and Qihai (Ren 6) and guide the channel qi to flow along the Spleen Channel of Foot—Taiyin and the Stomach Channel of Foot—Yangming to balance qi.

2. Qigong—Acupuncture

Insert the filiform needles into Guanyuan (Ren 4), Zhongji (Ren 3), Sanyinjiao (Sp 6) and Zusanli (St 36), and emit qi toward them with dragon— mouth hand gesture and pushing, pulling and rotating manipulations to get qi balanced between the points.

3. Self Qigong Exercise as Accessory Treatment

(1) The Automatic Qi Circulation Exercise

Take a lying posture relaxed and in quiescence with breath even and tongue stuck against the palate. Taking the navel as the centre of a circle, guide qi to rotate clockwise from the smallest cirle at the navel to the largest at the flanks of the abdomen, while saying silently "the white tiger hides in the east; the green dragon hides in the west" during every circle, for altogether 36 circles. Then guide qi to rotate counterclockwise from the largest circle to the smallest while saying silently "the green dragon hides in the west; the white tiger hides in the east" for also 36 circles. Patients with dysmenorrhea of excess type should guide qi to rotate counterclockwise round the navel for 81 circles before doing the above exercise, and those with dysmenorrhea of deficiency type should get qi to rotate clockwise for 81 circles. The exercise should be started 10 days before the menstrual period and continued until the end of it 2 – 4 times a day.

(2) The Exercise of Kneading the Abdomen

Rotate–knead Zhongwan (Ren 17) above the navel and the region below the navel counterclockwise 36 times each, then knead the navel clockwise and counterclockwise 36 times respectively.

(3) Rub the hands to get them warm and scrub the two sides of the waist with the hand till the waist feels warm.

Case

Zhao, female, aged 23, unmarried, came for the first visit on March 21, 1981.

Complaints   The patient complained of discomfort and pain in the lower abdomen beginning 4 — 11 days before every menstruation, which might be relieved after the period, for successively eight years, and delayed menstrual period, scanty thin blood, painful shock, cold extremities and aversion to cold. Constant administration of traditional and Western drugs yielded no apparent effect.

Examination   Physical examination found pale tongue proper with white, thin coating, deep, thready and feeble pulse, and retroversion of uterus with no inflammation and other abnormalities.

Treatment   Flat—palm hand gesture and pushing,rotating, quivering and leading manipulations were taken to emit qi toward Qihai (Ren 6), Guanyuan (Ren 4), Guilai (St 29), Shuidao (St 28), Mingmen (Du 4), Shenshu (UB 23) and Sanyinjiao (Sp 6).

Chronic Pelvic Inflammation

Etiology

It is chiefly caused by accumulation of dampness—heat or stagnation of cold— dampness in the uterus.

Symptoms

Patients with chronioc pelvic inflammation usually have the symptoms of pain in the lower abdomen, hypostatic distension, soreness in the lumbosacral portion, and pain and distension that may become worse during menstruation or after strain. If it is caused by damp—heat accumulation, there will be vaginal discharge, headache, fever, aversion to cold, and yellowish and greasy tongue coating. If it is caused by cold—dampness stagnation, vaginal discharge is white and stenchful, the tongue fur is white and greasy, and the pulse is deep and slow, or taut and slippery.

Treatment

1. Emission of Outgoing—Qi (Waiqi)

(1) Press—knead Zhongwan (Ren 12), Daimai (GB 26), Zhongji (Ren 3), Pishu (UB 20), Mingmen (Du 4), Shenshu (UB 23) and Sanyinjiao (Sp 6). Rub the abdomen on either sides.

(2) Emit qi with middle—finger—propping hand gesture and vibrating and quivering manipulations toward Zhongwan (Ren 12), Qihai (Ren 6) and Zhongji (Ren 3) for 8 or 16 respiratory cycles each. Then emit qi, with flat—palm hand gesture and pushing, pulling and leading manipulations toward Dantian, Qihai(Ren 6), Zhongji (Ren 3) and Tianshu (St 25), and guide qi to flow downward along the Stomach Channel.

(3) Emit qi, with flat—palm hand gesture and pushing, pulling and quivering manipulations, toward Mingmen (Du 4) and Shenshu (UB 23) for 8 or 16 respiratory cycles respectively, and regulate qi along the Dai Channel (the Belt Channel) to get the functional activities of qi normalized.

Modification: In case of dampness—heat accumulation, add emission of qi with cold— guidance of qi; in case of cold—dampness stagnation, add the heat—guidance of qi.

2. Qigong—Acupuncture

Insert the filiform needles into Zhongwan (Ren 12), Guanyuan (Ren 4), Zhongji (Ren 3), Sanyinjiao (Sp 6) and Zusanli (St 36), and guide the channel qi of the patient with dragon—mouth or bird—mouth hand gesture and pushing, pulling and rotating manipulations to get it balanced between the points.

3. Self Qigong Exercise as Accessory Treatment

(1) Practise the Inner Health Cultivation Exercise (refer to "Diabetes").

(2) Practise the Exercise of Kneading Dantian to Strengthen Qi as follows.

Overlap the hands and put them on Dantian and knead it clockwise and counterclockwise 36 times respectively. Then practise the Automatic Qi Circulation Exercise (refer to "Dysmenorrhea").

Hysteroptosis

Etiology

It is mainly caused by asthenia after delivery or by overstrain which leads to collapse of qi and dysfunction of the uterus.

Symptoms

The uterus may be found falling down to the vagina or to the lower vaginal orifice.There is often aching pain in the abdomen accompanied with listlessness. The pulse feels threadyand feeble and the tongue looks pale. Flat—palm detection often reveals scattered, stagnated and tingling qi at the lower abdomen.

Treatment

1. Emission of Outgoing—qi (Waiqi)

(1) Press—knead Baihui (Du 20), Zhongwan (Ren 12),

Qihai (Ren 6), Sanyinjiao (Sp 6) and Zhaohai (K 6).

(2) Emit qi with flat—palm hand gesture and vibrating manipulation toward Baihui (Du 20), then toward Zhongwan (Ren 12) and Qihai (Ren 6) for 48 respiratory cycles respectively.

(3) With flat—palm hand gesture and pulling and leading manipulations, emit qi toward Qihai (Ren 6) and Zhongji (Ren 3) and guide qi to the Middle Dantian.

2. Qigong—Acupuncture

Insert the filiform needles into Baihui (Du 20), Zhongwan (Ren 12) and Guanyuan (Ren 4), and emit qi toward the needles with flat—palm or dragon—mouth hand gesture and pushing, pulling and rotating manipulations for 14 respiratory cycles respectively.

3. Self Qigong Exercise as Accessory Treatment

(1) Practise the Inner Health Cultivation Exercise (refer to "Diabetes").

(2) Practise the Exercise of Rotation of Dantian and Baihui (Du 20) as follows.

Overlap the hands (the left above the right) with the Inner Laogong (P 8) of the left over the Outer Laogong (P 8) of the right. Put the hands on Baihui (Du 20) with the three points joining vertically and turn the hands clockwise and counterclockwise 36 times each, one time in one respiratory cycle. Contract the abdomen and lift the anus and perineum during inhalation and relax during exhalation. Rotate Dantian along with the rotation of Baihui (Du 20).

Section Three   Traumatological Diseases

Stiffneck

Etiology

It is often caused by improper sleeping posture, and invasion of pathogenic wind—dampness leading to obstruction of channels and collaterals.

Symptoms

It is usually noticed in the morning when the patient feels pain on one side of the neck, cervical immobilization and sometimes radiating pain in the shoulder and back. Cervical muscles are in a spasmodic state and local tenderness is obvious, but no local swelling and infammation can be found.

Flat—palm detection often reveals cold and densified sensation of qi at the painful area.

Treatment

1. Emission of Outgoing—Qi (Waiqi)

(1) Press—knead Tianzhu (UB 10) and the Urinary Bladder Channel on the two sides of the neck, then press—knead Fengchi (GB 20), Fengfu (Du 16), Jianzhongshu (SI 15), Jianwaishu (SI 4), Quchi (LI 11) and Hegu (LI 4), to open through the points and dredge the channels and collaterals.

(2) With flat—palm hand gesture and pushing, pulling and leading manipulations, emit qi towards the painful area on the neck, guide the channel qi to flow downward along the Urinary Bladder Channel and also guide it to flow to the upper arms along the Small Intestine Channel to get qi balanced.

(3) Apply the methods of rolling, tracting—countertracting and pulling—obliquely of the neck to help relieve the rigidity of the joints and to regulate the muscles.

2. Qigong—Acupuncture

Insert the filiform needles into Ashi point (pressure pain point), Tianzhu (UB 10), Fengchi (GB 20), Quchi (LI 11), Hegu (LI 4) and Xuanzhong (GB 39). Emit qi toward the needles with dragon—mouth hand gesture and pushing and pulling manipulations, and guide qi to flow from Fengchi (GB 20) to Xuanzhong (GB 39) with sword—fingers hand gesture to get qi balanced between the points.

3. Self Qigong Exercise as Accessory Treatment

(1) Dredging Fengchi (GB 20)

Knead the point Fengchi (GB 20) of both sides gently with the thumbs 5 times during each inhaling and each exhaling for altogether 14 respiratory cycles.

(2) Massaging Tianzhu (UB 10)

Bend the head forward slightly. Rub the back of the neck along its midline with the cushion of the four fingers of either hand from the top of the neck downwards 7 times during exhaling, and stop rubbing during inhaling. Do this for 7 respiratory cycles. Then massage the painful side with the same method for 9 respiratory cycles.

(3) Turning the Neck to Guide Qi

Turn the neck counterclockwise, for half a circle during inhalation and half a circle during exhalation for altogether 8 circles. Turn it clockwise in the same way for another 8 circles.

(4) Pulling the Neck

Cross the fingers of the two hands to hold the back of the

neck and pull the neck forwards during inhalation, at the same time raise the head and look as backwards as possible. Relax during exhalation. Do this for 9 respiratory cycles.

Cervical Spondylopathy

Etiology

The disease is usually caused by pathogenic wind, cold and dampness, trauma, overstrain and, in the aged, failure of blood to nourish the tendons due to insufficiency of qi and blood.

Symptoms

Clinically, symptoms of cervical spondylopathy are miscellaneous; however, those such as pain or numbing pain in the neck, shoulders (including their periphery, upper part of the back and chest and upper extremities due to irritation or compression of cervical nerve roots are common.Cervical overstrain or exopathic cold may serve as factors inducing this disease or worsening its symptoms. If the spinal cord is irritated or compressed, symptoms of numbness and weakness of the lower extremities, and staggering gait may appear; while if vertebral artery is irritated or compressed, vertigo and dizziness may appear.

Flat—palm detection often reveals cold, densified, tingling and stagnated sensation of qi at the neck and the arm of the affected side.

Treatment

1. Emission of Outgoing—qi (Waiqi)

(1) Press—knead Fengchi (GB 20), Fengfu (Du 16), Tianzhu (UB 10),Jianzhongshu (SI 15), Jianwaishu (SI 14),

Jiquan (H 1), Quchi (LI 11), Hegu (LI 4), Shaohai (H 3) and Xiaohai (SI 8).

(2) Emit qi, with flat–palm hand gesture and vibrating and quivering manipulations, toward Dazhui (Du 14) for 16 respiratory cycles, and with flat– palm hand gesture and pushing, pulling and leading manipulations, toward Fengchi (GB 20), Dazhui (Du 14) and Ashi points. Then guide qi to flow to the fingertips along the Three Yang Channels of Hand.

(3) Again press–knead the points mentioned in (1). Then conduct patting, hitting, rocking rubbing and tracting–countertracting hand manipulations to end the treatment.

2. Qigong–Acupuncture

Insert the filiform needles into the Ashi point, Fengchi (GB 20), Tianzhu (UB 10), Quchi (LI 11) and Hegu (LI 4), then emit qi with dragon–mouth hand gesture and pushing, pulling and rotating manipulations toward the needles to get qi balanced between all the points.

3. Self Qigong Exercise as Accessory Treatment

(1) Practise the Exercise of Stroking the Ball to Lead Neck Movement as follows.

Take a sitting or standing posture. Set the left hand at the height of Tanzhong (Ren 17) and the right at the height of Dantian with the centre of the two palms facing each other as if holding a ball. When qi is felt between the palms, abduct the left hand and adduct the right as if stroking a ball, with the head following the movement of the left hand, 9 or 18 times. Exchange the positions of the hands and the direction of their movements and stroke the "ball" 9 or 18 times, with the head following the movements of the right hand. (2) Practise the Exercise of Dredging Fengchi (GB 20), Massaging Tianzhu (GB 20) and Pulling the Neck (refer to "Stiffneck").

Case

Ying, male, 40, a Britishman studing in China, came for the first visit on January 20, 1983.

Complaints   The patient complained of pain in the neck and radiating pain in the left—upper arm for a year accompanied by stiffness of the neck and numbness of the fingers. Traction treatment, acupuncture and treatment with Western and traditional drugs yielded no apparent effect. The pain was aggravated in the last thirty days, which affected his sleep and study and urged him to seek Qigong treatment.

Examination   There was tenderness in the 4th, 5th and 6th cervical vertebral processes, along their sides and at Bingfeng (SI 12), Quyuan (SI 13), Tianzong (SI 11), Quchi (LI 11) and Shaohai (H 3). Anvil test and cervical root tension test were positive. X—ray film showed disappearance of the physiological radian of the normal anterior process (lordosis) of cervical vertebrae and mild osseous proliferation at the posterior aspect of the 4th and 5th vertebrae. Flat—palm detection revealed cold, tingling and distending sensation of qi at the neck and the left—upper arm.

Diagnosis   Cervical spondylopathy (Shoulder—arm pain).

Treatment   Points applied to treatment were Fengchi (G.B. 20), Tianzhu (UB 10), Bingfeng (SI 12), Jianwaishu (SI 14), Jianzhongshu (SI 15), Tianzong (SI 11), Quchi (LI 11), Hegu (LI 4), Shaohai (H 3) and Xiaohai (SI 8). Hand manipulations of rolling, pressing, kneading, digging—grasping, rocking and flicking were carried out first, followed by emission of qi with flat–palm hand gesture and pushing, pulling and leading manipulations.

Course of Treatment On receiving outgoing–qi, the patient felt a flow of warmth rushing from the neck and shoulder down to the hands along the Yangming, Taiyang and Shaoyin Channels of Hand, which made the upper arm warm and comfortable. The disease was cured with all the symptoms disappeared after 8 times of treatment.

Omalgia

Etiology

Three main factors may contribute to the origination of the disease: failure of nourishment of the channels and collaterals due to asthenia at old age; obstruction of the vessels due to trauma in the shoulder; and stagnation of qi and stasis of blood in the vessels and muscles leading to difficulty in stretching the arm due to the effect of pathogenic wind, cold and dampness.

Symptoms

The main symptom is aching pain in one of the shoulders which is often more severe during the night and can be aggravated by activity, accompanied with stiffness and mobility dysfunction of the shoulder joint. The pain may radiate to the neck and the upper limb. Delayed treatment may lead to joint adhesion and anergasia, and atrophy of the shoulder muscles or spasms.

Flat–palm detection may reveal a sensation of densified,

cold and tingling qi at the shoulder and neck of the affected side.

Treatment

1. Emission of Outgoing—Qi (Waiqi)

(1) Conduct rolling and kneading massage manipulations on Jianyu (LI 15), Binao (LI 14), Jianzhen (SI 9), Tianzong (SI 11), Quchi (LI 11), Shousanli (LI 10) and Hegu (LI 4).

(2) Emit qi with spread—plaw hand gesture and vibrating and quivering manipulations around the shoulder joint for 48 respiratory cycles. Then with flat—palm hand gesture and pushing and pulling manipulations, emit qi toward Dazhui (Du 14) and Jianyu (LI 15) and guide the channel qi to flow along the Small Intestine Channel of Hand—Taiyang and the Large Intestine Channel of Hand—Yangming to the fingertips to balance qi.

(3) Apply pressing, flicking, patting and rocking manipulations to the shoulder joint to lubricate it. Then conduct rubbing and shaking to end the treatment.

2. Qigong—Acupuncture

Insert the filiform needles into Tianzhu (UB 10), Jianyu (LI 15), Tianzong (SI 11), Jianzhen (SI 9), Quchi (LI 11) and Hegu (LI 4). Then emit qi toward them with dragon—mouth hand gesture and pushing, pulling and quivering manipulations to get qi balanced.

3. Self Qigong Exercise as Accessory Treatment

(1) The Exercise of Stretching the Arms by Climbing the Wall.

Stand facing the wall. Place the hand of the affected side on the wall. Take in a breath. During inhaling, raise the affected side of the arm to climb the wall as highly as possible. Do this for 9 or 18 respiratory cycles.

(2) Carry out movements of the shoulder joint such as bending, stretching and abducting to increase the degree of mobility of the shoulder joint.

Prolapse of Lumbar Intervertebral Disc

Etiology

The disease is due rupture of the fibrous ring of vertebral disc caused mostly by sudden or repeated sprain, overstrain on lifting heavy things, lumbar sprain or invasion of the waist by pathogenic cold.

Symptoms

The most prominent symptom is pain, which goes from the waist via the hip, the posterior aspect of the thigh, the lateral—posterior aspect of the shank, the heel, the sole and the lateral—dorsal aspect of the foot to the toes. The pain may be aggravated with the increase of the abdominal pressure due to, e.g., cough or defecation. There are obvious tenderness along the sides of the lumbar vertebral process, stiffness and dysfunction of the waist which often lead to difficulty in walking, and muscular atrophy of the lower limbs in cases with long course of the illness.

Flat—palm detection often reveals densified, stagnated and cold sensation of qi at the waist and the affected leg. X—ray examination may show lateral prolapse, narrowed and unequal interspaces and variation of the physiological radian of the lumbar vertebra.

Treatment

1. Emission of Outgoing–Qi (Waiqi)

(1) Apply rolling, pressing and kneading massage to Shenshu (UB 23), Yaoyangguan (Du 3), Huantiao (GB 30), Yanglingguan (GB 34), Weizhong (UB 40) and Chengshan (UB 57).

(2) With flat–palm hand gesture and pushing, pulling and leading manipulations, emit qi toward Mingmen (Du 4), Shenshu (UB 23) and Ashi point (pressure pain point) and guide qi to flow down to the lower limbs along the Urinary Bladder Channel of Foot–Taiyang to get qi balanced.

(3) With flat–palm hand gesture and pulling and leading manipulations, emit qi to Huantiao (GB 30) and guide the channel qi to flow down to the lower extremities along the Gallbladder Channel of Foot–Shaoyang to get qi balanced.

(4) Apply pulling–obliquely and patting manipulations to the lumbar region and passive movement of the waist, hip and knee to lubricate the joints and remove qi stagnation and blood stasis.

2. Qigong–Acupuncture

Insert the filiform needles into Houxi (SI 3), Ashi points, Yaoyangguan (Du 3), Shenshu (UB 23), Huantiao (GB 30), Weizhong (UB 40), Yanglingguan (GB 34), Xuanzhong (GB 39) and Kunlun (UB 60) of the affected side. Then emit qi with dragon–mouth or flat–palm hand gesture and pushing, pulling and rotating manipulations toward the needles to get qi balanced between all the points.

3. Self Qigong Exercise As Accessory Treatment

(1) Scrub Shenshu (UB 23) with the hands till the region is hot. Then scrub Yongquan (K 1) in the same way.

(2) To dredge the channels of the lower limbs, push—rub with the two palms from the lumbar region to the sole along the Three Yang Channels of Foot during exhaling, then back to the waist along the Three Yin Channels of Foot during inhaling, for altogether 7—9 respiratory cycles.

(3) Sit on bed with legs straight. Push the palms out to touch the toes and then pull them back. Do this 21 times.

Case

Li, female, aged 29, came for the first visit on June 13, 1983.

Complaints   Pain in the waist and the left lower limb for nine months, which was more severe on coughing and defecating and became worse in the last two months, resulting in great difficulty in walking. Treatment with traditional drugs, blockage therapy, acupuncture and massage (Tuina) yielded no apparent effect.

Examination   There were tenderness and percussion pain in the interspace of lumbar processes and the left side. Straight elevation test of the left leg showed an angle of 35 degrees. There were weakened dorsiflexion of the left toe and reduced reflexion of the knee jerk and Achilles tendon. X—ray film showed narrowed lumbar vertebral interspaces.

Diagnosis   Prolapse of lumbar intervertebral disc (waist—leg pain).

Treatment   Flat—palm hand gesture and pushing, pulling, quivering and leading manipulations were taken to emit qi to Dachangshu (UB 25), Shenshu (UB 23), Weizhong (UB 40), Chengshan (UB 57) and Kunlun (UB 60), followed by acupuncture of the left Shangliao (UB 31) with a filiform needle and emission of qi to it with dragon—mouth hand gesture and pulling, rotating and leading manipulations.

Course of Treatment   During emission of qi, synchronized movements of the hips and the left leg of the patient such as quivering, stretching and flexing appeared. The radiation pain in the leg diminished. The disease was cured after 8 times of treatment.

Sprain of the Elbow Joint

Etiology

The sprain often results from impact by external force, palm—supporting of the body on falling, or over—traction.

Symptoms

The main symptoms are swelling and pain in the elbow with dysfunction of the joint.

Treatment

1. Emission of Outgoing—Qi (Waiqi)

(1) Apply rolling, pressing and kneading manipulations on Quchi (LI 11), Zusanli (St 36), Shaohai (H 3) and Xiaohai (SI 8) first.

(2) Emit qi toward the painful place with flat—palm hand gesture and vibrating manipulation, then toward Quchi (LI 11) with the same gesture and pushing, pulling and leading manipulations and guide qi with the same method to the fingertips along the Large Intestine Channel of Hand—Yangming.

(3) Rub and rock the elbow joint to end the treatment.

2. Qigong—Acupuncture

Insert the filiform needles into Quchi (LI 11), Shousanli

(LI 10), Ashi points and Hegu (LI 4). Then emit qi with dragon—mouth hand gesture and pushing and pulling manipulations toward the needles to get qi balanced.

3. Self Qigong Exercise as Accessory Treatment

Practise the Exercise of Raising the Arm and Bending the Elbow as follows.

Stretch the affected arm at the shoulder level along with inhaling, with the back of the hand upward and the abdomen buldged. Abduct the hand and withdraw the elbow to the hypochondrium. Do this for 9 respiratory cycles.

Sprain of the Knee Joint

Etiology

The sprain is commonly caused by impact from external force or by over—abduction, over—adduction and over—rotation.

Symptoms

The main symptoms are swelling and pain in the knee joint, dysfunction of the joint manifested as inability to stand or as limping. Flat—palm detection often reveals densified, stagnated, tingling and distending sensation of qi.

Treatment

1. Emission of Outgoing—qi (Waiqi)

(1) First, press—knead and push—rub the affected region and its periphery. Then knead with the fingertip Xuehai (Sp 10), Liangqiu (St 34), Xiyan (Extra 36), Yinlingquan (Sp 9) and Yanglingquan (GB 34) to open through them and dredge the blood vessels.

(2) With flat-palm hand gesture and pushing, pulling, quivering and leading manipulations, emit qi toward the painful area and guide the channel qi to flow to the foot along the Three Yang and Three Yin Channels of Foot to get qi balanced.

(3) Rock and press-knead the knee to end the treatment.

2. Qigong-Acupucture

Insert the filiform needles into Xiyan (Extra 36), heding (Extra), Liangqiu(St 34), Xuehai (Sp 1), Yinlingquan (Sp 9), Yanglingquan (GB 34), Zusanli (St 36). Then emit qi with dragon-mouth hand qesture and pushing and pulling manipulations toward the needles to balance qi.

3. Self Qigong Exercise as Accessory Treatment

Practisè the Exercise of White Crane Turning Its Knees as follows.

Stand with feet close to each other and knees slightly bent, the knees and feet being on a vertical line. Place the palms on the knees with the thumb and the index and middle fingers on the two depressions at the knee-lap respectively. Turn the knees clockwise and counterclockwise 10 times each with the speed of the movement synchronized with the rate of respiration and qi sent down into Dantian.

Sprain of the Ankle Joint

Etiology

It is due to the over-adduction of the ankle joint resulting from loss of one's footing when walking, running or jumping.

Symptoms

The main symptoms are swelling and pain in the ankle, dysfunction of movements such as standing and walking.Flat—palm detection with outgoing—qi often reveals stagnated and densified qi sensation at the affected region.

Treatment

1. Emission of Outgoing—Qi (Waiqi)

(1) Press—knead the pressure pain point and its periphery; knead Qiuxu (GB 40), Shangqiu (Sp 5), Jiexi (St 41), Yanglingquan (GB 34), Zusanli (St 36), Kunlun (UB 60) and Taixi (K 3).

(2) Emit qi with flat—palm hand gesture and vibrating and quivering manipula— tions toward the affected aspect, then tract and rock the ankle joint.

(3) Guide the circulation of qi along the Stomach Channel of Foot—Yangming and the Spleen Channel of Foot—Taiyin to get its flow smooth and its activities balanced.

2. Qigong—Acupuncture

Insert the filiform needles into Jiexi (St 41), Kunlun (UB 60), Taixi (K 3), Shangqiu (Sp 5), Qiuxu (GB 40), Yanglingquan (GB 34), Yinglingquan (Sp 9) and Zusanli (St 36), then emit qi toward them with dragon—mouth hand gesture and pulling and leading manipulations to get qi balanced between them.

3. Self Qigong Exercise As Accessory Treatment

Practise the Exercise of Rolling the Wooden Rod as follows.

Sit on a stool with feet put on a round rod. With the point Yongquan (K 1) as the centre, roll the rod to and fro 81 times.

Section Four   Disorders of the Eye, Ear and Nose and Pediatric Diseases

Myopia

Etiology

Myopia is common in youngsters. It is believed that this disease is related to improper lightening, improper posture and successive long–time reading.

Symptoms

To victims of myopia, all objects in distance are blurred although nearby objects are clear.

TREATMENT

1. Emission of Outgoing–Qi (Waiqi)

(1) Press and knead Jingming (UB 1), Qiuhou (Extra 4), Yintang (Extra 1), Taiyang (Extra 2), Fengchi (GB 20) and Hegu (LI 4).

(2) Emit qi toward Jingming (UB 1) and Fengchi (GB 20) with one–finger–meditation or sword–fingers and pushing and pulling manipulations, then emit qi toward Ganshu (UB 18) and Shenshu (UB 23) with flat–palm hand gesture and vibrating and quivering manipulations for 11 or 22 respiratory cycles respectively.

(3) Emit qi, with flat–palm gesture and pushing and leading manipulations toward the eyes, then guide qi to flow to Xuanzhong (GB 39) along the Gall–bladder Channel, to make the functional activities of qi normalized.

2. Qigong–Acupuncture

Insert the filiform needles into Jingming (UB 1), Qiuhou (Extra), Taiyang (Extra 2), Xuanzhong (GB 39) and Hegu (LI 4) and emit qi toward the needles with dragon—mouth or bird—mouth hand gesture and pushing, pulling and leading manipulations to make qi balanced between the needles.

3. Self Qigong Exercise As Accessory Treatment

Practice the Exercise of Soothing the Liver and Improving Acuity of Vision as follows.

(1) Preparation

Stand relaxed and quiet, place the feet apart as wide as the shoulders, drop the hands naturally at the sides of the body, picture supporting an object on the head, pull in the chest and straighten the back, relax the waist and knees, look straight forward, and breathe naturally.

(2) Vision Regulation

Look straight forward first, and then look farther and farther until unable to see farther. Stare at a point for a moment and draw the vision gradually back to the nearest. Do this 4 times.

(3) Turning the Neck and Moving the Eyeballs

Look in the distance, turn the neck clockwise and counterclockwise 4 times each, with the eyes following the movement of the neck. Inhale when the neck is turned backwards and exhale when it is turned forwards.

(4) Throwing Out the Chest and Relaxing the Back

Raise the arms to the chest with the elbows bent and palms towards the breasts. Draw the elbows backwards to throw out the chest and inspire at the same time; then relax the back and expire. Do this for 8 times.

(5) Pressing Jingming (UB 1) and Guiding Qi

Press with the thumbs the point Jingming (UB 1) near the inner canthus while concentrating the mind on the eyes. Press toward the orbits and then backwards during inhalation; squeeze the eyeballs gently during exhalation while uttering "xu".

(6) Regulating Qi

Close the eyes lightly, bent the elbows and raise the hands in front of the abdomen, palms upward. Lift the palms slowly to the level of the eyes. Concentrate on the eyes during inhalation, the two hands lifted a fist from the eyes; then begin exhalation while still concentrating on the palms, the two hands descending to the level of the abdomen. Do this 8 times before dropping the hands at the sides as described in the preparatory posture to end the exercise.

Case

Dai, female, aged 15, came for the first visit on November 17, 1981.

Complaints   The patient complained of suffering from short sight for three years manifested as blurred vision of subjects in distance which turned worse gradually. There was no family history of myopia.

Examination   The vision of the left eye was 0.2, the right 0.4. There was tenderness in the area of the 3rd and 4th cervical vertebral processes.

Diagnosis   Myopia.

Treatment   Emission of qi was performed with middle-finger-propping hand gesture and pushing, pulling and rotating manipulations toward Jingming (UB 1), Qiuhou

—431—

(Extra), Sizhukong (SJ 23), Tongziliao (GB 1), Fengchi (GB 20) and the pressure pain point. The vision was improved after treatment for twice to be 0.4 of the left eye and 0.5 of the right, and further improved to be 1.2 and 1.5 after 15 times of treatment. Follow—up visit in Febrary, 1983 found no aggravation.

Tinnitus and Deafness

Etiology

The diseases are most commonly caused by stagnation of qi of the Shaoyang Channels due to adverse rising of the liver wind—fire induced by violent rage and terror, by obstruction of the orifices on the head due to exopathic wind affection, or by failure of the kidney essence to reach the ears due to kidney deficiency.

Symptoms

1. Excess Type

Sudden deafness or distending pain in the ear with noise as chirping. Adverse rising of liver wind—fire or gallbladder wind—fire is often manifested as flushed face, dry mouth, vexation and irritability and taut pulse; while affection by exopathic wind, as chills and fever and headache. Flat—palm detection usually reveals densified, tingling and distending sensation of qi at the affected area.

2. Deficiency Type

The deafness and tinnitus occur constantly or intermittently and may be aggravated by over—strain and relieved by hand pressure, often accompanied by dizziness, soreness of the waist, seminal emission, leukorrhea and feeble and thready pulse. Flat–palm detection may reveal densified, tingling and distending sensation of qi.

Treatment

1. Emission of Outgoing–Qi (Waiqi)

(1) Press–knead Tinggong (SI 19), Yifeng (SJ 17), Hegu (LI 4) and Zhongzhu (SJ 3).

(2) Emit qi toward Dantian with one–finger–meditation and sword–fingers hand gestures, pushing and pulling manipulations and the qi–guiding method of making three points linear.

(3) With flat–palm and pulling and leading manipulations, emit qi toward the affected ear and guide qi to flow to the ends of the extremities along the Sanjiao Channel of Hand–Shaoyang and the Gallbladder Channel of Foot–Shaoyang to balance qi.

Modification: In case of adverse rising of the liver wind–fire, add flat–palm hand gesture and vibrating and quivering manipulations to emit qi to Ganshu (UB 18) and Danshu (UB 19) for 14 respiratory cycles, and in case of kidney deficiency, add the same to emit qi toward Shenshu (UB 23) for 14 respiratory cycles to balance qi.

2. Qigong–Acupuncture

Insert the filiform needles into Tinggong (SI 19), Yifeng (SJ 17), Zhongzhu (SJ 3) and Xuanzhong (GB 39), then emit qi toward the needles with dragon–mouth hand gesture and pulling and rotating manipulations to get qi balanced between the points.

3. Self Qigong Exercise as Accessory Treatment

(1) Striking the Heavenly Drum

Press the ears with the palms, the point Inner Laogong (P 8) aiming at the ear orifice and the fingers resting on the back of the head. Put the index fingers on the top of the middle ones and then slip them down forcefully to tap the back of the head lightly 24 times. One can hear rat—tat when doing this.

(2) Pressing the Ears to Guide Qi

Press the ear orifices tightly with the palms and release them to compress qi in the inner ears 10 times. Be sure to avoid forceful and violent pressing or releasing. Though the pressing should be tight and releasing rapid, they must be done gently and moderately.

(3) Massaging the Auricles

Pinch the top of the auricles gently with the thumbs and the index fingers and massage the auricles from the top downwards repeatedly 24 times to get them warm.

Case

Zhang, male, 34, came for the first visit on October 31, 1987.

Complaints   Loss of hearing of the right ear for three days accompanied with bitterness in the mouth, dry throat, flushed face, vexation and dark urine. The patient had, before deafness, a noise in the ears like wave roaring for ten days.

Examination   There were no abnormal findings in the right ear, the drum membrane was perfect and the deafness was believed to be nervous. The tongue was reddened with thin and yellow coating, and the pulse taut and rapid. Flat— palm detection with outgoing—qi revealed tingling, distending and tractive sensation of qi.

Diagnosis   Deafness (fulminant deafness).

Treatment   Acupuncture was conducted on Tinggong (SI 19), Zhongzhu (SJ 3) and Xuanzhong (GB 39) and qi was emitted toward the needles with dragon—mouth hand gesture and pushing, pulling, quivering and leading manipulations.

Course of Treatment   The patient could answer telephone calls after treatment for 3 times. Hearing of the right ear recovered after 9 times of treatment.

Sinusitis

Etiology

The nose is the orifice of the lung. Invasion of pathogenic wind—cold into the lung brings about accumulation of heat and obstruction of the lung—qi, which further impair the purifying and descending function of the lung. The pathogenic evil may then come into the air passage and accumulate in the nose, giving rise to sinusitis.

Symptoms

Sinusitis is manifested by constant yellowish and foul nasal discharge and impairment of smell, accompanied with cough, dull pain in the sinciput, rapid pulse, reddened tongue and thin, white and greasy tongue coating.

Treatment

1. Emission of Outgoing—Qi (Waiqi)

(1) Press—knead Yingxiang (LI 20), Yintang (Extra 1), Fengchi (GB 20), Hegu (LI 4) and Lieque (Lu 7) first.

(2) Emit qi toward Yingxiang (LI 20) with one—finger —meditation or sword— fingers hand gesture and pushing, pulling and leading manipulations and guide the channel qi to flow downward to Zusanli (St 36) along the Stomach Channel

of Foot—Yangming to get qi balanced between the upper and lower.

2. Qigong—Acupuncture

Insert the filiform needles into Yintang (Extra 1), Yingxiang (LI 20), Fengchi (GB 20), Hegu (LI 4), Lieque (Lu 7) and Zusanli (St 36), then emit qi toward the needles with dragon—mouth hand gesture and pushing and pulling manipulations to get qi balanced between the points.

3. Self Qigong Exercise As Accessory Treatment

(1) Bathing the Nose

Rub the dorsal sides of the thumbs against each other till they are hot. Rub with them the sides of the nose gently up and down. Rub 5 times during each inhaling and exhaling for altogether 10 respiratory cycles.

(2) Kneading the Nose Apex

Put the tip of the middle finger of the right hand on the nose apex and knead it clockwise during inhaling and counterclockwise during exhaling 5 times each. Do this for 10 respiratory cycles.

Infantile Convulsion

Etiology

Infantile convulsion is usually caused by fright.

Symptoms

The disease is characterized by disphoria, listlessness, night crying, poor appetite, diarrhoea and fever.

Treatment

(1) Knead Xiaotianxin (a massage point, at the root of the

palm and the depression between the thenar eminence major and thenar eminence minor) and pinch the points for child massage of Xinjing, Ganjing and Wuzhijie (the joints of the five fingers) of each hand and the points Yintang (Extra 1) and Baihui (Du 20).

(2) Use flat-palm gesture and pushing, pulling and leading manipulations to emit qi towards the fontanel and Baihui (Du 20) and then, to guide qi to flow to Dantian along the Ren Channel to "get qi back to its origin" as it is called. (2) Use middle-finger-propping hand gesture and vibrating and quivering manipulations toward Dazhui (Du 14), Xinshu (UB 15) and Ganshu (UB 18) and then, regulate qi of the Urinary Bladder Channel and the Du Channel to smoother its circulation.

Section Five   Qigong Deviations

Deviations of qigong refer to the adverse reactions of qigong exercise which make the practitioner uncomfortable and uncontrollable. Such reactions are physically and mentally harmful. They may even lead to confinement of the practitioner to bed or mental disorders. So the qigong therapist should attach great importance to such deviations by providing timely instructions and proper treatment.

From our experiences in rectifying deviations in 68 cases (53 cured, 10 improved and 5 with no effect), we believe that qigong deviations can be cured very quickly provided timely instructions in exercise and proper retifications are given. Delayed treatment or treatment with careless emission of outgoing-qi should be avoided, otherwise the patient's qi activities may be disturbed and the deviation exacerbated other than improved.

Etiology

(1) Failure to obey the principle of "exercising in light of concrete conditions", for example, those who are not fit for the exercise of intrinsic qi circulation force themselves to do it.

(2) Exercising or practising without instructions of an experienced practi- tioner, or practising unduly for quick results.

(3) Being overly suspicious, some people may fail to respond to the tiding and qi effect in the correct way. And those who are mentally weak may have too heavy a psychological burden in the course of qigong practice so that they gradually fall into victims of deviation.

(4) Some practitioners often fail to master the principle and methods of the "three regulations" (regulation of posture, respiration and will), fail to exercise in accordance with the given instructions, or change their styles now and then. All these may get themselves confused mentally and physically.

Symptoms

1. Deranged Flow of Qi and Blood

Qi may get deranged and out of self control during or after qigong exercise, which usually gives rise to dizziness, vertigo, panic, chest distress, short breath, uncontrolled movement of the extremities, or syncope. In most cases, patients are able to tell the location and direction of qi flow.

2. Stagnation of Qi and Stasis of Blood

During or after qigong exercises, disorder of qi may occur,

causing qi stagnation and blood stasis in a certain location accompanied by the symptoms of pain, heaviness, sore and distending sensation and sensation of compression, which can not disappear automatically.

3. Leaking of Genuine Qi

During or after qigong exercise, one may feel leaking of qi from the external genitals, anus and some points, which can not be controlled by oneself. Leaking of genuine qi may lead to wasting,weakness of the extremities, pale greyish and dark complexion, vexation, failure of mind concentration, hypomnesis,spontaneous perspiration, night sweat, seminal emission, insomnia and reluctance to speak or move.

4. Mental Derangement

During qigong exercises, a phenomenon of mental derangement, also called "being infatuated" (Ru Mo), may appear in some practitioners who regard the illusion emerging during or after qigong exercise as true, and this often leads to mental derangement manifested as uncommunicative and eccentric in disposition, withered and dull in expression, idle in movement, and apathy and trance. Some even lose their confidence of living and want to commit suicide; others suffer from continuous auditory hallucination and visual hallucination which are similar to that seen in psychotics. These symptoms are summarized as ten devils in Zhong Lu Chuan Dao Ji (Works of Zhong and Lu's Taoist Doctrine), which are the devil of six thieves, devil of wealth, devil of aristocracy, devil of six passions, devil of love, devil of adversity, devil of saints, devil of fight, devil of amusement with women and devil of sexuality.

5. Unchecked Flow of Pathogenic Qi

In practitioners suffering illnesses, there may be struggle between the healthy qi and pathogenic qi during exercises. And because the healthy qi is reinforced owing to Qigong exercise, the pathogenic qi may flow unchecked to a certain location and cause pain, soreness, distention, heaviness, coldness and hotness.

Treatment

1. Treatment of Deranged Flow of Qi

(1) Emission of Outgoing—Qi (Waiqi)

Regulate the activities of the Eight Extra—channels in accordance with the "Eight Methods of Intelligent Turtle", the technique of point selection, and with the principle of "opening the points on time".

Then select points in the location and along the channels where functional activities of qi have been in a state of disorder. Flat—palm or sword—fingers hand gestures and pushing, pulling and quivering manipulations may be used to activate the channel qi, then guide qi with leading manipulation to the related channel or organ, or back to Dantian.

(2) Daoyin Massage Based on Symptoms

First, dizziness or vertigo may be treated by pressing—rubbing Baihui (Du 20), Hanyan (GB 4), Shuaigu (GB 8) and Xuanlu (GB 5), followed by pushing—opening Tianmen (Extra), pushing Kangong (Extra), kneading Taiyang (Extra 2), digging—pressing Fengchi (GB 20) and pressing Mingmen (Du 4).

Second, chest distress and shortness of breath may be treated with finger—kneading Tanzhong (Ren 17), Rugen (St 18), Rupang (Extra), Yunmen (Lu 4) and Zhongfu (Lu 1), pushing–kneading Tanzhong (Ren 17) and pressing–kneading Neiguan (P 6).

Third, uncontrolled movement of the extremities can be treated by calling the patient by name and by saying some proper words to get the movement holted, followed by patting Dazhui (Du 4) and Mingmen (Du 4) and then pressing Mingmen (Du 4) digitally.

Finally, syncope should be treated by pressing Yintang (Extra 1) and Renzhong (Du 26), digging–grasping Quchi (LI 11), Hegu (LI 4), Weizhong (UB 40) and Chengshan (UB 57), and guiding qi back to Dantian.

(3) Self Qigong Exercise as Accessory Treatment

Stop doing the Qigong exercise which has caused the symptoms.

Then conduct self patting on the head, back and chest, and carry out self Daoyin massage along the Three Yang Channels of Hand, the Three Yang Channels of Foot, the Three Yin Channels of Hand and the Three Yin Channels of Foot based on their courses and directions.

(4) Treatment with Traditional Drugs

The following ingredients may be described with modification, and decoctd in water for oral administration.

Radix Angelicae Sinensis (Danggui)	12 grams
Magnetitum (Cishi)	30 grams
Radix Achyranthis Bidentatae (Niuxi)	18 grams
Fructus Corni (Shanyurou)	15 grams
Os Draconis (Shenglonggu)	30 grams
Concha Ostreae (Shengmuli)	30 grams

2. Stagnation of Qi and Stasis of Blood

(1) Emission of Outgoing–Qi (Waiqi)

In accordance with corresponding channel point selection, select certain points in and around the location where qi stagnation and blood stasis exist. Rub, press and knead the points along the channel.

Then emit qi with flat–palm hand gesture and pushing, pulling and quivering manipulations so as to activate the channel qi. Then guide the channel qi to flow along the channels to dredge them.

(2) Daoyin Massage Based on Symptoms

Depression sensation on the head may be treated by pressing–kneading Baihui (Du 20) and Fengchi (GB 20), pushing–opening Tianmen (Extra), pushing Kangong (Extra) and kneading Taiyang (Extra 2) and Dazhui (Du 14), and by patting along the Du Channel and the Ren Channel.

Tightness and compression sensation at the forehead may be treated by pushing–opening Tianmen (Extra), pushing Kangong (Extra), kneading Taiyang (Extra 2) and Baihui (Du 20) and pressing Jingming (UB 1), as well as patting the Ren Channel from the upper to the lower.

Distending pain in Dazhui (Du 14) can be treated by pressing–kneading Dazhui (Du 14), Fengfu (Du 16), Fengchi (GB 20) and Jizhong (Du 6), and by patting along the Du Channel and the Urinary Bladder Channel of Foot–Taiyang. (3) Self Qigong Exercise as Accessory Treatment

Stop doing the exercises which have caused the symptoms.

Carry out constant pushing–rubbing, kneading–suppressing and patting on the painful and discomfortable places.

(4) Treatment with Traditional Drugs

The following ingredients may be described and decocted in water for oral administration.

Radix Angelicae Sinensis (Danggui)	12 grams
Semen Persicae (Taoren)	9 grams
Flos Carthami (Honghua)	9 grams
Rhizoma Corydalis (Yuanhu)	12 grams
Fructus Liquidambaris (Lulutong)	30 grams
Radix Achyranthis Bidentatae (Niuxi)	18 grams
Retinervus Luffae Fructus (Sigualuo)	9 grams

3. Leaking of Genuine Qi

(1) Emission of Outgoing—Qi (Waiqi)

Emit qi with flat—palm gesture and pushing, pulling and quivering manipula— tions toward Dantian and Mingmen (Du 4), and again to Dantian with flat—palm hand gesture and vibrating and quivering manipulations for 9 or 18 respiratory cycles.

(2) Daoyin Massage Based on Symptoms

Push—open Lanmen (Extra), knead Zhongwan (Ren 12), Qihai (Ren 6) and Guanyuan (Ren 4), push and rub the abdomen and knead Shenshu (UB 23) and the first collaterals of the Du Channel and the Urinary Bladder Channel.

(3) Self Qigong Exercise as Accessory Treatment

Practise the exercises of mind—concentrating on Dantian, anus contracting, teeth tapping and saliva swallowing among other techniques.

Pat the torso and the extremities.

(4) Treatment with Traditional Drugs

The following ingredients may be decocted in water for oral administration.

Radix Rehmanniae Praeparatae (Shudi)	30 grams
Fructus Corni (Shanyurou)	30 grams
Radix Ginseng (Renshen)	9 grams
Magnetitum (Cishi)	30 grams
Radix Achyranthis Bidentatae (Niuxi)	18 grams
Cortex Cinnamomi (Rougui)	6 grams
Os Draconis (Shenglonggu)	30 grams
Concha Ostreae (Shengmuli)	30 grams
Cinnabaris (Zhusha)	1 gram (taken following its infusion)

4. Mental Derangement

(1) Emission of Outgoing-Qi (Waiqi)

Open the point of the Eight Extra-channels in accordance with the "Eight Methods of Intelligent Turtle", the technique of point selection, and with the principle of "opening the points on time".

Press and knead the points Baihui (Du 20), Dazhui (Du 14), Lingtai(Du 14) and Feishu (UB 13); then use the flat-palm or sword-fingers hand gesture and pushing, pulling and vibrating manipulations to emit qi and guide qi to flow along the channel.

Press-knead Baihui (Du 20), Yintang (Extra 1), Shangen (radix naxi), Renzhong (Du 26), Tinggong (SI 19), Jiache (St 6), Quchi (LI 11), Hegu (LI 4), Weizhong (UB 40) and Chengshan (UB 57).

Middle-finger-propping hand gesture and vibrating and quivering manipulations are used to emit qi toward Jiuwei (Ren 15) and Zhongwan (Ren 12) for 27 respiratory cycles, then guide qi to flow along the Ren Channel back to Dantian.

(2) Daoyin Massage Based on Symptoms

Push—open Tianmen (Extra), push Kangong (Extra), Knead Taiyang (Extra 2) and Baihui (Du 20), pat along the spinal collumn and push the Urinary Bladder Channel from the upper to the lower, and pat the back and the extremities.

(3) Self Qigong Exercise as Accessory Treatment

Practise Automatic Qi Circulation Exercise as described below.

While saying "the white tiger hides in the east and the green dragon hides in the west", guide qi to rotate with the navel as the centre clockwise and counterclockwise 36 times respectively.

Carry out self massage and patting.

(4) Treatment with Traditional Drugs

The following ingredients may be described to be decocted in water for oral administration.

Radix Rehmanniae Praeparatae (Shudi)	30 grams
Bulbus Lilii (Baihe)	30 grams
Os Draconis (Shenglonggu)	30 grams
Concha Ostreae (Shengmuli)	30 grams
Radix Achyranthis Bidentatae (Niuxi)	15 grams
Radix Polygalae (Yuanzhi)	12 grame
Semen Ziziphi Spinosae (Chaozaoren)	12 grams
Magnetitum (Cishi)	30 grams
Fructus Corni (Shanyurou)	30 grams
Cinnabaris (Zhusha)	1 gram (taken following its infusion)

5. Unchecked Flow of Pathogenic Qi

(1) Emission of Outgoing—Qi (Waiqi)

Determine the Jing point (well point, one of the five shu points located at the tips of the fingers and toes. Each of the Twelve Regular Channels has such a point). Push—knead the affected place to open the point and guide the channel qi along the course of the channels.

With flat—palm hand gesture and pulling and leading manipulations to pull and guide the pathogenic qi, or to open the point to dispel it.

(2) Daoyin Massage Based on Symptoms

Push—rub, tab digitally and rotate—flick the affected region to relax it fully.

(3) Self Qigong Exercise as Accessory Treatment

Practise the exhaling exercise to dispel pathogenic qi. Inhale naturally and exhale to lead qi by will to the affected location, imagining qi is being expelled. Do this for 49 respiratory cycles.

Apply medication treatment in the light of the principle " Excess Syndrome should be treated with the method of purgation and reduction".

Case one

Li, male, aged 28, came for the first visit on April 18, 1983.

Complaints The patient complained of rushing of qi to the top of the head and suffering from headache and dizziness for two months.

The patient felt motion of qi in the Lower Dantian 20 days after he began to practise Qigong independently. A few days later he felt qi rushing toward the lower limbs, the back and the head, which gave him a feeling of heaviness and compression on the head as if holding a heavy cap, followed successively by dizziness, headache, stiffness of the back and shoulders, numbness of the legs and unckecked and continuous flow of qi in the lower limbs, waist and head which turned worse gradually, accompanied with palpitation, terror, insomnia and listlessness. The condition was diagnosed as "neurosism" in a hospital but treatment with Western and traditional drugs failed.

Examination   No abnormalities were found in the head and extremities. The pulse was deep and thready, and tongue coating thin and white. Flat–palm detection revealed densified and disordered qi at the head and back.

Diagnosis   Qigong deviation (deranged flow of qi and blood accompanied by stagnation of qi and blood).

Treatment   Flat–palm hand gesture and pulling and leading manipulations were applied to emit qi toward Baihui (Du 20), Yintang (Extra 1), Fengfu (Du 16), Dantian and Hegu (LI 4).

Course of Treatment   All the symptoms improved after 3 times of treatment. The condition was corrected completely after 9 times of treatment.

Case Two

Wang, male, 66, came for the first visit on February 3, 1983.

Complaints   The patient complained of a sensation of depression on the left shoulder for 10 days.

The patient began to practise qigong twice a day in order to cure his romote myocardial infarction. Spontaneous movements occurred during practice and the primary symptoms of the disease were relieved gradually. But two months later when he was doing the qigong exercises, he suddenly felt an egg–sized mass rushing out from his heart toward the back and lingering in the left Quyuan (SI 13) and Bingfeng (SI 12), followed by heaviness, soreness and immobility of the shoulder and restless sleep at night.

Examination   Physical examination found swelling of the left Quyuan (SI 13) and Bingfeng (SI 12) with mild tenderness. Flat–palm detection revealed densified and cold qi at the affected region and at the point Xinshu (UB 15).

Diagnosis   Qigong deviation (Unchecked flow of pathogenic qi).

Treatment   Flat–palm hand gesture and pulling and leading manipulations were used to emit qi to Jianwaishu (SI 14), Bingfeng (SI 12), Quyuan (SI 13), Tianzong (SI 11), Quchi (LI 11), Xiaohai (SI 8) and Hegu (LI 4) once a day.

Course of Treatment   After the second treatment, the patient felt that the qi mass was removed to the elbow manifested by heaviness and discomfort of the elbow joint and disappearance of the symptoms of the shoulder. The condition was cured completely after the fourth treatment.

Case Three

Zhang, male, 60, came for the first visit on December 20, 1984.

Complaints   The patient complained of suffering from auditory hallucination for three months.

Spontaneous movements appeared for successively ten months with practice of the Crane Qigong Exercise

(Hexiangzhuang Qigong). One night when he was practising static exercise, he heard a man say to him, "Go straight to the gate and you can get through the grill". He did so, bumped against the door, fainted and was rushed to the hospital. Examinations gave no positive findings. There were no headache and dizziness, but the auditory hallucination became more severe. It was surprising that when the patient wanted to know something, the voice would come and tell him, which could not be interfered with at all even the sound volume of the radio or television set was turned to the highest. The patient and his relatives were greatly frightened. Treatment with Western and traditional drugs, acupuncture and outgoing-qi therapy in a hospital of mental diseases failed.

Examination The tongue coating was white and thin but yellow at the root; the pulse was thready and deep-sited. The patient looked mentally normal and could cooperate with the doctor in inquiry and physical examination. Flat-palm detection with outgoing-qi found densified, stagnated qi at the back of the head and the ears.

Diagnosis Qigong deviation (Mental degrangement).

Treatment Pressing and nipping were applied to Yintang (Extra 1), Tinggong (SI 19), Yifeng (SJ 17), Hegu (LI 4) and the ear orifice first, followed by emission of qi toward them with flat-palm hand gesture and pulling, rotating and leading manipulations.

Course of Treatment When the author said to the patient, " You have developed specific physiological function. You needn't worry and need no treatment. Don't follow the voice. You'll be all right if you continue to practise Qigong as usual". But the patient answered, "My family and I are frightened. I will practise no more Qigong if you can cure me." The author had no choice but treating him with the methods mentioned above. During the first treatment, the patient heard creaking sound on emission of outgoing-qi toward his ears and the hallucination improved markedly. The hallucination disappeared after the third treatment and the patient recovered completely.

ANNEX: Selected Treatises on Experimental Studies of the Effect of Outgoing—qi (Waiqi)

Experimental studies on the effect of outgoing—qi (waiqi) emitted by the author were carried out by the specialists form the Channel, Collateral and Acupuncture Department, Physiology Department and Anatomy Department of Shandong Traditional Chinese Medicine College. The experiments have proved that outgoing —qi has obvious regulating function on the skeletal muscles of the human body, the heart of toad and the Oddi's sphincter of rabbit, and that the needles inserted into the points can conduct outgoing—qi to the related organs and regulate the physiological function of them. The achievements in these experiments have shown that the existence of outgoing—qi as a substance is an objective reality, which has provided reliable experimental and theoretical basis for clinical application of outgoing—qi therapy. Selected hereof are four treatises representative of the effect of outgoing—qi.

The Influence of Qigong Outgoing—qi on the Cardiac Functions of Toad

Previous experiments have proved the dilation of the peripheral blood vessels and the reduction of the heart rate in qigong practitioners, and it is believed that these changes are relative to the decrease of sympathetic excitability and the increase of parasympathetic excitability. However, there had been no reports on the effec of outgoing–qi on the heart of animals. Our study was designed for observation of the functional changes of the heart of toad under the effect of outgoing–qi.

1. Materials and Methods

Fifteen healthy toads were prepared for tests of the effect of outgoing–qi and another fifteen were used as controls. The experiments were done at a room temperature of $13 - 15°C$. After the toad was washed with running water, a needle probe was inserted vertically into the cranial cavity of the toad through the great occipital foramen and then was moved left and right to stir the brain tissue. The probe was then withdrawn and inserted into the spinal canal through the great occipital foramen to stir the spinal cord. The softness of the extremities and the disapperance of breath meant that the pithing was succeeded. The chest cavity was opened and the cardiac cytomembrane removed to expose the heart, on which Rinne's fluid was dropped. The apex of the heart was clipped with frog heart clips, and was connected to the multichannel physiological recorder (RM–6000) by means of a dynamic transducer for oscillography and tracing of the heart beat with a paper speed of 25 cm / second.After the recording, outgoing–qi was emitted with the selected hand gesture (10–20 cm away from the heart of the toad) toward the heart of the toad for 10 minutes. And recording was done for one minute each time right at the emission of qi and at $2'30''$, $5'$, $7'30''$ and $10'$ after the qi emission was started, and at $2'30''$, $5'$, $10'$ and $20'$ after it was discontinued. The mean of the width of the ventricular systolic wave in the 10 successive cardiac cycles and the heart rate were taken as indicators in the experimental group (Group A). In the control group (Group B), emission of qi was simulant, done by one who had not practised qigong but the method of recording and detection was as same as that taken for the experimental group.

2. Results

1 The effect of qigong outgoing—qi on the ventricular systolic wave width of the toad is shown in Table 1.

In the experimental group, the ventricular systolic wave was widened after the heart of the toad received outgoing—qi from $2'30''$ after beginning of qi emission to $20'$ after the discontinuance of emission compared with that recorded before the emission of qi was started, and the difference was significant ($p < 0.01$), indicating that the ventricular systole time was prolonged under the effect of outgoing—qi.

Table 1   The Effect of Qigong Outgoing—qi on the Ventricular Systolic Wave Width (Per Second) of Toad

Group of Toad	No. Toad	Before Emission of qi	During Emission of Qi					After Emission of Qi			
			Start	2.30min	5min	7.30min	10min	2.30min	5min	10min	20min
A	15	2.98 ± 0.06	0.93 ± 0.07	1.02 ± 0.09	1.19 ± 0.12	1.27 ± 0.12	1.29 ± 0.12	1.27 ± 0.12	1.29 ± 0.013	1.27 ± 0.12	1.26 ± 0.12
P			> 0.05	< 0.01	< 0.01	< 0.01	< 0.01	< 0.01	< 0.01	< 0.01	< 0.01
B	13	0.96 ± 0.08	0.99 ± 0.08	0.09 ± 0.09	1.02 ± 0.08	0.99 ± 0.10	0.99 ± 0.09	1.02 ± 0.09	0.98 ± 0.09	1.00 ± 0.06	0.98 ± 0.09

Table 2 Effect of Outgoing–Qi on the Heart Rate of Toads

Group of Toad	No.	Before Emission	During Emission of Qi					After Emission of Qi			
			Start	2.30min	5min	7.30min	10min	2.30min	5min	10min	20min
A	15	65.5 ± 1.99	65.0 ± 2.56	62.7 ± 3.62	60.7 ± 4.55	58.2 ± 4.55	57.9 ± 4.46	57.3 ± 4.35	57.3 ± 4.39	56.8 ± 4.02	56.9 ± 4.23
P		70.05	>0.05	<0.01	<0.01	<0.01	<0.01		<0.01	<0.01	<0.01
B	13	63.2 ± 3.19	62.8 ± 3.10	62.1 ± 3.35	61.1 ± 3.52	61.8 ± 3.49	61.1 ± 3.48	61.7 ± 2.87	61.1 ± 3.68	61.1 ± 3.48	60.8 ± 3.29

(2) The effect of qigong outgoing–qi on the heart rate of the toad is shown in Table 2.

In the experimental group, the heart rate of the toad was slowed down after the heart received outgoing–qi form $2'30''$ after the beginning of qi emission to $20'$ after the discontinuance of qi emission compared with that recorded before emission of qi was started, and the difference was also significant ($p < 0.05$).

The results show that the ventricular systole time of the toad in the experimental group was prolonged and the heat rate was accordingly slowed down significantly.

3. Discussion

It has been observed that there are certain changes of cardiovascular functions in those who have practised qigong to a certain extent or in those who have entered qigong "quiescence", and it is believed that the entering into a qigong state can regulate the functional state of the human organism. Viewed form the results of observations on the decrease of the sympathetic excitability and the increase of the parasympathetic excitability, the regulation of the balance of yin and yang of the human organism is considered as a process of energy accumulation. However, no observations have been reported on the effect of outgoing—qi on the functional changes of the heart of animals.

In our studies, observations were made on the functional changes of the toad, whose serebrospinal cord was destroyed, under the effect of outgoing—qi. The results preliminarily show that in the experimental group the heart rate of toads is markedly slowed, and the ventricular systole wave is significantly widened after the heart of the toad has received outgoing—qi, while in the control group, there are no significant changes, proving that outgoing qi can slow the heart rate and prolong the ventricular systole time. This indicates that the slowing down of the heart rate may reduce the per minute output and the prolongation of the ventricular systole time may increase the per minute output, and the regulation of the per minute output may result in reduced energy consumption during the period of cardiac systole. Nevertheless, the effect of outgoing—qi on the peripheral nervous knots of the heart or the working cell of the cardiac muscles, and on the muscular conduction system remains to be studied.

(Participants: Cao Zhenhua, Bi Yongsheng and Zhao Luming).

Effect of Qigong Outgoing-qi on the Tensityf the Oddi's Sphincter of Rabbit

A number of reports on the curative effect of outgoing-qi (waiqi) in clinical treatment of diseases of the liver and gallbladder system have proved that outgoing-qi is quite effective for treatment of chronic cholecystitis and cholelithiasis, especially for relieving symptoms and allaying pain. This indicates that outgoing-qi can improve the functional status of the Oddi's sphincter. So in our study, electromyogram of the smooth muscles of Oddi's sphincter is taken as an indicator for observation of the tensity changes of the sphincter under the influence of outgoing-qi.

1. Materials and methods

Twenty healthy male and female rabbits (2.5–2.9 kg) were anaesthetized by intravenous infusion of urethane (0.1g / 1 kg body weight) after being starved for 15 hours. With endotracheal intubation, lateral median abdominal incision was made to open the abdominal cavity and expose the duodenum, Oddi's sphincter and choledochus. An obligue incision was made in the choledochus 1 cm from the sphincter to allow an insertion of a plastic tube (2 mm in diameter) toward the liver into the choledochus. The tube was withdrawn immediately when there was discharge of bile and was quickly replaced by another plastic tube, which had the same diameter and was filled with adhesive 502. This tube was inserted 5 mm deep into the choledochus, its end was made adhesive with the tissues round the incision and its top was clipped tightly with hemostatic forceps to cause choledochus obstruction. With reference to Sahli's method, sphincter myoelectric signal was induced with a pair of hornskin copper coils (with the cornskin at the two ends removed), which served as copper electrodes. The myoelectric signal was put into the Y—axis amplifer of a JD—2 myoelectric apparatus with the parameters of: interference inhibition ratio 49.5, frequency 2 Hz — 2 kHz, sensitivity 5 mm / cm. The magnified myoelectric signal was put into the rear amplifier of a SJ—41 multichannel physiological recorder and was recorded by the tattooing needle with a paper speed of 1.25 cm / sec. The indifferent electrode was placed subcutaneously left to the abdominal incision. The temperature of the abdominal cavity was kept a. 38.2—40.2°C by means of an operating light (60 W) hanging a ove the rabbit table and two lights (15 W) setting at the downside of the table. Sodium chloride fluid 0.9% in concentration and 38°C in temperature was dropped into the abdominal cavity before the recording was started. The sphincter myoelectric potential was recorded for 10 minutes first for auto— control. After that, qi was emitted by the author toward the Oddi's sphincter of each of the 10 rabbits in the experimental group (Group A) for 30 minutes with fixed hand gesture and with the hand 10 — 20 cm off the sphincter. Observations were continued up to 30 minutes after the stoppage of qi emission. The sphincter myoelectric frequency was recorded at the 0 — 10, 10 — 20 and 20 — 30 minutes from the start and stoppage of qi emission respectively. As to the 10 rabbits in the control group, the same procedures were performed except the emission of outgoing—qi.

2. Results

The results of statistical analysis of the data gained prior to the emission of qi and those gained during or after that showed significant difference (p < 0.05) in the experimental group and no statistical significance in the control group, demonstrating that under the influence of outgoing—qi, the frequency of myoelectric potential of the Oddi's sphincter was reduced and the tensity of it was decreased (Table 3).

Table 3   Effect of Outgoing Qi on Myoelectric Frequency (Times) of Oddi's Sphincter$\overline{X}\pm$ SD

Group	10min before Emission of Qi	During Emission of Qi			After Emission of Qi		
		0−10min	10−20min	20−30min	0−10min	10−20min	20−30min
A	109.9 ± 26.1	37.4 ± 13.1	28.9 ± 14.0	22.0 ± 96	35.3 ± 18.7	33.5 ± 15.3	39.0 ± 17.6
P		<0.05	<0.05	<0.01	<0.05	<0.05	<0.05
B	82.5 ± 21.7	81.6 ± 20.61	81.1 ± 21.4	80.8 ± 21.0	80.9 ± 22.13	78.4 ± 21.29	76.6 ± 20.57

3. Discussion

Qigong was found to be effective for chronic cholecystitis and cholelithiasis in the previous clinical and experimental studies of the effect of qigong in treatment of diseases related to the liver and gallbladder. Wang Jisheng et al have confirmed the tranquilizing effect of qigong outgoing—qi through experimental researches. In our study, the effect of qigong was observed with the results of myoelectric activity of the Oddi's sphincter as the indicators, which was achieved when the gallbladder was at a hypertensive state reduced by blocking the cholechus of rabbits. A direct relationship between the myoelectric activity and the tension of the smooth muscles was observed in animal tests done by others. Wang Yiding and Liu Kan et al believe that the reduction of the myoelectric discharge to the Oddi's sphincter might reduce the tensity of the sphincter, which in turn might facilitate the drainage of bile and gallstones. The results of our experiment showed marked drop of the myoelectric frequency of the sphincter potential beginning at 10 minutes after the start of qi emission till 30 minutes after the stop of the emission ($P < 0.05$), which indicated the reduction of the sphincter tensity. And because of the tensity reduction, the drainage of bile and gallstones was promoted, leading to alleviation of pain and other symptoms of cholecystitis.

(Participants: Zhang Shiping, Cao Zhenhua and Bi Yongsheng)

Myoelectrographic Observations on the Dynamic Phenomenon Induced by Qigong Outgoing-Qi

From 1981 to the end of 1984, qigong outgoing qi (waiqi) was applied to tremtment of over 400 patients,among which over 60 presented dynamic phenomenon. For further investigation, myoelectric observations were carried out in 3 of them who had recovered from their illnesses.

1. Patients and Methods

Patients: Li, female, aged 29, had suffered from pain in the waist and the left lower limb for nine months. X—ray film showed narrowed interspace between the 4th and 5th lumbar vertebrae. The diagnosis was prolapse of lumbar intervertebral disc. Jiang, female, aged 48, had suffered from sciatica for two years. And Cheng, male, aged 29, had suffered from vegetative nerve functional disturbance for three years. All the patients were cured with outgoing—qi therapy.

Detecting methods: Detection was carried out stage by stage with a RW − 600 multichannel physiological recorder. The patients were asked to assume a sitting or lying posture. Myoelectric needles were inserted into the left—side long palmar muscle of Cheng, the right—side gastrocnemius muscle of Jiang and the left side greatest gluteal muscle of Li, and the electrode was inserted into the AB—600 bioelectric amplifier. The myoelectric changes were recorded and at the same time observed through a screen. Detection was carried out at three stages: on emission of qi, on stop of qi emission and on closing of the qi emission procedure. One acupoint was selected in each patient for insertion of the filiform needle. Qi was emitted near the needles. As a control, electric stimulation was conducted with a electro—therapeutic apparatus manufactured in Shanghai Third Electro—Apparatus factory.

2. Results

(1) Dynamic Phenomenon in Patients duing Qi Emission

Before emission of qi, the patients were in a static state and the myoelectrogram showed static potential. When the doctor emitted qi toward the body surface of the patients with flat—palm hand gesture (hand 30—100 cm away from the pa-tients' body surface) and pushing, pulling, quivering and leading manipulations, the action of qi on the channels and points was manifested by motion of the muscles and by the persistent occurrence of single and mixed modes of electric potential and then interference mode potential in the myoelectrogram with the amplitude of vibration gradually augmented. The high amplitude interference mode existed after the emission of qi. When the doctor closed the qi emission procedure, the amplitude of interference mode reduced immediately and turned into mixed, single, and finally static.

(2) Dynamic phenomenon in Patients during Emission of Qi toward the Needles

Three filiform needles were inserted respectively into the left Ciliao (UB 32) of patient Li, the right Shangliao (UB 31) of patient Jiang and the left Jianshi (P 5) of patient Cheng as the receivers of outgoing–qi. Prior to the emission of qi, the patients were at a static state and the myoelectrogram showed static potential. When the doctor emitted outgoing–qi with dragon–mouth hand gesture (hand 2–3 cm off the needles) and pulling and quivering manipulations, the myoelectrogram presented paroxysmal interference mode potential. The fasciculated electric change was consistent with the frequency of the hand manipulations of the doctor, and the myoelectrogram showed static potential immediately when the doctor ended his qi emission procedure.

(3) Myoelectrographic Changes Induced by Electric Stimulation

Two filiform needles were inserted into the body of each patient near the three myoelectric needle electrodes as the electrodes, and electric stimulation was performed by means of a electric therapeutic apparatus. Before the stimulation, the patients were static and the myoelectrogram presented static potential. When the stimulation reached a certain extent of intensity, the muscles of the patients began to contract and the myoelectrogram showed changes. The frequency of the electric potential was coincident with that of electric stimulation.

3. Discussion

(1) The Evocation of Outgoing—qi Message and Uncontrolment Outgoing—qi, acting on the channels and points of the patient, can activate his qi activities and make the circulation of qi and blood smooth. One of the manifestations is the contracting movements of the muscles, which may be very marked in some cases. Once this strong effect is triggered, the patient will not be able to control it voluntarily.

(2) The Synchronism between Outgoing—qi Message and the Triggering Effect

When the therapist emits qi rhythmically toward the patient, the muscles of the patient will present rhythmic contration correspondingly, and paroxysmal interference mode can be observed on the electromyogram.

(3) Outgoing—qi in Control of the Triggering Effect

The effect triggered through emission of outgoing—qi can be controlled by the therapist though it can not be controlled by the patient himself. Once the therapist stops emission of qi, the contracting movements of the muscles will disappear.

The mechanism of the dynamic effect triggered by outgoing—qi awaits for further studies.

(Participants: Bi Yongsheng, Cao Zhenhua, Zhao Luming and Zhang Liancai)

Myoelectrographic Observation of the Influence of Outgoing—Qi on the Oddi's Sphincter of Rabbit via Needles

There have been abundant reports on clinical application of outgoing—qi to treatment of cholelithiasis. However, no facts had been mentioned about the actual effect of outgoing—qi on the needles and its acting mechanism. This study was done with rabbit. The choledochus of the rabbit was obstructed artificially, then filiform needles 3 cun long were inserted into the two Zusanli points(St 36) and outgoing—qi was emitted toward the needles. The control group was given no needling and emission of outgoing—qi. Observation was made on the changes of the myoelectric frequency of the Oddi's sphincter. Effect of outgoing—qi on the needles and its subsequent cholagogic function were analysed.

1. Materials and Methods

(1) Experimental Animals and Method of Choledochus Blockage

Thirty—two male and female rabbits with a mean body weight of 2.53 + 0.47 kg were divided randomly into three groups: qigong—acupuncture group (A), acupuncture group (B) and control group (C). All the rabbits were anesthetized intravenously with urethane (1g / 1kg body weight) after being starved for 14 — 20 hours.

An incision was made in the middle of the upper abdomen to expose the choledochus and the Oddi's sphincter, with no injury to the blood vessels and nerves. An oblique incision 1 cm away from the Oddi's sphincter was made on the choledochus. A plastic tube 2mm in diameter, which had been soaked in adhesive 502, was inserted into the choledochus. The tube adhered with the surrounding tissues immediately. The residual end of the tube was cut off and the tube was clipped tightly with hemostatic forceps so that the opening of the tube can be sealed by the adhesive to prevent the outflowing of bile.

After the choledochus had been blocked for 2.5 − 5 hours, the upper part of the choledochus above the blockage thickened and congested obviously. The choledochal pressure of the 25 rabbits in Group A was 2.35 + 0.24 kPa (21.44 + 2.42 cm / water column). This was significantly higher than that of the common rabbits, which was usually 690 − 1470 Pa (7 −15 cm / water column), indicating that the choledochuses of rabbits of Group A were blocked and were at a state of hypertension.

(2) Leading Electrodes and Apparatus

Improved Sahli's method was adopted. A pair a copper coil electrodes (200 um in diameter) were placed at the Oddi's sphincter to lead myoelectricity. The indifferent electrode was placed subcutaneously at the left abdomen. As the sphincter of the rabbit was stable when the peritoneal temperature was at 38.3 + 0.9℃, an operating light (60 W) was put above the abdominal cavity and two common lights (15 W) were put below it. The peritoneal temperature was then increased to 38.7 + 0.48℃ . Before the experiment, some saline water (38℃) was dropped onto the tissue to moisten it. The abdomen was cut open to get ready for the experiment.

The electric signal was put into the Y−axil amplifier of the electromyograph (Type JD—2) with the parameters of: interference inhibition ratio 49.5, frequency range 2—2000 Hz, and sensitivity 1mv / cm. When the electric signal had been amplified, a post—amplifier of polygraph (Type SJ—41) was inputted to record the myoelectricity. The standard voltage of the amplifier was 0.2 mv / 10—20mm; the paper speed was 2.5mm / s or 5mm / s.

(3) Division of Groups and Methods

Group A: This group included 12 experimental rabbits. Filiform needles were inserted into the point Zusanli (St 36) of both legs and was left still (with no stwisting or lifting and thrusting manipulations) for 10 minutes. Then dragon— mouth hand gesture and pushing, pulling and rotating manipulations were taken to emit qi, with the hand 3—5mm off the needles, toward the needles for 30 minutes. Then record and observation were made for 30 minutes. The whole process took 70 minutes. Myoelectric frequency of the sphinter was recorded at:10 minutes before emission of qi; 0—10, 10—20, and 20—30 minutes during it; and 0—10, 10—20, and 20—30 minutes after it.

Group B: This group had 10 experimental rabbits as controls, which got only acupuncture as mentioned in Group A without outgoing—qi. Myoelectric frequency was observed and recorded once every 10 minutes for altogether 70 minutes.

Group C: This group was taken as the common control, with 10 rabbits. No stimulation (acupuncture, outgoing—qi, etc.) was given yet the same observation and record as mentioned above were made .

2. Results

Myoelectric frequency was recorded for 70 minutes after

the choledochus was blocked for more than one and half hours when the myoelectricity got stable. Analysis of the 32 electromyograms revealed two wave types: single wave potential, and multi—continuous wave potential with resting intervals. The wave amplitude was ranged 0.02—1.10mV. With the myoelectric frequency as the indicator, the results showed a significant difference in Group A between the periods of 10—30 minutes during emission of qi and 30 minutes after it and the period 30 minutes prior to it (p<0.05; p<0.01). No statistical difference was found in Group B and C. The stimulation of outgoing—qi to the sphincter via the needles and further the points and channels relieved the tension of the sphincter and reduced the myoelectric frequency (Table 4).

Table 4 Effect of Outgoing—qi on the Needles and Its Subsequent Influence on the Myoelectric Frequency of Oddi's Sphincter

Group	10min Before Emission of Qi	During Emission of Qi			After Emission of Qi		
		0—10min	10—20min	20—30min	0—10min	10—20min	20—30min
A	92.7±63.4	55.2±108.4	29.6±45.5	17.7±22.4	26.5±32.3	28.2±31.4	43.2±50.5
(n=10)		(9>0.05)	(p<0.05)	(p<0.01)	(p<0.05)	(p<0.05)	(p<0.05)
B	124.4±73.7	93.4±85.4	91.0±80.6	102.6±81.3	102.2±79.4	104.3±84.6	106.3±82.1
(n=12)		(p>0.05)	(p>0.05)	(p>0.05)	(p>0.05)	(p>0.05)	(p>0.05)
C	82.5±65.2	81.6±61.85	80.8±63.5	80.9±66.4	78.4±63.8	76.6±61.7	76.6±61.7
(n=10)		(p>0.05)	(p>0.05)	(p>0.05)	(p>0.05)	(p>0.05)	(p>0.05)

Note: Myoelectric Frequency (Time / 10m) x SD

3. Discussion

There have been no reports about the physiological effect induced by outgoing —qi conducted via the needles, points and channels. Our study was made on the basis of the marked achievements in the authors' clinical application of qigong–acupuncture to treatment of liver and gallbladder diseases.

In our study, observation was made on the effect of outgoing–qi which was emitted to the needles inserted into the two Zusanli (St 36) points of the rabbits, taking the myoelectric activity of the Oddi's sphincter, which was artificially blocked in order to give high tension to the gallbladder, as the indicator.The results showed that ten minutes after the beginning of qi emission toward the needles, the myoelectric frequency of the Oddi's sphincter slowed down markedly ($p < 0.05$), and after $20 - 30$ minutes, it slowed down most significantly ($p < 0.01$). Such effect was also observed half an hour after emission of qi ($P < 0.05$). This shows that outgoing–qi can reduce the tension of the gallbladder, and the needle (filiform) can transmit outgoing–qi via the points and channels to the Oddi's sphincter. As the reduction of tension of the sphincter is helpful to discharge of bile and gallstones and alleivation of pain and gallbladder inflammation, the results gained in our study have provided experimental base for treatment of diseases with qigong–acupuncture.

(Participants: Zhang Shiping, Cao Zhenhua and Bi Yongsheng)

中国气功外气疗法

毕永升　著

于文平　译

山东科学技术出版社出版

中国济南玉函路 16 号　邮政编码 250002

山东莒县印刷厂印刷

中国国际图书贸易总公司发行

中国北京车公庄西路 35 号

北京邮政信箱第 399 号　邮政编码 100044

1997 年　（大 32）　1 版 2 次

ISBN7—5331—1041—2/R·277

04800

14—E—2649P